Body, Mind, and Spirit
"Vitamins"
for Your Whole Health

Body, Mind, and Spirit
"Vitamins"
for Your Whole Health

Gary D. McKay, Ph.D.
W. F. Peate, M.D., M.P.H.
Erik Mansager, Ph.D.

***Impact Publishers*®**
ATASCADERO, CALIFORNIA

ATTENTION ORGANIZATIONS AND CORPORATIONS:
This book is available at quantity discounts on bulk purchases for educational, business, or sales promotional use. For further information, please contact Impact Publishers, P.O. Box 6016, Atascadero, California 93423-6016.
Phone: 805-466-5917, e-mail: info@impactpublishers.com

Library of Congress Cataloging-in-Publication Data

McKay, Gary D
  Body, mind, and spirit : "vitamins" for your whole health / Gary D. McKay, Erik Mansager, and Wayne F. Peate.
    p. cm.
  Includes bibliographical references and index.
  ISBN 978-1-886230-81-1 (alk. paper)
  1. Medicine, Psychosomatic. 2. Health. 3. Well-being. I. Peate, Wayne F. II. Mansager, Erik. III. Title.
  RC49.M365 2009
  613—dc22

                                                                2008039910

Publisher's Note: This publication is designed to provide accurate and authoritative information in regard to the subject matter covered. It is sold with the understanding that the publisher is not engaged in rendering psychological, medical, legal, or other professional services. If expert assistance or counseling is needed, the services of a competent professional should be sought.

Impact Publishers and colophon are registered trademarks of Impact Publishers, Inc.

Cover design by Gayle Downs, Gayle Force Design, Atascadero, California
Composition by UB Communications, Parsippany, New Jersey
Printed in the United States of America on acid-free, recycled paper
Published by **Impact Publishers**®
POST OFFICE BOX 6016
ATASCADERO, CALIFORNIA 93423-6016
www.impactpublishers.com

CONTENTS

Introduction 1

The Cree Shield 11

PART I: THE THREE DIMENSIONS OF HEALTH: BODY, MIND, AND SPIRIT 13

1. First Dimension: Body 15
   WAYNE F. PEATE

   Meditation and Movement 41
   BILL W. HILLMAN

2. Second Dimension: Mind 43
   GARY D. MCKAY

3. Third Dimension: Spirit 63
   ERIK MANSAGER

   "You'll Live Longer If You Die Laughing":
   The Value of Humor 89

PART II: APPLICATION TO THE CHALLENGES OF LIVING 111

4. De-stressing Yourself 113

5. "Who's on Top?": Aggression and Anger 133

6. In the Mood: Depression 159

7. The Sun Will Rise Tomorrow: Addiction 185

8. When Life Seems Too Much: Chronic Illness 221

   The Aging Cure: Making It Worth the Wrinkles 249
   JAMES R. HINE

9. See What Tomorrow Brings: Aging and Planning
   for the Future 255

Appendix: Recommended Books, Articles, and Websites 285

References 291

Index 301

DEDICATIONS

To my wife Joyce for putting up with me all these years!

GARY D. MCKAY

To Lynn, Lauren, Marissa, and Elise who have touched my soul.

WAYNE F. PEATE

To Pudge. Debt lovingly repaid.

ERIK MANSAGER

ACKNOWLEDGMENTS

Many have contributed in different and unique ways to the development and publication of this book. We wish to acknowledge the following with deep appreciation.

First, thanks to the staff at Impact Publishers, especially our editors Kelly Burch and Robert Alberti, whose critique, suggestions, and edits were invaluable to this project.

Next we'd like to thank some of the wonderful Adlerians in our lives — James Bitter, Oscar Christensen, Rudolf Dreikurs, Don Dinkmeyer, Sr., Albert Ellis, Bill Hillman, Jane Griffith, Leo Gold, Jim Hine, Richard Royal Kopp, Al Milliren, Harold Mosak, Bill Nicoll, Walter "Buzz" O'Connell, Robert L. Powers, Henry Stein, Wes Wingett, and Vicki and James Straub — have been our teachers and colleagues whose work and friendship have inspired and enriched our knowledge and careers.

The only people in our lives we're more grateful to are our wives and partners in life — Joyce L. McKay, Ph.D., Lynn Struthers Peate, M.D., and Jane Pfefferlé-Mansager, M.A., M.C. — for their love, encouragement, support, and patience with us as we spent many hours writing this book.

Gary wishes to give a special thanks to Lyric Peate (Wayne's niece and Gary's honorary adopted granddaughter) for her assistance in data entry and the editing process. Erik would like to acknowledge Jos Corveleyn at Katholieke Universiteit Leuven, who is a personal and professional exemplar of holistic psychology and spirituality.

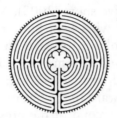

BODY, MIND, AND SPIRIT: "VITAMINS" FOR YOUR WHOLE HEALTH

Remember the past, but don't dwell on it. Look toward the future, but don't count on it, and always enjoy every single second of the present.

— MATTIE J. T. STEPANEK

Zooming down a Chicago hotel hall in his wheelchair — like any other boy running on legs — a quick pass and look around the gift shop and off down the hall again. That was our first encounter with the late Mattie J. T. Stepanek, then the twelve-year-old international ambassador for the Muscular Dystrophy Association and an inspiration to us all. Mattie was at the 2002 annual convention of the North American Society of Adlerian Psychology with his mother and counselor to receive a recognition award and make a presentation.

Born with a rare dystrophic disease — mitochondrial myopathy — Mattie lost two siblings from the same disease before his birth and another one when Mattie was two. Mattie wasn't supposed to last very long either, but at that time he was still going. He was attached to a tube in his windpipe — a "trach" for oxygen — and of course he moved around by

1

wheelchair. Yet this didn't slow him down. His stunning personality and brilliant mind kept him going and inspiring others with his poems and interviews. When we met him, Mattie had published four books of poetry (see the appendix for his website address) and was working on a book about world peace with former U.S. president Jimmy Carter.

On the Larry King Live show (2003), Mattie answered questions from callers. When asked what kept him going, he replied: "Friends, family, and God and looking forward to what's going to happen tomorrow." He then quoted some lines for the caller from that inspirational poem he had written in 2002: "Remember the past, but don't dwell on it. Look toward to the future, but don't count on it, and always enjoy every single second of the present." He went on to say: "It's really tough sometimes to stay positive. . . . Sometimes I say, 'Why me; why am I even doing this'? But it's important not to give up. If you give up there's nothing to live for. . . . You can say, 'I don't care if I have one hour or a millennium to live, I'm gonna live it to the fullest'. I stay positive by praying and talking with my family and friends."

Mattie wrote about and worked for peace. On Larry King's show he said: "If we spent as much time advocating peace as we do war, we'd have peace." Ah, the wisdom of youth! His sense of humor was priceless. One April Fools' Day he was in the hospital and full of tricks. I felt sorry for the doctors and nurses; they didn't know what hit them! Mattie wanted to be a father some day. On Larry King's show he also said: "I don't want to die anytime soon. I've got a lot to do while I'm here and I hope I can do it."

Mattie died on June 22, 2004 — just a few weeks short of his fourteenth birthday. What gifts he gave us while he was with us! His poems, his peace-making efforts, his charm, and his wonderful spirit will live forever. Mattie's positive attitude toward life, his faith, his relationships, and his contributions most likely aided in his living as long as he did.

What's Happening in Your Life?

Are you stressed, depressed, angry, fed up with what's going on in your life? Or, are things mostly okay, but you'd like your life to be better — more fulfilled? This book will help you make the most of your life. You can learn — as did Mattie Stepanek in his short fourteen years — to "add years to your life and life to your years."

Body, Mind, and Spirit: "Vitamins" for Your Whole Health addresses the "whole you." Your physical well-being, your mental state, and how you answer the big questions, such as "What's it all about?" are all interrelated.

We live in a fragmented world, with "experts" everywhere on every conceivable topic. It's nearly impossible to get a "big picture" look at issues today; when people go to the many sources available to them for input they find more contradiction than consensus. The experts are often more into promoting their own views or specialties than on seeing the matter as a whole.

Our approach, in contrast, celebrates the big picture. We are a physician, a psychologist, and a spiritually oriented clinical counselor who live and breathe a belief in the importance of the whole. We believe that sharing our knowledge and blending our approaches produces a result that is greater than the sum of the parts. In the chapters that follow, we intertwine our experiences and what we've learned to show that there is no disparity among the physical, mental, and spiritual aspects of health; that all aspects are interrelated; and that it's powerfully helpful to see health this way.

In this book, you'll learn how the health of your body affects your mental health and spiritual health and how to take better care of your body. You'll discover how your mind affects your physical health and spiritual health and how to take care of your mind. And you'll be shown what impact your beliefs about the meaning of life — your spirituality — have on body and mind and how to nurture your spirituality.

We address many life issues in this book, including stress, depression, aggression, addiction, chronic illness, and aging. You'll learn techniques to help you manage these challenges and others. You'll laugh and cry with the stories of unique people who've dealt with life's obstacles. You'll learn to identify how you're functioning and what you can do to improve. And you'll discover how to examine, plan, and track your progress.

Body, mind, and spirit are not separate parts but integrated, interwoven dimensions — like a "human quilt" — that contribute to a healthy, satisfying life. As you will see in this introduction and as you proceed through the book, the central, driving force of all three dimensions is our marvelous human brain. As you learn to change your perceptions and thoughts about your life, you will affect your physical, psychological, and spiritual health. For example, deciding to exercise will increase your energy. An increase in energy will, in turn, affect your outlook on life. Similarly, deciding to let go of negative thoughts and concentrate on what you can change benefits your physical health. Becoming involved in spiritual activities, such as prayer or nontheistic approaches to spirituality, will change the way you think and help you feel better physically and psychologically.

Negative thoughts — "I'm stupid." "Nobody cares about me." "I never do anything right." — are associated with such unhealthy conditions as depression, anxiety, heart disease, and even suicide. Can you recall times when you've harbored such negative thoughts? How did you feel? Maybe, at times, you've expected the worst and you got it! The late famed New York psychologist Dr. Albert Ellis coined the term "awfulizing" to describe the way many people exaggerate how bad a situation really is. The fact is things usually are not as awful as you think! (Remember Mattie.)

Okay, you can see the power of negative thinking. What about *positive* thoughts? Barbara Fredrickson, professor of psychology at the University of North Carolina, is one of hundreds of psychologists who have shown that such thoughts foster greater well-being and creativity (Fredrickson, 2004). In fact, "positive psychology" has become a promising and popular new field of study.

Journey with us as we explore how to access this storehouse of vitality for a better life.

The Secret to Well-Being Is Inside Your Head

Wayne F. Peate, M.D., M.P.H.

> *The brain is the largest secreting gland in the human body, and these secretions are the psychochemicals.*
>
> — PAUL PEARSALL

Although we have the power to create positive thoughts, many of us spend our time dwelling on what we have to do — or *think* we have to do — worrying about what's left to do, or what we haven't gotten done. Sound familiar? We may suffer from a condition I call "modernitis."

Modernitis

Modernitis refers to the physical effects of stress so frequently encountered in our hectic "instant everything, get it done yesterday" (that is, "modern") world (Peate & Hine, 1997). Natalie is one of many that I encounter every day with this condition.

> *One day in the clinic, a young saleswoman named Natalie had blood pressure that was on the boil. If her pressure had stayed in the stratosphere, she might have had a stroke — a*

destruction of brain cells that could put her in a wheelchair. She didn't have a history of heart symptoms or past medical conditions. None of her tests showed any signs of abnormality. So, I asked her: "Is there anything going on in your life?"

"I've been under a lot of stress lately," she admitted. She was working twenty hours of overtime a week to earn money to start her own business. She was not sleeping well. Her breakfast that morning had been two cups of black coffee and a nonprescription stimulant.

Natalie had modernitis. Her self-inflicted stress was destroying her. Where does stress really come from: other people, the job, traffic, the news? In fact, stress comes from none of these. Its origin is in the brain's perception of life events. Chronic stress from the pressures of modern living causes the release of a tidal wave of stress hormones that can damage your body. When you are under stress, the hypothalamus in the brain instructs the adrenal glands to release catecholamines (epinephrine and norepinephrine) and glucocorticoids (cortisol and cortisone), which, if elevated too long, weaken your immune system and increase your risk of obesity, insomnia, digestive problems, heart disease, depression, and memory impairment. In short, excessive stress isn't good for you!

There are many nutrients we must have to be healthy: water, essential fatty acids, essential amino acids, dietary minerals, and vitamins. Humans require thirteen vitamins: four that are fat soluble (A, D, E, and K) and nine that are water soluble (vitamin C and the eight B vitamins). Vitamins are essential for normal growth and development and for the healthy maintenance of the cells, tissues, and organs; we also need them to efficiently use the chemical energy that food provides and to process the proteins, carbohydrates, and fats required for respiration. Prolonged vitamin deficits may result in painful and potentially deadly diseases. Because our bodies don't store most vitamins (vitamins A, D, and B12 are exceptions), a well-balanced, vitamin-rich diet is necessary to optimize health (for a list of vitamins, their functions, and results of vitamin deficiencies, see http://dietary-supplements.info.nih.gov).

Like the rest of our body, our brain needs certain "vitamins" (neurochemicals) for optimal function. Here are just a few examples of chemicals under the control of the brain and their effects on our bodies:

- dopamine — affects attention, motivation, pleasure
- serotonin — affects mood, sleep, libido
- glutamate — affects alertness learning, memory

Can We Control Our Body Chemistry?

Ever have a near miss on the highway and feel that surge of adrenaline? The oldest part of the brain, known as the brainstem, releases chemicals that help us escape danger — and destroy us, if we let them. Our ancestors developed the "fight or flight" response to help us deal with danger. Because this response originates in the ancient prerational brain, it takes over the more rational, more developed, calmer brain we call the neocortex.

Once I lost my young child in a shopping mall. Fear flooded all thoughts. When I found her, anger erupted: "Where have you been? I've been looking everywhere." Certainly you've experienced simultaneous fear and anger like this. Everybody does at some point or other; it's part of being human.

Fear and anger have similar chemical pathways. When fear begins, it controls the emotions, the heart, and other muscles; we're tense, make bad decisions, lose sleep. The rational voice that urges us to use our heads gets lost in the roar of rage. Is this loss of control inevitable? Are the "fear and rage" chemicals supreme? No. Research has shown that focusing on nonfearful calming thoughts soothes our "savage breast."

> *Jack was a patient of mine with "rage syndrome" — uncontrolled fear and anger. I asked if there was one joyful moment that might counter his reoccurring negative emotions. "My wedding" was his response (Jack was recently married). I suggested that when he's ready to blow his top, he focus on thinking about the wedding and the joy it brought to his life. He reported to me that my suggestion worked.*

When I was discouraged in medical school, I listened to an upbeat Scottish tune — Sir Harry Lauder's Keep Right on to the End of the Road — to keep my spirits up. Music has a powerful effect on our emotions.

Positive emotions knock out health-sapping negative thoughts. In chapter 2, you'll learn more about how to take charge of your thoughts and emotions. But first, in the next section of this introduction Gary will introduce the power of the mind and perception.

Using Your Head

Gary D. McKay, Ph.D.

Wayne has explained how our minds influence our health. Our perception is the key because what we perceive, we believe. As the following old joke illustrates, it's not so much what is, as what we see.

Sherlock Holmes and Dr. Watson are going camping. They pitch their tent under the stars and go to sleep. In the middle of the night Holmes wakes Watson up.

Holmes: *"Watson, look up at the stars, and tell me what you deduce."*

Watson: *"I see millions of stars and even if a few of those have planets, it's quite likely there are some planets like Earth, and if there are a few planets like Earth out there, there might also be life."*

Holmes: *"Watson, you idiot, somebody's stolen our tent!"*

— ANANDAPPA

Just as Watson overlooks the obvious, we can, too. We can see either possibilities or restraints in life. It's up to us: we can choose to dwell on the minus side or the plus side.

As Wayne pointed out earlier in this introduction, focusing on the positive side of life can directly and powerfully influence your health. If you're going to make the most of your life — no matter what its boundaries — like Mattie, you have to "think outside the box" (or the tent, as the case may be). It's amazing what we can make out of what we have. Our thoughts, goals, and purposes enrich our lives or make us miserable — the choice is ours.

In chapter 2 you'll discover how you actually think yourself into strong, negative feelings that impact the quality of your life and health and how you can think yourself out of them. You will learn that as Dr. Harold Mosak, Adlerian therapist, teacher, and writer, says: "Believing is seeing." You'll see that your emotions serve a purpose; they provide the fuel for your actions. Throughout the book you'll learn how to apply what you learn about thinking and emotions to the challenges you face in life.

Other techniques for changing thinking, feelings, and actions will be introduced in chapter 2 and used throughout the book. These techniques include reframing — seeing the positive or opportunity in a situation you judge as negative — finding laughter and humor in the challenges of life, and using relaxation and imagery to deal with disturbing issues.

The last section of the introduction presents the value of spirituality for physical and mental health. Spirituality is prevalent among humans because everyone ponders the meaning of life and the universe. The popular theme song from the 1966 movie *Alfie* (featuring Michael Caine) put it this way: "What's it all about . . . ?"

Let's see what Erik has to say about the importance of spirituality.

Getting in the Spirit

Erik Mansager, Ph.D.

What is spirituality anyway? Tough question. And if there isn't a *final* answer (and there probably isn't), there are still some pretty good ones to get us started. Final meaning is the meaning of things at the end, the "real" meaning. We can never know this end, we go on trust; and spirituality is the attempt to make final meaning out of life experiences.

So much happens in life — so much good and so much bad — we thirst to understand and make sense out of it all. One way or another, we're on our way to quenching this thirst, to figuring it all out. The way you do that is your spiritual path.

Now here's an insight that we'll go deeper into later but that I want to introduce you to early: This "path"— whether you're religious or not — has two primary movements: *inward* and *outward*. The movements are something like the air we breathe (inhale/exhale, inhale/exhale . . .), the beating of our hearts (lub/dub, lub/dub . . .), or our gait when walking (left foot/right foot, left foot/right foot . . .). You'll soon see how interconnected, or holistic, these movements really are. One of the most common ways to understand the movements is to think of one of them as leading inward (*intra*-personal, inside yourself) and one as leading outward (*inter*-personal, between you and others).

The *inward movement* starts when you find yourself among others and progresses to finding yourself alone with your thoughts, desires, hopes, fears, and the like. Some people call this the movement to know yourself better, or to discover "authenticity," or to find your "truer self." It's about being connected, really rooted to your deepest convictions. With so many different people saying so many different things (including how to get salvation accomplished), it's very normal to try to figure things out for yourself. We humans work quite naturally to find a way to personally respond to it all. For at our "center," we act on our convictions and truest beliefs; that's who we are, it is our "I am."

The *outward movement* goes from within yourself out to the world and beyond. It's about being connected to something greater than yourself, understanding that you're not the center of the world (though some people act as if they are!), understanding that you're somehow part of something quite a bit greater. This can involve a personal god or some other higher power, or it can be quite secular in nature and involve whatever you value most dearly. And, naturally, some believers describe their god as their "ultimate value."

So here's another insight: "It's not just about me." Both parts of the spiritual movement are, instead, connected to "the other." Spirituality, the search for meaning, is a sense of connectedness with humanity, whether through a god, nature, or both. However you connect with others is certainly a matter of personal choice and conviction; but because we humans are social beings, it's vital to be connected to humanity in some way. We live in groups. Even hermits who live apart from others have to locate somewhere near a community where they can get food and other essentials to sustain their lives.

We've understood for a long time that "the punishment worse than death" is solitary confinement. Although we can choose to isolate ourselves for a time — after all, each of us can appreciate quiet time alone for reflecting or relaxing — choosing to isolate ourselves altogether does us more harm than good. We're not going to find enduring happiness or good health there.

So how are you connected to others? Your community? Your intimate connections? We'll explore these and lots of other questions later; but here you have the appetizer. Your unique spiritual breath, or heartbeat, or gait — or however you will come to make sense of it for yourself — forms the quest to make meaning out of life. In chapter 3 you'll learn all about this along with some "spiritual vitamins" that help you keep this process on track. Enjoy the stroll.

A Look Ahead

Okay, there you have it, the three dimensions of health: body, mind, and spirit. Here's a brief overview of what's in store for you in the book. *Body, Mind, and Spirit: "Vitamins" for Your Whole Health* has two parts:

In part I, "The Three Dimensions of Health: Body, Mind, and Spirit," we explain the three dimensions and how they interact to affect physical, psychological, and spiritual health. Thus, the first three chapters provide a detailed look at each dimension and how they interweave to make us "totally" human.

Between the parts we offer some ideas on how to apply perhaps the most beneficial human asset — a sense of humor — to your daily challenges.

In part II, "Application to the Challenges of Living," we apply the three dimensions to common human conditions or challenges: stress, aggression and anger, depression, addiction, chronic illness, and aging. As a bonus, you'll find a guide to recommended resources in the appendix.

You'll receive lots of ideas and food for thought in this book. In addition, we'll provide many suggestions for how to "healthy-up" your life. Learning to use these skills will take commitment and practice. Take it a step at a time, stick to it, and you'll find your life increasing in vitality. And don't forget Mattie's prescription:

". . . always enjoy every single second of the present."

Vitamins for Your Whole Health: Introduction

- Body, mind, and spirit are not separate parts but integrated, interwoven dimensions (like a "human quilt") that contribute to a healthy, satisfying life.
- Although we have the power to create positive thoughts, many of us spend our time worrying: a condition called "modernitis."
- Chronic stress from the pressures of modern living releases a tidal wave of stress hormones that can damage your body. Positive emotions can knock out health-sapping negative thoughts.
- Perception is key: what we perceive, we believe. We can see either the possibilities or the restraints in life.
- "Believing is seeing." Our thoughts and purposes can enrich our lives or make us miserable — the choice is ours.
- Although god is at the heart of many religions, god isn't necessarily at the heart of spirituality for many.
- Spirituality is our attempt to make meaning, final meaning, out of life experiences. The way we do that is our spiritual path, which has two primary movements: inward (intrapersonal, inside yourself) and outward (interpersonal, between yourself and others).
- Spirituality is a sense of connectedness with humanity and that which is greater than ourselves-whether through god, nature, or both.

When we discuss "God" in this book, we fully respect that many don't believe in a god. Our goal is to include believers and nonbelievers alike, and our intent is to explore spirituality irrespective of religious affiliation.

THE CREE SHIELD

Consider the Shield

Recently, Wayne had the opportunity to learn more about how indigenous people of North America utilize the three dimensions in healing. Marylyn Cook, M.D., a member of the Cree Nation who works for the Mohawk Council of Akwesasne, Quebec, Canada, described her approach. The Cree Shield (see illustration) has "the Creator" — that is, your highest value — in the center, surrounded by

Cree Shield

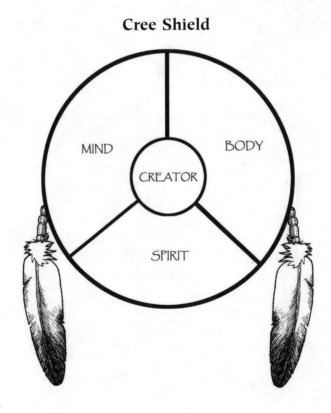

three segments. One stands for the spirit, another for the body, and the third for the mind. When she sees patients for an illness, she not only asks about their physical health, but also about what they are doing to improve their mind and spirit. For the mind, she might ask if they are learning anything new, if they are teaching others, such as their children or grandchildren, or whether they have any emotional issues. For the spirit, she asks if they would like any spiritual support for their health issues or other challenges in their lives. Her patients thrive because she understands the benefits of a holistic approach.

As you proceed through the book and learn more about the three dimensions, use the Cree Shield to "analyze" your progress. Consider each of the three dimensions and decide how you're doing and what you can or are willing to do to improve your health and your life.

PART I

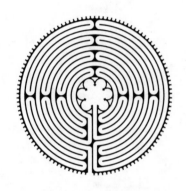

THE THREE DIMENSIONS
OF HEALTH: BODY,
MIND, AND SPIRIT

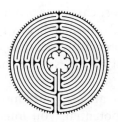

FIRST DIMENSION: BODY

Wayne F. Peate

*The best six doctors anywhere
And no one can deny it
Are sunshine, water, rest, and air,
Exercise, and diet.
These six will gladly you attend
If only you are willing.
Your mind they'll ease
Your will they'll mend
And charge you not a shilling.*

— NURSERY RHYME QUOTED
BY WAYNE FIELDS

I n this chapter, I discuss the tremendous influence of physical well-being on mental and spiritual well-being as well as behaviors that will help you improve and maintain your health. Let's start with a little "pretest" to focus our attention.

Which of the following is the cause of half the deaths in industrialized countries?

1. Heart disease

3. HIV/AIDS

2. Cancer

4. Behavior

The answer is 4. In most cases, according to research by Bill Foege and Mike McGinnis (1993), former heads of the Centers for Disease Control and Prevention, premature death is caused by what our brain tells our body about what to eat, smoke, or inject or with whom to copulate.

Physical health greatly affects your emotional health. If you want to reach your happiness potential, you must take care of your brain and body. People who modify their behavior in response to a disease or other physical disorder always report being happier, less stressed out, and less irritable. This improvement in mood is not simply the result of being free from the serious health problem: the less irritated your body is, the less irritated you are; the less burdened your body is, the less emotionally burdened you are; the happier your body is, the healthier your mind and spirit are. Health and happiness are mutually dependent.

You Won't Have to Fix It if You Don't Break It

An ounce of prevention is worth a pound of cure.

— BENJAMIN FRANKLIN

When it comes to your health, prevention is the easiest, most effective, least expensive, and least painful way to go. The quality of health care in the Western world is truly amazing, and yet a healthy lifestyle beats anything that medicine can offer. Prevention means taking an active role in your well-being. Prevention is as much about what you do as what you don't do. Prevention is exercising the brain, watching what you eat, making sure to get enough vitamins and minerals, exercising the body, getting adequate sleep, seeing your doctor for routine check-ups, avoiding tobacco and illicit drugs, and drinking only in moderation. Prevention is about taking responsibility for your current and future states of health. Living a healthy life does not mean you will never get sick; but it does ensure that if you do, your body will have a far better chance of recovering.

When was the last time you got a shot? Did you know that your need for immunizations doesn't end when you get your high school diploma? In fact, it never ends. According to a survey by the Centers for Disease Control and Prevention (2007), more than 80 percent of adults don't know this. Most adults don't realize there are vaccinations for adults other than those for the flu. However, immunizations can prevent serious illness and death. They save you money and, besides, when you keep up with your vaccinations, you're being a good example to your kids or grandkids.

Shots recommended for adults include those against pneumonia, hepatitis A, hepatitis B, tetanus, diphtheria, pertussis, bacterial meningitis, the human papillomavirus, shingles, and, of course, the yearly flu. Check the Centers for Disease Control and Prevention website to see their recommended adult immunization schedule (http://www.cdc.gov).

All adults need routine exams to check on the health of their heart, colorectal tract, ears, eyes, teeth, and reproductive tract and to check for diabetes and skin cancer. Women, in addition, need their thyroid health, bone density, and breast health checked. Go to the website of the U.S. Department of Health and Human Services to see their recommendations on when to go to your doctor for testing and what to be tested for:

> For women:
> http://www.womenshealth.gov/screeningcharts/general/general.pdf.

> For men:
> http://www.womenshealth.gov/screeningcharts/men/men.pdf.

Exercise for the Brain: Keep Learning

I think it keeps the little gray cells "a-perking" and "a-firing" away.

— JAN HENRIKSON (REGARDING SAGE, A LEARNING-IN-RETIREMENT PROGRAM)

To keep your brain healthy, exercise it and your body. Decreased blood flow to the brain and loss of brain cells lead to an ebbing memory and diminished ability to concentrate. Physical exercise helps the brain work better by causing nerve cells to multiply, strengthening their interconnections and protecting them from damage. Regular cardiovascular exercises, including brisk walking, slow jogging, biking, or swimming, improve circulation to the brain and can help improve memory 20 to 30 percent.

To flex your brain "muscle," incorporate mind-rousing games into your daily life that keep your mind working and energized. Listen intently and memorize names. Memorize shopping lists and poetry.

Figure out what change the cashier should give you every time you buy something even though you don't need to. Do sudoku and other puzzles. Use your left hand (or your right if you're left-handed) to eat and write. Learn new card games and play them with your friends.

Brain Food

A balanced diet rich in essential amino acids, omega oils, minerals, and vitamins ensures a vibrant, sharp memory. Make sure to eat some form of protein with every meal, such as nuts, seeds, beans, legumes, or animal products. Fish, especially deep ocean fish, is a good source for the essential oils that our brain cells need to function optimally. Some other foods especially good for our brain are apples, bamboo shoots, beets, bell peppers, celery, yams, squash, snow peas, pumpkin, potatoes, parsley, mushrooms, berries, papaya, pineapples, raspberries, oats, black beans, chestnuts, sesame seeds, and (black) walnuts.

Drinking green tea is thought to benefit the brain by lowering the activity of monoamine oxidase (an enzyme that contributes to Alzheimer's). Also, green tea is rich in polyphenols — antioxidants that help prevent premature brain aging (Graham, 1992; Yokogoshi et al., 1998). Herbs especially good for the brain are dill, clove, oregano, cilantro, rosemary, sage, fennel, anise, cardamom, garlic, onion, ginger, leek, scallion, pepper, chive, cinnamon, basil, and coriander.

The Sleep Factor

A good night's sleep is crucial for mental energy because our body regenerates during sleep. When you feel tired, take a fifteen-minute power nap.

Use It or Lose It

Education is not the filling of a pail, but the burning of a fire.

— WILLIAM BUTLER YEATS

Consider Alzheimer's disease, which has devastated millions with its crippling effects on the brain. Everywhere you turn, you hear about the dread effects of Alzheimer's on the body, from the late former president Ronald Reagan to the elderly next-door neighbor who can't remember your name. There is no cure, and available medication only slows the effects — until now. It's been discovered that keeping the mind active, working out the brain, can mitigate the effects of Alzheimer's, even in people who already have the disease. I say more on Alzheimer's in chapters 8 and 9.

Although the brain is an organ, it is much like a muscle in that it needs exercise to stay in shape. Continuing to learn throughout life provides that exercise.

The "Keep Learning" pyramid. You've probably seen the FDA food pyramid that illustrates the major food groups and the amount of each you should eat each day. I've followed that model for several similar pyramids you'll encounter throughout this chapter.

The first is a pyramid of mental activities that help prevent Alzheimer's disease and related conditions. For those who don't enjoy school, especially at a mature age, fear not! As Mark Twain quipped, "Never let school interfere with your education." Even activities like crossword puzzles have been shown to help. The secret is to keep the brain exercising. You choose the method. Be sure to make it fun! One grandfather plays chess via the Internet with his grandson 2,000 miles away. Another loves astronomy and volunteers to teach teens about his passion. The following graphic will guide you on the number of "mental workouts" you should have each day. The plus side is that, unlike the food pyramid, overdoing one item won't put you into diabetic coma or harden your arteries.

The pyramid begins by advising you to "watch TV sparingly." Why? Well, a couch potato is like any other potato — if it sits around too long, it rots! So the important thing is to keep your mind active — and there are many activities presented in the pyramid that do that. Of course, there are educational programs on TV that are valuable if they engage your thinking or promote a discussion with others. Good old-fashioned conversation also helps fire up those little gray cells.

In the second cell from the top, you're asked to "count your blessings," "identify what you are thankful for," and "thank those who help you." You may wonder what these activities have to do with exercising your brain. Simply, it reminds you that, as Erik said in the introduction: "It's not all about me!" You're connected to others and to the greater meaning of life. Doing these things will help you focus on "what it's all about."

As you study this pyramid, in addition to activities that will "strengthen your brain" you'll find ways that help maintain your mental health. Charles Berde, professor of anesthesiology and pediatrics at Boston's Children's Hospital, has conducted groundbreaking research on mind-body approaches to health for children with headaches. A six- to eight-week behavioral training program that focused on decreasing negative attitudes was found to be as beneficial as medicine

(Koman, 2005). You can reduce your "headaches" — physical or psychological — by replacing your negative thoughts with the more positive activities listed in the lower part of the pyramid. (In chapter 2, Gary discusses more ways to examine and change your negative thoughts and emotions.)

The "Keep Learning" Pyramid, along with two others I discuss later in the chapter is adapted from my book *Native Healing: Four Sacred Paths to Health* (Peate, 2002).

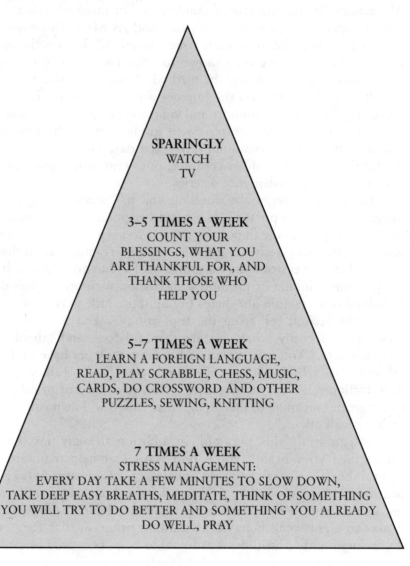

SPARINGLY
WATCH
TV

3–5 TIMES A WEEK
COUNT YOUR
BLESSINGS, WHAT YOU
ARE THANKFUL FOR, AND
THANK THOSE WHO
HELP YOU

5–7 TIMES A WEEK
LEARN A FOREIGN LANGUAGE,
READ, PLAY SCRABBLE, CHESS, MUSIC,
CARDS, DO CROSSWORD AND OTHER
PUZZLES, SEWING, KNITTING

7 TIMES A WEEK
STRESS MANAGEMENT:
EVERY DAY TAKE A FEW MINUTES TO SLOW DOWN,
TAKE DEEP EASY BREATHS, MEDITATE, THINK OF SOMETHING
YOU WILL TRY TO DO BETTER AND SOMETHING YOU ALREADY
DO WELL, PRAY

Brain Grooves

Imagine that you could look into the brain and see how it functions. Even better, what if you could guide the brain to heal itself of disorders such as Alzheimer's disease, schizophrenia, Parkinson's disease, insomnia, anxiety, and depression?

I'm reminded of my daughter's kindergarten teacher. She promised the parents that if we didn't believe half of what our kids said was going on in the classroom, she wouldn't believe half of what our kids said was going on at home! Until recently, what we know of the brain has been like that: we've only known half of what's going on.

fMRI (functional magnetic resonance imaging) reveals much about how the brain operates. It allows us to see what's happening in the part of the brain we haven't understood before and offers possibilities and opportunities to heal that might rival the discovery of antibiotics.

fMRI reveals which parts of our brains are active for different emotions, where we store certain types of memories, when we are attentive or creative, and how we are different from each other. For example, it has been shown to affect specific areas in the normal brain.

How does fMRI tell us what's going on? First some background on how the brain functions. The brain has about 100 billion neurons that together are similar to (although far more complex than) the hardware in a computer in that they store and process information. Most fascinating are the one to five quadrillion synapses that provide electrochemical connections between the neurons. These provide the "software" for the brain (Fields, 2008). Computers need power to run; so does the brain. It uses the energy stored in glucose that is delivered to the brain by the bloodstream. If your blood sugar is ever low, you'll recognize how poorly your brain works when it is starved.

Brain Triads

This brain triad that is similar to the three parts of a computer provides an infinitude of possibilities for new ideas and responses and for healing troubled brains.

Here's what scientists have learned about this topic of brain health using fMRI. When we are creative, telling a story, or daydreaming, the part of our brain called the dorsolateral prefrontal cortex shuts down and another part, the medial prefrontal cortex, fires up. The results are amazing. We suddenly have an increased ability to use our senses of touch, sound, sight, and smell (Limb, 2008).

The implications for human healing are profound. We already know that singing or humming can stop a stutter. Successful country singer and stutterer Mel Tillis is one of many examples. When he sings his stutter disappears. Likewise for stroke victims. Instead of having them rehabilitate their impaired speech with the current method of word repetition, perhaps we should have them also sing to fully activate their lost senses and brain function.

Similarly, now that fMRI has shown us that different parts of the brain turn on and off in a certain order, we might be able to use this knowledge to add to our treatment of schizophrenics, whose brains activate in a different order from those who don't have schizophrenia.

Can humans really rewire their brain for the better? Previously, it was believed that we couldn't change the structure of the brain, but strong evidence now exists that we can through an understanding of plasticity. An example of this concept is that pianists have more white matter — the myelinated axons or "connectivity" part of the brain that transmits brainwaves — than others. The longer one has played the piano, the greater the effect (Bengtsson, 2005; Fields, 2005).

If we can rewire the structure (or hardware) of the brain by playing a musical instrument, consider what we could do to repair brains damaged by the loss of myelin caused by multiple sclerosis. Maybe we can eliminate the chronic sleep loss caused by an overactive part of the brain by soothing it via guided brain therapy using fMRI to locate troublesome areas. Alzheimer's patients suffer from impaired thinking from poor brain transmission connectivity due to tangled brain fibers. Why not create new connections with a brain makeover with the help of fMRI?

Train Your Brain

Spirituality plays a fascinating role in our understanding of plasticity and the healing potential of the brain to change itself. Buddhist monks with 10,000 hours of meditation can slow their heart rate, alter their skin temperature, and turn on the positive thinking part of the brain in the frontal cortex where our greatest intellectual and mental potential resides. Dr. Richard Davidson and associates (2005), in cooperation with the Dalai Lama, are using fMRI to investigate which body functions and conditions, such as insomnia and depression, can be changed by meditation. Stay tuned.

Maybe you are intimidated by 10,000 hours as the admission price for meditation-induced healing. I certainly was. To attain this level would require one hour of meditation every day for thirty years! fMRI may provide a shortcut if we can find that activating certain brain areas through a selective meditative approach has a greater and quicker yield than routine meditation.

An example of such a fast track to reach a difficult goal is training for a marathon. Previously it was thought you had to run every day. A less time-consuming and equally effective strategy requires only three days of running a week. This homed in approach might work for brain workouts. A medical colleague of mine used meditation after knee surgery to manage pain so that he could avoid using painkillers. In his entire life he had used meditation for less than 100 hours, a far cry from the 10,000-hour master monk level.

The future for plasticity and brain rehabilitation looks bright. Just as we advise stretches and exercises after a shoulder injury, we might prescribe brain function "practice" to heal mental damage. "Synapse stretches" might replace mind-altering medications for depression, anxiety, and attention deficit/hyperactivity disorder. Teachers might use brain calisthenics to wake up student brains, and composers could use synapse strengthening to write the next award-winning musical.

Secret to Happiness?

Master monks can readily increase gamma wave activity in the prefrontal area of the left brain, an area that corresponds to happiness, kindness, willingness to help others, and a higher level of consciousness. At the same time, they decrease activity in the right prefrontal region that corresponds to anxiousness and negativity.

Just as we brush our teeth to remove plaque and to prevent cavities, so can we emulate the monks' "brain scrubbing" to reduce negative thinking and anxiety. You might even produce superathletes with brain imagery that teaches the brain to imagine and then achieve better performance on the athletic field by staying "on game" with all your mental power (Coyle, 2007).

Keeping Physically Fit

Okay, I've discussed how keeping mentally fit helps improve your health, but as you know, being physically fit is also important. So in the next section I discuss ways to keep your body — and your health — in shape. I begin by discussing food, vitamins, and minerals.

What about Diet?

Certainly, what you eat has an effect on your heart as well as your health in general. The food pyramid shows what kinds of foods to eat as well as suggested amounts (USDA, mypyramid.gov). You can learn more by visiting the recommended websites on healthy eating listed in the appendix.

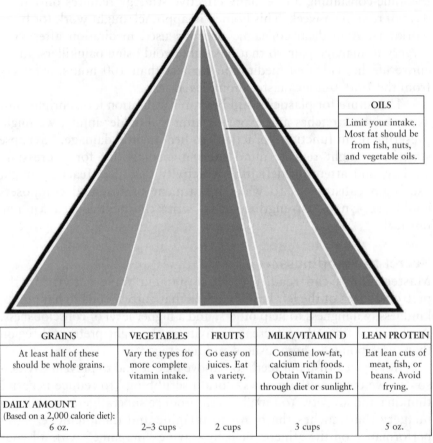

		OILS
		Limit your intake. Most fat should be from fish, nuts, and vegetable oils.

GRAINS	VEGETABLES	FRUITS	MILK/VITAMIN D	LEAN PROTEIN
At least half of these should be whole grains.	Vary the types for more complete vitamin intake.	Go easy on juices. Eat a variety.	Consume low-fat, calcium rich foods. Obtain Vitamin D through diet or sunlight.	Eat lean cuts of meat, fish, or beans. Avoid frying.
DAILY AMOUNT (Based on a 2,000 calorie diet): 6 oz.	2–3 cups	2 cups	3 cups	5 oz.

Remember to consume plenty of water. (Recommended amounts vary; 6–8 glasses is often suggested.) Sugar is not recommended, and consumption should be limited.

What about Vitamins?

You may have wondered, because the sub-title of this book begins with "Vitamins," just when we'd get around to talking about them. Well, the time has come. You're very likely aware that vitamins are natural substances found in plants and animals. Your body uses these substances to stay healthy and support its many functions. There are two types of vitamins: water soluble and fat soluble.

The water-soluble vitamins, vitamin C and the eight B-complex vitamins, are easily absorbed by your body. Your body doesn't store large amounts of these vitamins. Those you don't need right away are removed by your kidneys and come out in your urine. Water-soluble vitamins need frequent replacement in the body.

Fat-soluble vitamins. The fat-soluble vitamins are vitamin A, vitamin D, vitamin E, and vitamin K. A certain amount of fat is needed in the diet to help the body absorb these vitamins. Fat-soluble vitamins are found in the human liver. If the diet contains more fat-soluble vitamins than is immediately required, the surplus is stored in the liver and in fatty tissues. Fat-soluble vitamins are eliminated much more slowly than water-soluble vitamins.

What Are Minerals?

Dietary minerals such as calcium, phosphorus, iron, sodium, and selenium are the chemical elements our bodies need. Rich sources of calcium include dairy products and green leafy vegetables. Magnesium is found abundantly in nuts, cocoa, and soy beans. Legumes (for example, beans, peanuts, and peas), potato skins, tomatoes, and bananas are good sources of potassium. Sulfur (yes, you need it!) is found in meat, eggs, and legumes. Green leafy vegetables, fish, eggs, beans, and whole grains are rich in iron.

Do I Need to Take Vitamin and Mineral Supplements?

The best way to get the vitamins and minerals your body needs is from the food you eat. Most people don't need to take supplemental vitamins and minerals; you should not take them without consulting your doctor first. Your doctor may suggest taking vitamin or mineral supplements if you have certain health problems (for example, Crohn's disease and cystic fibrosis), smoke, drink excessively, or take certain medications that interfere with vitamin absorption. You need more vitamins and minerals at certain times in your life, such as the following:

- If you're a woman trying to get pregnant, your obstetrician will likely suggest you take a pill that contains folic acid. Women who don't get enough folic acid during pregnancy are more likely to have a baby with neural tube defects (serious problems of the brain or spinal cord). It's important to take folic acid before becoming pregnant because these problems develop very early in pregnancy.

- If you're pregnant or breastfeeding, your doctor may suggest that you take a prenatal mineral and vitamin pill that includes iron to protect you against anemia, calcium to keep your bones strong, and folic acid.
- If you're a man (currently there are 2 million men in the United States suffering from osteoporosis and another 12 million at risk for this disease) or woman at risk of osteoporosis, your doctor will suggest that you take a calcium supplement to support the health of your bones.
- If you eat a vegetarian or vegan diet (a diet that limits the animal products you eat), your doctor may suggest that you take supplements of vitamin B12, calcium, and vitamin D.

Can Vitamin and Mineral Supplements Be Dangerous?

Vitamins and minerals aren't dangerous unless you get too much of them. It would be hard to "overdose" on vitamins or minerals that you get from the foods you eat. But if you take supplements, you can get too much. There is a much greater risk of overdose with fat-soluble vitamins.

Taking too much of a dietary supplement can also cause problems with some medical tests or get in the way of how some drugs work. It's important to talk with your doctor before you take any vitamin or mineral supplement, especially if you take prescription medicines, have any health problems, or are elderly. You can learn more about vitamins and minerals by checking the recommended websites in the appendix.

Okay, so far we've discussed exercise for the mind as well as food, vitamin, and mineral intake. Let's move on now to more ways to stay healthy or improve your health beginning with physical activity.

Keep Moving: Physical Activity

The Centers for Disease Control and Prevention has provided conclusive evidence of the benefits of physical activity, including the prevention of diabetes, osteoporosis, heart disease, and even cancer.

One way to think about exercise is that it helps you avoid costly medicines. It makes your heart stronger, helping it pump more blood with each heartbeat. The blood then delivers more oxygen to your body, which helps it function more efficiently. Exercise also lowers blood pressure and reduces levels of LDL ("bad") cholesterol, which clogs the arteries and can cause heart attack, stroke, and peripheral vascular disease. At the same time, exercise raises levels of HDL ("good") cholesterol, which helps protect against heart disease.

Combined with a healthy diet, exercise speeds up weight loss. Regular exercise is also the best way to maintain weight loss. Regular exercise helps you burn calories faster even when you're sitting still — the extra muscle you've developed requires more calories even when you're at rest.

When the body is physically active, it produces endorphins — natural pain relievers. No drug allergies, known side effects, or FDA approval needed. Exercise reduces some of the effects of aging, contributes to your mental well-being, relieves depression, stress, and anxiety, increases your energy and endurance, helps you sleep better, and helps you maintain a healthy weight by increasing the rate at which you burn calories. Most health experts now agree that physical activity should be prescribed for nearly everyone.

How Much and What Kinds of Exercise Do I Need?

There are three types of exercise, and all are essential for achieving and maintaining health.

Aerobic exercise, also called cardiovascular or endurance exercise, includes brisk walking, dancing, swimming, hiking, bicycling, and playing tennis. Aerobic exercise involves physical activity that is rhythmic, repetitive, uses the large muscles, increases your heart and breathing rates (aerobic means "with oxygen"), and increases blood flow to the muscles for an extended period of time. Aerobic exercise reduces your risk of heart disease, high blood pressure, osteoporosis, diabetes, and obesity. For healthy people, the President's Council on Physical Fitness and Sports recommends a minimum of three twenty-minute sessions of continuous aerobic exercise per week.

Anaerobic exercise, also called strength training, includes lifting weights and doing push-ups, pull-ups, and sit-ups. The benefits of anaerobic exercise include the increase and maintenance of bone density and muscle mass and tone, increased tendon and ligament strength, improved physical performance and appearance, improved metabolic efficiency, and decreased risk of injury. Recommended is a minimum of two twenty-minute sessions per week that include exercises for all the major muscle groups (upper body: chest, upper back, arms, and shoulders; middle body: abdominals and lower back; and lower body: backside and legs).

Also essential to health, although often overlooked, is exercise that increases **flexibility**. This includes yoga, tai chi, and just plain stretching and benefits the range of motion of joints and muscles, reduces the risk of injuries during other activities, and decreases the probability that you will suffer from back pain and other postural types of pain syndromes. Keeping joints, tendons, and ligaments flexible makes it easier to move around. The President's Council on Physical Fitness and Sports advises ten to twelve minutes of daily stretching exercises performed slowly, without a bouncing motion.

It is important that your exercise routine include some weight-bearing exercises, that is, exercises that work against the force of gravity. Weight-bearing exercise is essential for building strong bones, which helps prevent osteoporosis and bone fractures later in life. Examples of weight-bearing exercises are walking, jogging, hiking, climbing stairs, dancing, and weight training.

It is wise to warm up before and cool down after your aerobic exercise sessions. For warm up, five to ten minutes of exercise such as walking, slow jogging, knee lifts, arm circles, trunk rotations, or low intensity movements that simulate movements to be used in the activity are effective. For cool down, you need a minimum of five to ten minutes of slow walking or low-level exercise combined with stretching, which can count as your flexibility exercise.

Tips You Can Use

Remember it's all about physical activity — not equipment or a skill. Gardening, hauling the laundry basket, and walking the dog all count. The key is to keep moving. At home avoid staying on the couch, do a chore, etc. Consider buying a treadmill or similar device: you won't be able to say it's too rainy to exercise!

Where exercise is concerned, one size certainly doesn't fit all. The "Keep Moving" pyramid offers options. In general, if you haven't been exercising, gradually work up to the exercise program that is ideal for you. Your doctor will help you decide what is best based on your health. As you're getting started, try to alternate exercise days with rest to prevent injuries.

I Know I Should, but . . .

Motivation, of course is an important factor in getting regular exercises. Let's say you decide to jog. Inevitably there will be times when you are too tired, too busy, just don't feel like it, or are bored with it. Or like many of my patients, you have a hard time getting started. I often hear comments such as

- "I'm too heavy to exercise."
- "I don't like health clubs, it's a meat market. They'll make fun of me."
- "I'm too tired at the end of the day to exercise, and too busy in the morning before work."
- "Exercise makes my knees (back, feet, etc.) hurt."

If you're prone to making excuses to not exercise (and most of us are), there's a solution. Read on.

Get Yourself an Exercise Buddy

Ever start on an exercise program or diet in January to shed some of your holiday-acquired weight? (You know, those good ole New Years' resolutions) Sometimes after a week or two of determination, your efforts fail. Consider the following to regain your resolve:

"No man is an island" goes the expression. Use the power of relationships in healing. Support groups for breast cancer and other illnesses and conditions have taught us that the power of one is greater when united with the whole. What does that mean for exercise?

Consider group exercise programs. Or, exercise with your spouse or partner, a friend, co-worker, or neighbor. If you do this, two amazing things may happen. First, the commitment to meet someone else for the designated activity will propel you to get out of bed, stop what you're doing, etc. When you're down, your exercise partner is likely to be up and vice versa; both of you are more likely to continue. Second, the psychological benefits are enormous. My wife and I, when our children were old enough, began to jog together again. It was like rediscovering an old friend, one to talk with (we jog slowly) without interruptions by children or phones (we leave our cell phones at home).

Having an exercise buddy is often the most effective motivator to get you going. Here are some other things to try (adapted from Pierson & Cloe) when your exercise buddy is out of commission:

- Build on success. Start with small goals that lead to larger goals.
- Find a role model. Find someone who started where you were. Get inspired by their success.
- Be realistic. Set attainable goals.
- Set well-defined goals and reward yourself for reaching them.
- Keep an exercise journal. You'll be able to see how far you've progressed and evaluate what works and what doesn't.
- Create variety. As you learn the basics add new exercises and activities into your program. This will help keep you from becoming bored with your routine.
- Don't make exercise just another item on your to-do list. Connect to it on a deeper level.
- Educate yourself. The more you know, the less likely you are to be injured or to get stuck in a rut.

- Know your limits and stay within your means. Fatigue, insomnia, irritability, and elevated resting heart rate are all signs of overdoing it.

"Keep Moving" Pyramid

As I said above, physical activity doesn't require membership in a health club or expensive equipment: walking, weeding, vacuuming, parking farther from your destination, taking the stairs instead of the elevator all count. Walk during a coffee break or lunch. Walk more briskly. Do housework at a quicker pace and more often (for example, vacuuming every other day instead of once a week). Rake leaves, push the lawn

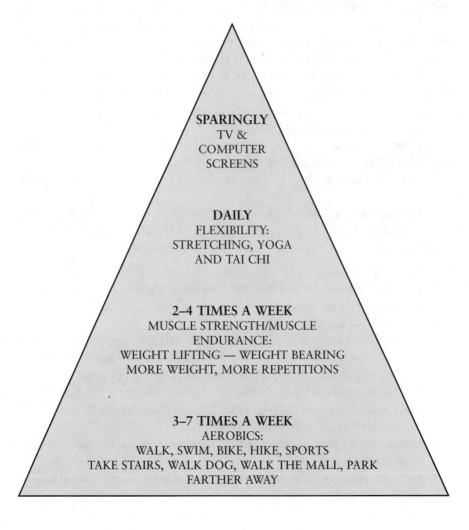

SPARINGLY
TV &
COMPUTER
SCREENS

DAILY
FLEXIBILITY:
STRETCHING, YOGA
AND TAI CHI

2–4 TIMES A WEEK
MUSCLE STRENGTH/MUSCLE
ENDURANCE:
WEIGHT LIFTING — WEIGHT BEARING
MORE WEIGHT, MORE REPETITIONS

3–7 TIMES A WEEK
AEROBICS:
WALK, SWIM, BIKE, HIKE, SPORTS
TAKE STAIRS, WALK DOG, WALK THE MALL, PARK
FARTHER AWAY

mower, trim the hedges. For those with special needs, disabilities, or injuries, alternative programs can be devised — see your doctor.

Much like the food pyramid, the "Keep Moving" (or physical activity) Pyramid provides a visual guide on the "portions" of activity to follow.

Sleep: Beyond Forty Winks

Early to bed and early to rise, makes [a woman and] a man healthy, wealthy, and wise.

— BEN FRANKLIN

Our good friend Ben Franklin apparently knew a thing or two about health and its impact on happiness. After all, he made it to the wise old age of eighty-four — not so common in eighteenth-century America.

For the average person, sleep consists of about five ninety-minute cycles during which we pass through rapid eye movement, or REM, sleep and four stages of non-REM sleep. Stages 1 and 2 sleep are considered light sleep and stages 3 and 4 are deep sleep. The REM and non-REM periods each have their own set of associated physiological, neurological, and psychological features. We spend 20 to 25 percent of our sleep time in REM sleep, during which we do most of our dreaming. According to the National Sleep Foundation (http://www.sleepfoundation.org), average, healthy adults need seven to nine hours of sleep each night from young adulthood through the later years.

And what's with all those weird dreams? Well, according to one theory, during the REM stage neurons in the pons fire at random. The forebrain then creates a story using these stimuli in an attempt to interpret the nonsensical sensory information it is receiving (Hobson & McCarley, 1977).

Widespread decreased sleep started with Thomas Edison and the invention of the light bulb. Previously, we went to bed when the sun went down and got up when the sun did. These days, due to modernitis, many of us feel that the bare minimum of sleep is sufficient, that sleep is a luxury to be caught up with on weekends or on vacation. Lack of sleep has a profound impact on our daily lives. Sleep is a major player along with exercise and proper diet to keep us alert and happy and living longer, higher quality lives.

Getting the optimal amount of sleep not only feels great, it is essential for our physical, and therefore mental and spiritual, health. During REM sleep the brain rebuilds itself. In stage 4 sleep, major healing occurs as the body rebuilds itself, regenerating cells and healing wounds.

Some large studies indicate that the recent increase in obesity seen in Westernized countries may be in part due to the decrease in the amount of sleep people are getting these days. Modernitis strikes again! These studies suggest that insufficient sleep increases appetite as well as decreasing our ability and motivation to make wise food choices. In deep sleep, growth hormone is produced in copious amounts. Muscle building requires growth hormone (at all stages of life, not just childhood). If you don't get enough deep sleep, your body doesn't make enough growth hormone, and the calories you've consumed during the day are made into fat instead (Hasler et al., 2004; Van Cauter & Spiegel, 1999). Diabetes is another concern for the sleep deprived. Sleep deprivation severely affects the body's ability to metabolize glucose, which can lead to early stage diabetes type 2 (Gottlieb et al., 2005).

Extreme sleep deprivation has been linked to the following problems: muscle aches, decreased mental activity and concentration, headache, daytime drowsiness (no surprise here), hyperactivity, irritability, memory lapses, blurred vision, depression, nausea, slowed reaction time, hypertension, impatience, a weakened immune system, and dizziness (Harvard Health Publications; Postgraduate Medicine Online; Read).

To decide if you have a sleep disorder, ask yourself these questions:

- Do you have problems staying awake doing routine things?
- Have you ever fallen asleep at the wheel or caught yourself dozing off while driving?
- Do you nap more than once a day?
- Do you feel tired after getting up?
- Does it take you more than a half hour to fall asleep?
- Do you have leg cramps or other leg symptoms at night? (If so you may have restless leg syndrome, a treatable condition. See your doctor.)
- Do others complain that you snore or have difficulty breathing at night? (You might have sleep apnea, another treatable condition that should be evaluated by a doctor.)

If you responded yes to any of these questions, you may find yourself in need of a sleep makeover. Follow these suggestions for better sleep, and you'll wake up feeling more refreshed.

- Set your bedroom temperature five degrees cooler than you are used to.
- Avoid beverages or foods with caffeine (coffee, tea, soda, and chocolate) at least four hours before bed.
- Cut back on nicotine intake.
- Avoid alcohol. It can make you sleepy, but it interferes with your REM sleep.
- If you exercise in the evening, make sure that you do it at least three or four hours before bedtime. (Exercise right before bed revs up the heart and makes it difficult to fall asleep.)
- Avoid heavy meals close to bedtime.
- Try taking a hot bath to relax before bedtime.
- Set up a regular sleeping and waking schedule. Going to bed at the same time each night (even on weekends!) and waking up at the same time each morning helps set your internal clock.
- Invest in a comfortable bed and pillow. You spend a third of your life in bed. It's worth the investment.
- Bed should be only for sleep and sex. Try to avoid doing anything else in bed.
- Avoid discussing or thinking about work and other life problems in bed.
- Avoid watching television and doing other stimulating activities right before bedtime.
- Try relaxation techniques such as breathing exercises or meditation. Several recordings are available.
- Keep the room quiet and dark. Invest in earplugs and an eyeshade if you need to.

If you work nights, try these suggestions:

- Eat your biggest meal when you wake up. You need the food for fuel. If most of your food intake is later in the day, the body stores it as fat and this leads to obesity, another risk factor for decreased sleep.
- Have caffeine-containing foods and beverages only before or early in your shift.
- Avoid fatty heavy foods toward the end of the shift. They take eight or more hours to digest.

Improving your sleeping habits will give you more energy and allow you to be more focused on your daily activities.

A Word on the Sun

The bottom line: get some, but not a lot. Ultraviolet rays from the sun activate vitamin D synthesis in your skin. Fifteen minutes of sunshine twice weekly will help you get your vitamin D, which is essential for musculoskeletal health and the immune system. Exposure to sunlight early in the day helps set our body clock (a control center in the hypothalamus region of the brain called the suprachiasmatic nucleus), which regulates our sleep/wake cycle. Sunlight may also boost mood by aiding in the production of serotonin (Lambert et al., 2002). But remember, skin cancers are the fastest growing type of cancer: use sunscreen!

Keep It Clean

Don't forget the impact of personal hygiene on your overall health. Wash your hands often and brush and floss your teeth daily. Recent research (Matthews, 2008) has indicated that those with poor oral hygiene are at an increased risk for heart disease. When our gums bleed, bacteria from the mouth enter the bloodstream. These bacteria irritate the lining of artery walls and cause them to inflame. The inflammation causes the formation of fatty plaques (artherosclerosis) and leaves the arteries vulnerable to ruptures, which lead to heart attack and stroke. Also atherosclerosis thus caused can block the artery, again leading to heart attack and stroke.

Moving On

I've discussed how taking good care of your body keeps us emotionally healthy. So now you know how to choose between eat, drink, and be merry for tomorrow we die and eat, drink, and be merry so that tomorrow *you can do it again!* Let's touch on the converse: how taking care of our emotional health keeps us physically healthy.

Head Trip to Health

While training as a physician, I met a patient whose body was sabotaging itself. Susan had rheumatoid arthritis, an autoimmune disease that cripples the joints. Her immune system — that wondrous mechanism that vigilantly defends our bodies against millions of bacteria, viruses, toxins, and parasites — was attacking the tissues of her joints as though they were foreign invaders. Her arthritis specialist taught me a lesson about the supremacy of the brain that I'll never forget. He drew fluid from one of Susan's swollen joints into a syringe. He filled another syringe with water.

He then dripped some of her fluid on her arm and said, "This fluid is from Susan's joint. It's filled with her own cells that are attacking her and causing her arthritis. Look what happens." Suddenly a red welt consistent with an allergic reaction appeared on her skin.

"I'm just allergic to myself," Susan said with resignation.

"Now watch the difference with water." He dripped an equal amount of fluid from the other syringe on her arm. Nothing happened. We said our goodbyes to Susan, and as we walked down the hallway, he told me that he had used fluid from the same syringe, the one with her joint fluid. Her belief that one syringe held only water made all the difference in her body's reaction.

We've all heard stories of how a frail elderly person lifted a car off a trapped victim. The only explanation was that the person's belief — like Susan's — made it possible. Does belief make a difference in your daily life? If you think you can do something, it's a whole lot more likely that you can.

Remember the first time you were deeply in love with someone who felt the same way about you? Remember how life's irritations just didn't seem to matter? A brain that's placed in a "positive gear" steers around bad emotions and circumstances.

Positive perceptions can even prevent heart disease. In this section, I show you how.

Healthy Heart or Mind?

The epidemiologist Michael Marmot (2003), who has conducted seminal studies of heart disease and stroke, points to two interesting factors that improve physical health: "enhancing the social and psychological resources of individual people, and improving the quality of neighborhoods and communal life" (p. 136). He goes on to say: "My own view is that the mind is a crucial gateway through which social influences affect physiology to cause disease. The mind may work through effects on health-related behavior, such as smoking, eating, drinking, physical activity, or risk taking, or it may act through effects on neuroendocrine or immune mechanisms" (p. 135).

Marmot affirms the power of the mind to help or hinder health through a variety of mechanisms. For example, two similar individuals with the same type and severity of disease can respond very differently to treatment. Attitude — the perception of events, even one's willingness to recover from an illness — is affected by the mind.

Is perception everything? What is the influence of your perception of your surroundings and your socioeconomic status? Which has the greatest effect on the differences in heart disease between rich and poor neighborhoods: income, education, occupation, smoking, physical activity, high blood pressure, type of cholesterol, weight/body mass index, or diabetes?

The answer, based on research in Britain and the United States, may surprise you. The answer is "all of the above" and more! Research suggests that there's something beyond genetics, lifestyle, behavior, income, and health care disparities that disrupt our health. For example, African Americans living in poor neighborhoods who have the *same* income, education, lifestyle, and risk factors as Whites in wealthier neighborhoods have more heart disease (Marmot 2003). Is it looking over your shoulder, comparing yourself to others, or lack of control that leads to health disparities? You're probably catching the pattern — the answer is "all of the above and more." What's inside your head — psychosocial factors — often trumps physical factors.

Think Yourself Happy

> Cogito, ergo sum. [I think, therefore I am.]
>
> — RENÉ DESCARTES

French philosopher Rene Descartes is credited with concocting the dualistic idea of separating the mind and body in Western thought. Modern research suggests that Descartes had it wrong. The mind and body are intimately intertwined.

Previously, illnesses of the mind were perceived as moral weaknesses. The mind was divorced from the body. Now, in many cases, disorders such as depression and anxiety are known to be the result of a body chemical imbalance. And the mind exerts a powerful influence on the production of body chemicals.

Present-day psychology and psychiatry often apply treatments that work synergistically with both the mind and the body. For example, depression is often effectively treated by combining antidepressants (body) with cognitive therapy (mind).

But can your mind heal your body and add vitality to your years? The answer is yes. As you explore the rest of this book, you'll discover

- that the body-mind-spirit connection has healing power
- that relaxation, hypnosis, volunteering, and physical activity should be prescribed as often as, or more than, drugs
- that "attitude is fortitude"

Now let's look at how the body and mind connect with the third dimension — spirit.

Body-Mind-Spirit Connection: Stay Connected

To emphasize that the three authors believe strongly in the holistic approach, as a physician I want to say some specific things about the interconnection of body, mind, and spirit. Numerous studies have demonstrated that people who pray regularly or who otherwise stay socially connected in a positive way live up to seven years longer than those who don't. In fact, the National Institutes of Health has funded a major study to assess the benefits of prayer, which Erik will address in chapter 8 on chronic illness.

For now I want to point out that the effect of social connectedness religion and spirituality offer is so profound that it can actually counteract some of the negative effects of smoking. Does this mean to light up? Hardly. What it suggests is that life is full of life-enhancing and life-diminishing choices that we have control over.

Several studies have demonstrated the growing body of evidence on the "stay connected" effect. Duke University conducted a study (Levin et al., 2006) of almost 4,000 older adults and found that regular worship can lead to a decrease in depression and anxiety and can improve the immune system. The social connections related to prayer have been shown to improve the quality of life for those with alcoholism, drug abuse, heart conditions, stroke, and rheumatoid arthritis. Prayer and the connective aspects of spirituality induce many other benefits as well.

And what if you're a nontheist and therefore don't pray? Whatever form your spirituality takes, as Erik will show you in chapter 3, it has an effect on your health.

The "Stay Connected" Pyramid

In the section on spirituality in the introduction, Erik pointed out that we humans are social beings and therefore need to be connected to others. This connection can be through work, social activity, volunteering, sharing spiritual activities, or all of the above. The "Stay Connected" Pyramid guides you on the amounts and types of social connection activities that add years to your life and life to your years.

At the top of the pyramid the advice "avoid self-pity" is given. It's important to do this because self-pity can isolate you from others or encourage you to seek others to feel sorry for you, which won't improve your relationships!

As you read through the pyramid, notice how different types of both social and spiritual suggestions are made. As Erik has pointed

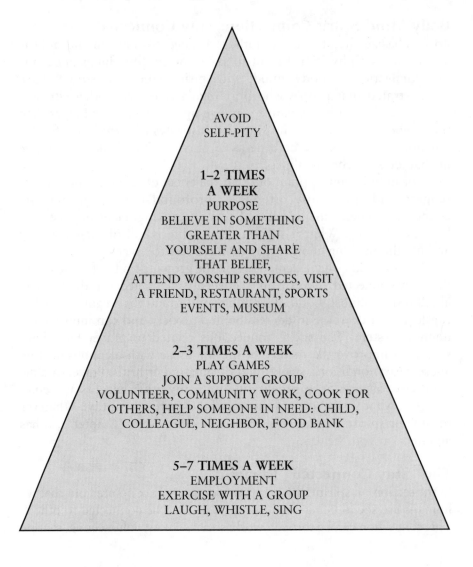

AVOID
SELF-PITY

**1–2 TIMES
A WEEK**
PURPOSE
BELIEVE IN SOMETHING
GREATER THAN
YOURSELF AND SHARE
THAT BELIEF,
ATTEND WORSHIP SERVICES, VISIT
A FRIEND, RESTAURANT, SPORTS
EVENTS, MUSEUM

2–3 TIMES A WEEK
PLAY GAMES
JOIN A SUPPORT GROUP
VOLUNTEER, COMMUNITY WORK, COOK FOR
OTHERS, HELP SOMEONE IN NEED: CHILD,
COLLEAGUE, NEIGHBOR, FOOD BANK

5–7 TIMES A WEEK
EMPLOYMENT
EXERCISE WITH A GROUP
LAUGH, WHISTLE, SING

out, it's important that you be connected with others or with god — if that's your belief — and that you recognize you aren't the center of the universe, that there is something greater, however you perceive it.

Pain — When Is It Physical and When Is It Psychological?

Physical symptoms like a headache or stomachache can be physical or psychological. How can you tell? Dr. Alfred Adler, psychiatrist and founder of Individual Psychology, used a diagnostic procedure to differentiate between somatic or physical causes of physical symptoms and psychosomatic or psychological causes of physical symptoms. He would ask his patient "The Question" (Adler, 1964; Dreikurs 1958, 1962; Mosak & Maniacci, 1998): "What would be different in your life if you didn't have this problem?"

If the person simply answered that he or she would not be in pain, then it was probable that the pain was somatic, or physical. If, however, the person's response indicated that without the pain she or he would be able to handle a particular task — such as completing a project, taking a certain job, or entering into a relationship — then it was probable that the pain was psychosomatic: the person's pain actually helped him or her avoid the task.

If you're experiencing a physical symptom such as a headache or stomachache and your physician can't find a physical cause, perhaps your pain has a purpose. You can ask yourself the same question: "How would my life be different if I didn't have this pain?" If your answer is simply that you wouldn't be in pain, then it's possible that your pain is somatic and your physician missed something.

If, on the other hand, your answer relates to being able to complete a particular task if you didn't have the pain, then it's possible that your pain is psychosomatic: your purpose is to avoid the task. If so, what is there about the task that's frightening? Are you afraid that you won't be able to do the task perfectly or at least well enough to satisfy yourself or others? If so, then you have a decision to make. You can decide to take the risk and do the task, even imperfectly, or you can decide not to do the task. With either decision, the pain no longer serves a purpose and will lessen or disappear. You could also decide not to decide: to leave things as they are, stay in pain so you can continue to avoid the task — or at least avoid making a decision.

"The Question" technique isn't intended to be used apart from a physician's care. So whenever you're in pain, even if you think you could be using the pain to avoid a task, make sure your physician thoroughly checks to see if it's somatic — physical — or not.

In this chapter I've discussed the power of the brain, the practice of maintaining your health through continuing to learn, eating right, exercising, sleeping better, and staying connected. In the next chapter, Gary will continue to discuss how what you choose to feel and believe impacts your physical, emotional, and spiritual health.

Vitamins for the Body

- When it comes to your health, prevention is the easiest, most effective, least expensive, and least painful way to go. A healthy lifestyle beats anything that medicine can offer.
- Staying healthy or improving our health involves exercising our mind, watching what we eat, making sure we get enough vitamins and minerals, exercising our body, sleeping adequately, and maintaining connections with others.
- What you eat has an effect on all the organs in your body as well as your health in general. Study the food pyramid to find proper foods and amounts.
- Physical activity doesn't require membership in a health club or even expensive equipment: walking, gardening, vacuuming, parking farther from your destination, and taking the stairs instead of the elevator all count.
- Getting proper amounts of quality sleep is shown to have a positive impact on mood, energy, and overall happiness. Making sure to get enough and the right kind of sleep will improve your physical, emotional, and spiritual health
- Numerous studies have demonstrated that people who stay socially connected live longer than those who don't.

MEDITATION AND MOVEMENT

Bill W. Hillman, Ph.D.

One example of a journey that incorporates the three dimensions of the mind-body-spirit connection is the labyrinth experience. "Labyrinth" is another word for "maze," only in the case of the labyrinth one not only finds an exit but also discovers something valuable inside.

The following labyrinth exercise, shared by another guest author, our mutual friend Dr. Bill Hillman, can be used by those of theistic beliefs to enter the presence of god or their spiritual deity or deities. For nontheists, the labyrinth exercise provides a time to explore their personal meaning of life — their sense of what it's all about. You'll see how Erik makes extensive use of this idea in chapter 3.

The Meditation Labyrinth as a Body-Mind-Spirit Metaphor

A meditation labyrinth, which is available in many faith communities, is a metaphor for the body, mind, and spirit connection. It involves activity of the body, stimulation of the mind, and transformation of the spirit. Labyrinths are often modeled after those at the Chartres Cathedral in France and Grace Cathedral in San Francisco. Walking the labyrinth is a very special experience for many people because it combines personal prayer and symbolic meditation with physical movement. The labyrinth takes the walker on a journey into a sacred space. The ordinary world is left behind for a time, the realm of the holy is entered, and then the ordinary world is reentered with the lingering scent of the sacred. Labyrinths aren't magical but are full of divine mystery that can be experienced on many different levels.

There are three movements in walking the labyrinth: going in, time in the center, and going out. The path into the labyrinth represents our spiritual journey to experience that which is most important to us and to renew our relationship with it. This can also be a time to transform

41

our negative thoughts and concentrate on seeing what's positive in our lives. It may be necessary to stop frequently along the way to eliminate being absorbed with ourselves. We may stop to be sure that we don't have unfinished business in our relationships with others. We may pause to examine any self-defeating behaviors that reduce our spiritual or mental effectiveness. We may stop to confess our part in perpetuating negative circular patterns in relationships with others and to ask forgiveness for wrongs we've committed.

Entering the center of the labyrinth is a time for personal transformation. It's an opportunity to enter the presence of "the Holy of Holies" and for "the spirit of god" to dwell within. This is a time for being aware of the mysteries of life and for experiencing its awesomeness. It's also a time to make a commitment to change things in our lives that aren't working. Traveling the path out of the labyrinth is a time for seeking guidance when we reenter the world and the complexities of modern society. It's a time to prepare for service to others who may be in need, and to develop a fuller awareness of the meaning of life.

It's not necessary to literally walk a meditation labyrinth located at a house of worship or retreat center if one is not readily available. The concept and potentially life-changing meaning of the labyrinth can be a part of your daily exercise and meditation program in your own neighborhood. You can walk around your block or exercise track three times. For the first lap, focus on the disciplines associated with entering the labyrinth. During the second lap, concentrate on the disciplines that are part of being in the center of the labyrinth. On the final lap, zero in on the disciplines of exiting the labyrinth and reentering the world of your daily routine. However you do it, symbolically walking a meditation labyrinth can vitalize your life and activate the body, mind, and spirit connection of holistic health.

CHAPTER 2

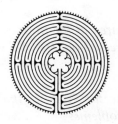

SECOND DIMENSION: MIND

Gary D. McKay

Man prefers to believe what he prefers to be true.

— FRANCIS BACON

BUILT LIKE A DEFENSIVE TACKLE, *thirty-three-year-old Garrett flopped down in the chair and with a big sigh said, "I've just about had it!"*

"Bad week, Garrett?" I asked.

"Oh you don't know the half of it." Another sigh.

"Tell me about it."

"Well, first my boss told me he has to cut the budget, which means my hours are cut back. And we need the money."

"That must be frightening."

"Yeah," he sighed again.

"And?" I asked.

"The kids are all upset and just driving me crazy and Kim is no help at all — she lets them do whatever they want!" he stressed.

"Sounds like you're pretty down."

"Yeah."

"Depressed?"

"Uh huh." He stared at the floor.

"Anxious and stressed out too, I'd guess."

"Oh, yeah!"

"Angry?"

He clenched his teeth. "You got that right!"

"Any physical problems?"

"Yeah, I don't sleep, my stomach is upset, and I get some monster headaches."

"So you're having a whole range of problems and it sounds like you're pretty miserable."

"Yeah, Doc, and I just don't know what to do."

"I hear your discouragement, but I think you will be able to handle these problems."

He perked up. "How?"

"I think we can start by investigating your psychological DNA."

Sitting straight up in his chair, Garrett exclaimed, "My DNA? You mean I inherited these problems; it's in my genes?"

"No, not your physical DNA, but your psychological DNA — your Discouraged Negative Attitude."

He folded his arms across his chest and said, "What do you mean my attitude? What's my attitude got to do with these problems? I didn't cause them!"

"I agree, you didn't cause the problems that others are putting on you, but how you respond, what you tell yourself about what's happening reflects your Discouraged Negative Attitude."

A fourth sigh. "What do you mean?"

"Well most of us would really like to have the power to change others, but really the only thing any of us has control over is our beliefs, our purposes, and our behavior. So, we can choose to respond in a discouraged way when bad things happen, or we can choose to respond in more self-encouraging ways."

Leaning forward in the chair, he asked, "How?"

Psychological DNA

Nothing is either good nor bad but thinking makes it so.
— WILLIAM SHAKESPEARE

As we said in the introduction and chapter 1, perception rules. What you believe, you see. Many of us see the minus side of issues that confront us. Our "psychological DNA" rules our perception.

Unlike physical DNA, psychological DNA is not inherited. It's just a term I use to explain a thinking process that gets us into trouble. It's certainly influenced by our parents, but not caused by them — we all are free to choose. May the "Poet's Society" forgive my feeble attempt at poetry, but "When life doesn't go your way, your PsyDNA comes into play."

When life gives us lemons, most of us don't make lemonade but end up with a bitter lemon instead! Most of us talk ourselves into bad feelings by demanding things be the way we think they should be, underestimating our ability to take life on its terms, maximizing discouraging situations by labeling them "catastrophes" or "awful," and blaming others, life, or ourselves for the problem. So, we engage in DUMB thinking: Demanding, Underestimating, Maximizing, Blaming.

I call this DUMB thinking because such beliefs create strong upset feelings that don't solve our problems. So our PsyDNA is just plain dumb!

Let's take a look at how we engage in DUMB thinking:

Demanding. We make demands on life, others, and ourselves. We proclaim things *should, must, have to,* or *always* happen or *shouldn't, mustn't,* or *never* happen. So when things don't go our way, we get very upset.

Underestimating. This involves discounting our ability to accept what's happening. We tell ourselves we just *can't stand it, handle it,* or *take it.* In this way, you excuse yourself from functioning.

Maximizing. You maximize the situation by judging it to be a catastrophe. You tell yourself that the event is *awful,* or *terrible,* or *horrible.* In other words, your world is coming to an end!

Blaming. You blame life, the person, or yourself for the problem. You judge life, others, or yourself as *totally* bad.

This kind of thinking discourages us. As long as we engage in DUMB thinking, the chances for effective solutions diminish.

As I helped Garrett explore his PsyDNA and look for his DUMB thinking, he discovered how he was discouraging himself. About his hours being cut back, he told himself: "This is awful. How will I pay the bills? I can't handle this. The boss is so stupid, if he'd planned better, this wouldn't have happened. He should've seen the problem coming!" About his wife and kids he thought: "The kids are so rotten. They know better than to behave like that, and Kim lets 'em get away with murder. I can't stand this. She should clamp down; after all, I'm going through hell here, trying to make ends meet."

Garrett's self-statements: "He (the boss) should've seen the problem coming" and "she (Kim) should clamp down" — are *demands* Garrett's making. And when these demands aren't met, he *maximizes* the situation by catastrophizing: "This is awful" and "I'm going through hell here . . ." He also *underestimates* his ability to handle the situations by proclaiming: "I can't handle" or "stand this." He *blames* his boss and his spouse, calling his boss "stupid" and implying that his wife is a lousy mother when he says: "She lets 'em get away with murder."

With this kind of self-talk, one can see why Garrett feels angry, stressed and anxious, and depressed. It's no wonder he can't sleep and has stomach upset and "monster" headaches. For, as Wayne pointed out in chapter 1, the mind has a powerful influence on our health. Garrett can take charge of his PsyDNA and dump his DUMB thinking so that he can get on with tackling his problems productively.

Okay, so *how* do Garrett and the rest of us get ourselves out of our DUMB ideas and create a more self-encouraging attitude? The following section gives you the road map.

Feng Shui for the Brain

> *It's strictly a case of mind over matter — if you don't mind, it doesn't matter!*
>
> — MARK TWAIN

Often you can't change things that happen in your life. As author Thomas La Mance said: "Life is what happens to us when we're making other plans." However, you can change how you respond. You can make life's happenings matter less, or not at all. You can, as TV's Dr. Phil says, "Get real." You get real by doing the following:

Reevaluate your demands. Just because you wish something to be the way you want it to be, as the late renowned psychologist Albert Ellis said, "What universal law says it should or must be your way?" When you place demands on others, life, or even yourself, you set yourself up for strong disappointment. The demand is the central cell of your PsyDNA. If you didn't believe that others, you, or life *should, must, ought, have to*, or *need to* be a certain way, or if you didn't engage in all or nothing thinking — *always, never, all, none* — you wouldn't create those strong upset feelings or discourage yourself. In other words, realize that your wishes are not your commands (McKay & Maybell, 2004).

Eliminate excuses. "I can't stand it; I can't take it" are just excuses for wallowing in our upset feelings. Where is the evidence that you *can't stand* something that has happened? You've probably stood many unpleasant things in your life; what makes the current situation any different? Believing that you can't stand something just puts you in the position of weakness. On the other hand, you can move from what Ellis called "can't-stand-it-itis" to what he called "I'll never like it but I can-stand-it-itis" (Ellis, 1998).

In my book *How You Feel Is up to You* (McKay & Dinkmeyer, 2002), I discuss other forms of excuses called "passive thinking." When we engage in passive thinking, we shift responsibility for feelings (and behavior) onto others or conditions. We say — and believe — such things as: "She (he/that) made me . . ."; "Something came over me"; or "I'm not myself today." Sometimes we give ethnic excuses like "We Irish (Italians, Jews, etc.) . . ." The point is by discounting our ability and making excuses, we excuse ourselves from responsibility.

Accept disappointments. Few things in life are catastrophes. Most of what happens can be frustrating, unfortunate, inconvenient, or disappointing — but seldom awful. Even if an event *is* catastrophic, how does it help you to dwell on that fact? Remember Mattie Stepanek from the introduction? You could say the condition that Mattie was born with and his early death were catastrophic, but how does that change anything? When Mattie was with us, he chose not to look at his condition as terrible and just went on with his life.

On a lighter note, you could become (if you're not already) a country music fan. Many country songs speak of the misery in life. But some of the lyrics give good advice in dealing with that misery. For example, Ray Stevens sang in an old country song: "I'm making the best of a bad situation." Johnny Cash put it this way: "I don't like it, but I guess things happen that way."

Let go of blame. We can't judge a person by his or her behavior. Each of us behaves in positive or negative ways. When we try to place blame, we end up judging the whole person. So, if you must judge, judge behavior not personhood. When you think someone has done you wrong, focus on the behavior — separate the deed from the doer. You wouldn't want to be judged by only one act; give others the same consideration. If you keep thinking the other person is a total jerk, how can you deal with him or her? You'll just continue to be angry and blame the person, which gets in the way of solving the problem.

If you're upset with yourself about something you've done, focus on that and how you can rectify the mistake, don't put yourself down. Life can throw you a curve, but don't totally degrade life either.

Let's go back to our example of Garrett and see how he changed his thoughts. As long as Garrett believes his situations are catastrophic, he won't be able to approach them in any positive way and will end up stuck in the rut he's thought himself into. But he doesn't have to stay in the rut; he can dig himself out by changing his beliefs.

Garrett began to get real by reevaluating his situation. Concerning the cutbacks at work, instead of demanding, underestimating, maximizing, and blaming, Garrett told himself: "This is frustrating and unfortunate. I don't like this but I can stand it. We'll have to trim our budget so we can ride out the loss of money. I think the boss could have made better choices, but that doesn't mean he's totally stupid — he's made other good decisions. Maybe he didn't realize there would be problems."

About his situation with the wife and kids, Garrett decided: "The kids are probably experiencing the tension and that's influencing their behavior. Kim's doing the best she knows how and I'm not helping by blaming her. I can take it — hard as it is — and I will pitch in more with the kids."

With these new beliefs came new feelings. Garrett was still frustrated and worried about the situation, but he was no longer angry and depressed. These milder feelings helped him get on with solving the problem. As long as he remained angry, stressed out, and depressed, solutions eluded him.

When we "make the best of a bad situation," it doesn't mean we immediately feel great and all our upset is removed. It means we lessen the upset, which allows us to think of solutions rather than wallowing in our strong upset feelings. Wallowing gets us nowhere. So, what I'm talking about here is a kind of "feng shui for the brain." You clean out those negative thoughts and make room for more positive ones.

You're Feeling That Way on Purpose

You've seen how you can think yourself into and out of strong upset feelings. But why do we have those feelings in the first place? What is their function? Alfred Adler said this about emotions: "In every individual, we see that feelings have grown and developed in the direction and to the degree which were essential to the attainment of his goal" (Ansbacher, 1956). Another Adlerian, Rudolf Dreikurs (1967), said that emotions ". . . provide fuel, the steam, so to speak, for our actions, the driving force without which we would be impotent." In other words, emotions serve a purpose.

Garrett's anger, depression, and anxiety actually kept him from solving the problem. Instead of creating movement, his anxiety stopped him in his tracks. His depression allowed him to take some time off and blame his wife for the problems with the kids. His anger served the purpose of getting even with his wife by withdrawing and with his boss by avoiding contact with him whenever possible.

When Garrett discovered the purpose of his upset feelings and saw how they were getting in his way, he decided to modify his purposes. He chose to use his anxiety to create movement — he began looking for another job. He realized that his taking time off by being depressed wasn't helping the situation with his kids or Kim. He dropped the desire to get even with Kim and his boss too because that wasn't helping either. And guess what — he slept better, his stomach got better, and he had no more headaches. See what your body can do when you put your mind to it!

Think Differently, Act Differently

When Garrett recognized his purpose and changed his thinking process, he was in a position to do some problem solving. As Garrett looked for another job, he and Kim took a good look at their budget to decide how they could survive until Garrett's situation improved. They talked about the kids' behavior and decided to take a parenting class at their church.

Although it's very important to look at your thoughts and the purpose of your emotions — how you create your feelings, how they serve your goals, and how you can modify your thinking and purpose — nothing will really change unless you act differently. So when you're looking at your thoughts and purposes, also consider how you can change your behavior.

The following chart helps you locate your DUMB thoughts and change them to REAL thoughts.

Managing Your Psychological DNA:
Moving from DUMB Thinking to REAL Thinking

DUMB Thinking	Examples	REAL Thinking	Examples
Demanding	Should, must, have to, need, always, never	Reevaluate your demands	I really want, prefer, wish
Underestimating	I can't stand, take, handle it	Eliminate excuses	I can stand it (take it, handle it) even if I don't like it.
Maximizing	Awful, terrible, horrible, a catastrophe	Accept disappointments	Frustrating, disappointing, inconvenient, annoying
Blaming	Jerk, stupid, rotten, bad	Let go of blame	Not a jerk, stupid, etc. Is okay despite this behavior.

Questions and Answers for Better Psychological Health

When you're facing a disturbing challenge, ask yourself: "What am I feeling?" Then consider: "What am I thinking?" (Your PsyDNA, your DUMB thoughts.) Ask yourself: "What might be the purpose of my emotion?" (We discuss the purposes of anxiety, anger, and depression in succeeding chapters.)

Next, revaluate your thoughts and purposes: "What new REAL thoughts will I develop?" "How will I modify my purpose?" Finally, ask yourself: "How will I behave differently?"

More Techniques for Changing Emotions

You can use the following techniques to help you change your thoughts and purposes. Experiment with each technique to see what works best for you. By experimenting, we don't mean just "trying" a technique. Trying isn't doing. Actor Gary Busey says that try means: "*Tomorrow*, I'll *remember* what I should have done *yesterday*." So don't try it, do it! And, like any good experiment, decide to do each technique for a period, withholding evaluation until your test period is finished.

Reframing: A Different Way to Think Differently

When we reframe an incident, we influence our emotions. Reframing involves changing perspective by finding what's positive in a situation — the opportunity in the obstacle, or what we can learn from a mistake (McKay & Dinkmeyer, 2002).

> *A real estate sales representative was working on his first sale. He took a couple out to show them a house listed by his agency. The agent thought he would best impress his clients by being honest.*
>
> *The agent told the couple, "I want to be honest with you about this house. I will tell you all the negative aspects and then I will tell you what's positive about the property. To the north are the stockyards. To the south is a fertilizer plant. On the east is a slaughterhouse and to the west, the city dump.*
>
> *The couple frowned and was about to walk out the door when the agent said, "Wait, don't you want to hear what's positive about the property?"*
>
> *"What could possibly be positive?" asked the wife.*
>
> *The agent replied, "You can always tell which way the wind is blowing!"*

Finding the positive in the negative is a powerful way to change one's thoughts and feelings. What could Garrett find that's positive in his reduced work hours situation? He could see it as an opportunity to do some things he didn't have time for in the past. He could use some of the time to pay positive attention to his kids — maybe they wouldn't be as interested in driving him crazy. Think of a negative situation in your life. What's on the other side of the coin?

As mentioned earlier, blaming people gets you nowhere fast. When we blame, we often use labels such as stubborn, picky, irresponsible, and stupid. But there's another side of the coin here too. The stubborn person is also determined; the picky one is also selective. Someone you see as irresponsible could also be spontaneous. And what about someone you label stupid? This often means the person just sees things differently from you! Think of labels you put on people, what are the "flip sides" of these labels? (McKay et al., 2001.)

Sometimes reframing involves learning from your mistakes. Garrett used reframing this way when he decided that blaming his wife for the kids' misbehavior wasn't helping the situation and decided to concentrate on discussing the issue and getting help. What are some mistakes in your life you can learn from?

Lighten Up: Laughter and Humor

Humor helps heal. We discuss humor throughout the book as well as devoting an entire chapter to it. For now, let's say that if you can find humor in a situation, you can survive it.

> *A man suffered a potentially fatal gunshot wound. As the team of pessimistic surgeons wheeled him into the operating room, the anesthesiologist asked him if he had any allergies. "Just to bullets," he gasped. The room erupted with laughter. The levity transformed the spirits of the doctors from discouragement to positive possibility. The man survived surgery.*

Humor has many health benefits, including helping control diseases like diabetes (Hayashi et al., 2007). It has been said that laughter is like jogging in place (Greenwood). Most health practitioners and patients often do not fully appreciate its physical benefits. Author Norman Cousins reported that his recovery from a serious connective tissue disease was due to his watching Marx brothers' movies and vitamin C (Cousins, 1991).

Humor is another way to reframe an unpleasant event. Perhaps Garrett could infuse humor into his situation by thinking about how it might play out if it were a sitcom. Think about unpleasant events you have in your life. What humor can you find? (Make sure you're laughing at yourself or the situation, not at the other person as this will only keep you from seeing the other person in a positive way.)

Posting your favorite cartoons in places where you'll see them frequently helps you bring humor into your life as well. Choose cartoons that help you laugh at yourself.

Take a Deep Breath: The Benefits of Deep Breathing

When you're under stress, anxious, or angry, your breath often comes in short bursts. You can concentrate on slowing down your breathing, which will help you relax. In *Native Healing: Four Sacred Paths to Health* (Peate, 2002), Wayne describes the following breathing exercise:

> *Exhale completely — push out bad thoughts. Inhale deeply and slowly through your nose, expanding your ribcage and then your chest. Count one ... two ... three ... four, and pause*

to breathe in good thoughts. Exhale completely and slowly through your mouth, count one ... two ... three ... four, and pause.

Silently repeat a phrase or sound. I usually advise the word "relax".... Allow other thoughts to enter and exit your mind, without focusing on them. Whenever other thoughts intrude, return your focus to the repetition of the word you've chosen. Later, if you're in a stressful situation, simply repeat the chosen word for a calming effect.

Mellow Out: Relaxation

When you're experiencing disturbing feelings, you're naturally "uptight" and tense. Relaxation helps you mellow out and prepare yourself to handle your upset thoughts and emotions.

People have all kinds of ways to relax. Some choose alcohol. Although a glass of wine or beer or a shot of whisky may help you relax, depending on alcohol for relaxation can turn to thinking "I need a drink," which of course can lead to dependence. Some take a nap. Although a short nap is relaxing and energizing, long naps can lead to sleep problems. Others fake illness to take a day off from work to relax or to take time for themselves. And although a few mood disorders are physiologically based, some people become depressed as a way to remove themselves from the demands of everyday life.

Relaxation is important, but to be helpful it needs to be healthy relaxation. Taking a bath, reading, watching a favorite TV program, and exercising are all relaxing. In addition to these kinds of activities, relaxation exercises help you rethink your situation and energize you to solve problems.

A simple relaxation exercise is to use the breathing exercise described above. You can add your favorite mantra to the exercise or count slowly to ten. Some examples of mantras are "I am relaxed," "I can solve this problem," "I'm in charge of me." Some people find humming a mantra relaxing.

When we're upset, our muscles are often tense. You can use progressive relaxation exercises to reduce this tension. Sit in a comfortable chair, close your eyes, and begin to breathe deeply. Begin by tightening the muscles in your feet — hold for fifteen seconds, then relax that set of muscles. Progress to your legs, abdomen, chest, hands, arms, neck, face, and head — tightening-releasing, tightening-releasing (Peate, 2002).

There are many books and tapes on relaxation. A trip to the bookstore or searching the Internet can help you locate resources.

Imagine That: Using Imagery

You can use imagery for a variety of purposes, such as relaxing, preparing for a challenging event, and helping with the healing process when ill. Combining imagery with deep breathing and relaxation techniques produces a soothing effect. Choose an image that's relaxing to you such as a lake, the beach, or the forest. Involve as many of your senses as you can — see it, hear it, smell it, taste it, touch it. Some people have trouble with visual images. If you do, that's okay; you can still use imagery by concentrating on the senses you can experience.

Concentrate on the image as you're relaxing. If other images intrude, let them pass and return to your relaxing image. You can use this technique when you find yourself becoming tense. In addition, relaxing imagery helps you fall asleep.

If you're facing a challenging event, you can "rehearse" with imagery. Suppose there's an upcoming event at work that you think may be difficult to deal with. You can rehearse your responses by getting yourself relaxed and then imaging the event. For example, see the people involved, including yourself. See how they are likely to act. Hear the words. See the faces and body language. Use positive self-talk. See yourself handling the event effectively. Practice the visualization for ten minutes, three times a day (McKay & Dinkmeyer, 2002).

Move It *and* Lose It: Exercise

Exercise helps you drain away stress, anxiety, and depression and lessen your anger. As Wayne said in chapter 1, people have all kinds of excuses for not exercising. Yet exercise is a solid method for changing your PsyDNA. Remember we said that emotions are a form of energy. The physical energy of exercise helps relieve the psychological energy of strong upset feelings. Although you're exercising, you can examine the situation and your discouraged negative thoughts. You can practice new ways of thinking and, as a consequence, experience a new way of feeling. You can think of ways you can reframe the situation. You can look for the humor. The energizing effects of the exercise will help you think, and feel, more clearly.

Share It, Don't Stuff It: Talk about Your Feelings

Talking about your feelings helps you get in touch with exactly how you're feeling and gain new insight. Choose someone who's a good listener and can see different perspectives. It could be your spouse, a friend, a relative, a clergyperson, or a professional therapist. Although talking about your feelings helps you feel better for the moment, in most cases, if you are to change the feelings and solve the problem, you'll also need to work on changing them by using the techniques discussed in this chapter.

Get in the Spirit: Seek Meaning

Depending upon your view of spirituality, you can use prayer or meditation to assist you in gaining guidance and strength to deal with the problem. Erik will be dealing with the Big Picture in some detail in the next chapter, but for now ask yourself: "How does this challenge fit with my view of the greater scheme of things?" Based on your spiritual beliefs, what thoughts and behavior are called for here? (McKay & Maybell, 2004)

Psychological Vitamins

All the ways to change your thinking, purposes, and behavior that I've discussed above are based on what I call "psychological vitamins." The following three vitamins are used to vitalize your psychological DNA:

Vitamin C: Choices

We humans are choice-making animals — nobody makes us do anything, we make our own decisions. We decide how to think, feel, and act. In early childhood, we make decisions about life and our place in it based on our influences, largely from our family. Because we have limited experience during these times, we often make erroneous decisions, yet these decisions map our lives. For example, oldest children often decide they must be first, on top, in charge. They can make good leaders, but they can also be bossy and put people down based on their decisions.

So, a good dose of vitamin C: choices from the "bottle of positive thoughts" helps us manage our lives effectively. In the example of being first, on top, in charge, a positive choice would involve leadership rather than dictatorship. There are many other examples of positive choices, such as deciding not to label things as awful when things happen that you don't like. Or if someone tries to get even with you, you can decide to be hurt and get even in return or you can decide to be empathetic and see if you can figure out why that person feels the "need" to hurt you and see if you can improve the relationship.

Don't fool yourself by blaming others or life for your problems and feelings. Realize that although you may not be able to control the situation, you do have a choice as to how you respond.

Vitamin E: Encouragement

Encouragement is vital to a fulfilled life and positive relationships. Think of your positive traits, look for your strengths, don't dwell on the negative or on your weaknesses. Have faith in yourself. If you don't believe in yourself, who will? Accept yourself despite your faults. We're all fallible, that's what being human is all about. Imagine how boring you would be if you were perfect! Decide to learn from your mistakes, not dwell on them.

Looking at the positive, focusing on strengths, having faith, and accepting others as they are, not just as they could be, are crucial for good relationships. Your spouse may not always please you, but that's not his or her job. You can think of her or his good side. You can appreciate his or her strengths. You can show that you believe in him or her, and you can accept your spouse "as is" despite her or his faults. Think how anger and stress will decrease if you have this attitude toward your spouse. This attitude toward a spouse works with a significant other for those who aren't married. It also keeps friendships and work relationships productive.

Encouragement is especially important for children. "A child needs encouragement like a plant needs water," said psychiatrist Rudolf Dreikurs, student of Alfred Adler and one of my teachers. Look for the plus side of your kids, see how they can use their strengths to contribute to the family — this helps build their self-esteem. Believe in them and accept them as worthwhile people even though you don't accept all of their behavior.

Vitamin R: Responsibility

You know that you make your own choices; be willing to accept responsibility for them. If you've done something distressing or hurtful to another, own up. Change your beliefs, purposes, and behaviors toward that person.

Be responsible to others. This involves making contributions, doing your share. If you're married or live with someone, make sure you're pitching in to maintain the relationship: do your share of household chores, childcare, errands, initiating affection, etc.

Being responsible to others doesn't mean taking responsibility from others. This shows disrespect and often creates resentment. Just as you take responsibility, let others do the same. Again this is especially important for children. Kids learn responsibility when parents let them be responsible for the things they are old enough to be responsible for.

For example, instead of nagging your four-year-old about picking up his toys — or picking them up for him — set up a lost and found box. Tell him that if he leaves his toys lying around, you'll assume he doesn't want them right now and you'll place them in the lost and found box, so if he's missing them, he may want to look there. You're still picking up the toys, but you aren't returning them to his room. Most likely, he'll get tired of rummaging through the box and put them away instead — especially as the box begins to fill up!

Healthy, daily doses of vitamin C: choices, vitamin E: encouragement, and vitamin R: responsibility help you maintain your sanity — and the sanity of those around you. They'll improve your PsyDNA. Now let's look at Psychological DNA and illness.

Psychological DNA and Illness

If you're ill — with a cold or cancer — although you can't cure your condition with the techniques we've suggested, you can make the situation more tolerable. You don't have to have a discouraged, negative attitude. As Wayne has pointed out, the mind is very powerful. In this section, you'll see how people have used that power to help them with their health.

Vicki Straub, Ph.D. of Columbia, Missouri, professor at the University of Missouri Medical School, and an old friend of mine, told me her story of using deep breathing, relaxation, and imagery to prepare for and recover from surgery.

Vicki's Story: "A Doctor Who Practices What She Preaches"

VICKI STRAUB, PH.D.

I had a full hysterectomy that included abdominal surgery along a previous C-section scar. To prepare for the surgery, I listened to and followed the instructions on the tapes of Emmett E. Miller, M.D.: Successful Surgery and Recovery: Conditioning Mind and Body: Guided Imagery and Music for Use Before Surgery and During Recovery. I followed instructions once or twice daily. I focused on breathing, then created a relaxing scene. Then I moved ahead through imagery to the future, feeling and being healed. I listened to the music that seemed to enhance all my senses: seeing, feeling, hearing, and smelling.

My relaxing scene involved a tree located by a beach with sand, water, and blue sky. I used this scene pre- and postsurgery;

seeing myself in the future (looking the way I want to look, feeling the way I want to feel, doing the things I want to do); going inside to where the sutures were beginning to heal (seeing the cells knitting together, making a strong connection, the scar tissue being as strong as, if not stronger than, before.)

To enhance my images, I told myself calming, healing self-talk: "I am relaxed, focused and alert; I see the cells knitting together, becoming stronger and stronger; I feel the breeze in my face as I walk down the beach; I feel the energy within; I feel confident, calm and relaxed; I am doing the things I want to be doing; my forehead is smooth and cool; the branches are budding and growing with new leaves."

On the morning of the surgery, I was very excited, pumped, and ready to get this surgery done! I actively visualized being wheeled down to the surgery room, down the halls feeling ready, curious, and excited. I told myself: "I am on the gurney going to the OR, feeling calm and relaxed; I feel the support of the gurney; I allow others to do their work."

I was given a spinal injection of a drug that caused amnesia both times I have had it with surgical procedures. So, I do not remember any of the surgery and some of the recovery. I don't recall any pain. Apparently, I was also given some morphine over the next hours, and by the next morning I was very nauseated. I believe there was no reason to have the morphine, but that the administration of pain medication was so second nature and business as usual for the anesthesiologist and gynecologist that it was given to me (and adjusted to a smaller dose due to my history of sensitivity/nausea/vomiting to pain medications). The most uncomfortable aspect of the operation was the nausea.

During the hospital stay, I was active once I got on the other side of the nausea. I expected to feel discomfort when taking the first steps, doing the walks in the halls of the hospital, but none of that was difficult.

I was surprised at the amount of bruising along the surgery line and that any sneeze or digestive activity could cause discomfort. As a matter of fact, four days after the surgery I recall feeling as though I had been beat up, I looked so black, blue, and cut. My anger was irrational (I had a surgery I wanted to have and the gynecologist even apologized for the amount of bruising), but I found it was important for me to verbalize these feelings to my husband. Once I did, I felt as though I moved through to the other side of those particular feelings.

Another surprise was the effort and pain associated with getting up and down. I had imagined the pain would be more like during my previous C-sections; however, I had forgotten that organs that had been in place a long time were being removed. So, whereas I used virtually no pain medications and did enlist the relaxation and imagery tools, rest and walking exercise, I did experience pain. The pain was tolerable and I felt in control. I used pain as feedback to move a bit more slowly, to rest, or to use breathing and imagery. In other words, the pain was appropriate pain and useful as a guide. I didn't feel reactively anxious, helpless, or discouraged by the pain.

During the recovery process, I called forth my images and told myself: "I am relaxed, safe, and healing; with every breath the swelling is subsiding; I am comfortable, relaxed; I see the cells knitting together; the cells are strong, resilient; I am healing rapidly." I stepped into the future image — feeling and looking the way I wanted to feel and look.

What has been the most profound aspect of this process I described above has been the active decision to take control over the things over which I have control. At another time when I was scheduled for this same surgery (it was canceled due to another risk factor for surgery at that time), I had not been actively involved in these techniques.

From the time of the first canceled surgery, I had been responding to a lot of uncertainty about a newly diagnosed serious chronic illness. Through that period of time (about a year), I eventually did make adjustments, sorted through a variety of feelings, and by the time of the current surgery was much more ready to claim control in very conscious, active ways.

I currently use imaging techniques to deal with my chronic illness — a liver disease called autoimmune cholangitis. My image is a tree with branches that are beginning to bloom with new leaves, new branches growing, seeing myself trimming the dead branches away so that new ones can grow. The liver is often described as a tree and seems to be a useful metaphor for me. I've become very attuned to trees, their branching system, especially in the spring of the year.

Through imagery, I sense a living, growing tree within my liver and I tell myself: "The branches are sprouting new growth — see the new leaves and new branches growing and spreading; I'm pruning the old branches, so new growth takes place." In addition to imagery and self-talk, using relaxation techniques has also been extremely important.

During the spring of 2002, I was very aware of the trees surrounding our home and the prolific growth taking place all around me. As I did yard work, picked up dead branches in the yard, trimmed old branches off bushes and small trees to allow for growth, I often "went inside" imaging the same process going on within myself. This spring of 2003, I have been much less consciously involved in imagery for this illness, but I believe I am still paying attention, just not so consciously.

Vicki's experience shows the power of the mind to help in the healing process. With situations like Vicki's, although it may not all be in your head, some of it obviously is!

Don't Become the Illness

What about a terminal illness? Life is over soon. How do "vitamins" for the body, mind, and spirit help? Wayne relates the story of Mary, a seventy-one-year-old with end-stage breast cancer whose life was slipping away. Cancer was consuming her body.

"I feel like a piece of Swiss cheese," she told me. "The cancer keeps punching out holes in my body."

"It must be tough. How are you handling it all?" Wayne asked.

"I've decided not to become my disease — and that has helped. I used to think 'I'm a breast cancer victim'. But that made me feel down all the time, like I was always the victim. Now I repeat to myself: 'I'm Mary. I'm not a disease. My life may be short, but my enjoying what I have left will be full of living.'"

I told Mary how impressed I was at her ability to use her mind to reframe the devastating predicament her body had placed her in.

(No PsyDNA here!) Wayne goes on to say:

Mary's story reminded me of my wife's grandmother Lucia, who had many hard knocks in life, including the crippling of her husband at an early age by rheumatoid arthritis and her own severe asthma. Despite her troubles, she was the most positive person I've ever met. Her secret was to take delight (and relief from the burdens of her world) in simple pleasures. During many a dinner she would exclaim: "Look at the beautiful sunset; we must go out and have a long look at it," and she and the family would.

I confess I used to think this was a frivolous waste of time. But then I saw its effects. As she seemed to breathe in the palette of colors of the setting sun, her own labored breathing improved. Lucia was able to draw up the good in the world around her, and in so doing do good for her chronic illness. She would beam around a baby the same way. Did she stop taking her asthma medicine? No way. Did using her attitude — a conscious effort to uplift her state of mind — alleviate her body's symptoms? I believe the answer is a resounding "YES!"

Did her faith and spirituality help her make the best of her time? Also affirmative. Even in the midst of terminal or chronic physical illness, mind does matter, and spirit does relieve.

Join Together — Support Groups

About support groups and illness, Wayne says:

> So often the psychological effects of chronic or terminal illnesses like cancer are as devastating as the physical. Feelings of loss, abandonment, concerns about untreatable pain and loss of appearance can debilitate. Support groups have also been found to counteract these psychological burdens and to improve the quality, if not the quantity of life for those with chronic or terminal illness. It appears that the opportunity to share and empathize is powerful. (Winzelberg et al., 2003)

Your physician or local hospital can help you locate support groups in your community. You'll notice that we suggest support groups throughout this book. Because we humans are social beings, joining with others really helps us gain that support and solve problems.

Change What You Can Change, Accept What Can't Be Changed

Sometimes you can change a disturbing situation, as Garrett did when he sought another job. When you can't change a situation, learn to accept it using the techniques we've discussed in this chapter. Remember the Serenity Prayer (Reinhold Neibuhr, 1926):

> *God, grant me the serenity to accept the things I cannot change, courage to change the things I can, and wisdom to know the difference.*

Even when you can change a situation, you may still have some strong upset feelings about the event that can interfere with your efforts to do so. If you're going to succeed in changing a situation, you must first change your thoughts, feelings, and purpose.

This chapter has covered the power of the mind to decrease or increase the vitality of life. The choice is yours. Throughout the book you'll see how you can think your way through the challenges in your life. In the next chapter, Erik further discusses the power of the spirit and its relationship to fuller living — adding life to your years.

Vitamins for the Mind

- Most of us talk ourselves into bad feelings by DUMB thinking: Demanding, Underestimating, Maximizing, Blaming. These beliefs lead to PsyDNA — Discouraged Negative Attitude.
- Often you can't change things that happen in your life, but you can change how you respond. You get REAL when you: Reevaluate your demands, Eliminate excuses, Accept disappointments, and Let go of blame.
- Emotions serve a purpose. In general, they give us the energy to act; but they can also keep us from solving problems.
- Although it's important to take a look at your thoughts and the purpose of your emotions, nothing will really change unless you act differently.
- You can "cure" your PsyDNA by applying "psychological vitamins": Vitamin C: choices; vitamin E: encouragement; and vitamin R: responsibility.
- Change what you can change; accept what can't be changed.

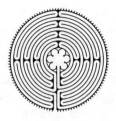

THIRD DIMENSION: SPIRIT

Erik Mansager

The Pope was engaged in an official and very tense ecumenical discussion with high-ranking officials of the Protestant and Orthodox churches when a breathless courier interrupted the meeting. Unable to contain himself, he blurted out: "Your Holiness, I have good news and bad news!"

"What's the good news?" the pontiff asked.

"The Lord has returned and he would like a word with you!" exclaimed the page.

"That's good news, indeed, my son!" The pope continued: "Fear not! What could possibly be the bad news?"

"Well, Holiness," replied the page: "He's calling from Mecca, and he sounds a little miffed!"

It's been five centuries since the Protestant Reformation and over a thousand years since the bishops of Rome and Constantinople mutually excommunicated one another. It's been a long time since Christians could agree on who really got it right! But some still hold on to hope that one or another of the camps in the age-old argument will actually have the final say. Many people wish someone could offer an answer really worth clinging to. "Back to the Bible!" cries one group. "Long live authority!" shouts another. "Tradition!" reply still others. And although none would deny that the others have a point, each group is just as likely to hold its own "truth" to be THE truth!

Christians hardly have a monopoly on family in-fighting, of course. Sunni and Shiite Muslims have been engaged in their own deadly battles for over 1,300 years. And, despite at least a couple of millennia since Moses received the tablets containing the Ten Commandments, the arguments that erupt between Hassidic and Reform Jews are almost as virulent, although not as deadly. You need only scratch a bit beneath the pious veneers to find humanity acting out, no matter the religion.

Such human arguments surely don't mean that the religions have nothing to offer. Most of the world religions came about to help a people transcend this tendency to argue and fight, to help find a better way. But religion is not the only spiritual path. In this chapter, I take on the differences between religion and spirituality — indicating that spirituality is, by and large, the way we make meaning in our lives. This sets the stage for understanding how a person can be spiritual with or without being religious or believing in a supreme being who governs the universe. Rather than identifying that universal being within a specific religious tradition, we simplify our discussion by using the term "god" throughout. I move from there into just how spirituality contributes to our overall health and well-being.

The Meaning of Meaning

Have you ever pondered the meaning of life? You'd be unique if you didn't! For many, the quest for meaning ("What's it all about . . . ?") generates more questions than answers.

Natural disasters — the 2007 cyclone in Bangladesh, the 2004 tsunami that devastated parts of Indonesia, Hurricane Katrina, and earthquakes in Pakistan and India in 2005 — or inhumane crimes — kidnapping and murdering children, school shootings, from the University of Texas, Austin massacre of August 1966 to the recent Northern Illinois University shooting in February 2008, call into question for some the very existence of god: "How could a 'loving God' let this happen?" For other believers, such disasters strengthen their faith: "God's ways are mysterious and it isn't ours to question," whereas still others sense: "This is the hand of the Evil One!" Either way, they develop a stronger connection to god, who lets nature take its course and lets humans work out their own problems. For those who don't believe in a personal god — let's call them "nontheists" — such events are also powerful happenings: things that happen either in nature or by our human nature. For them, "what is" simply and powerfully "is." And "what is" neither proves nor disproves the existence of a god.

All this is to say that god is an important *question* today and to some is an important *answer*. But although god is at the heart of many religions, god isn't at the heart of spirituality. Actually, spirituality comes up today in many contexts: in the context of whether one can be *free* of a god-concept and still be considered spiritual as well as in the context of how believers today manifest their spirituality. So in this chapter I explore the essence of spirituality. I encourage you to look again and see yourself as a spiritual person. And I discuss how you can focus on this dimension to enrich both your physical life and your mental well-being — whether you are Buddhist, Christian, Jewish, Muslim, Hindu, belong to another faith community, or belong to none.

Once when asked about the important question of "truth" as a religious quest, Deepak Chopra, the best-selling spiritual author, commented: "You know, God gave humans the truth, and then the Devil came and he said, 'Let's organize it — we'll call it religion'" (*Larry King Live*, 2005). It's in this sense that my exploration attempts to differentiate between religion and spirituality. I certainly don't contend that all religion is "of the Devil." Those who are comfortable believing in tried-and-true religious concepts will continue to experience their faith in a manner that enlivens their beliefs and helps them make sense out of life today. But there is also the need for exploring spirituality in today's world that involves making room in the discussion for those who no longer are able to believe in God, let alone the Devil.

To do this right, I write in harmony with what you've already read about the body and mind from Wayne and Gary. Like them, I have drawn from the work of social psychologist Alfred Adler as well as classic and contemporary spiritual writings. In the labyrinth exercise, we make three primary movements — one from the outside to the inside of the labyrinth, then one into the labyrinth's "sacred center," and finally one coming out into the world renewed and refreshed. Each of the movements is made up of two parts however you choose to describe them: steps, breaths, or even heartbeats.

First Movement — into the Labyrinth

When we have truly the taste for adventure we become as a child. Confident, we advance step by step and leave the dark forest in direction of the radiant light, guided toward the unknown by our capacity to marvel.

— OSHO RAJNEESH

The movement *into* the labyrinth differentiates spirituality from religion. This movement focuses on the importance of the meaning-making function of spirituality. In the first part, we explore how religion and spirituality are related but also how they don't have to be tied together anymore. In the second part of the inward movement, I expand on this idea by talking about "Big Questions" and "Big Answers."

Religion vs. Spirituality?

Religion is taking a real beating nowadays. Within the first decade our new century there have already been holy wars, sex abuse scandals, and unchecked misuse of church donations (Bergin, 2002; Küng, 2003; Wooten, Coker, & Elmore, 2003). It's enough to crush your faith. And for some, it has. Others are downright brokenhearted over distrusting a faith that used to sustain them in the crazy outside world.

Then you get a glimpse at the other side and see how some fundamentalists approach their faith — some by condemning others, some by killing them. What a quirk of fate that some see fundamentalism as the answer to today's problems and others think it's the cause of those very problems. Is religion altogether disgraced, or is it staging a comeback?

I know it's not that simple, but these extremes hint at the difficulty of the problem. Here in North America, attendance at Sunday services in Christian churches is dropping and dropping among the young. And in Europe — where they measure attendance with official records — the numbers of young refusing to claim church affiliation is at its highest since they started keeping records. So it goes in North America and Europe; but the commotion in the southern half of our globe is just as crazy, albeit in another direction. In Central and South America, Catholics are flocking to the evangelical Protestant Christian denominations in numbers close to those during the Reformation (Hallum, 1996; Stoll, 1991). Yet in Africa, Catholicism is the fastest growing religion going (Reuters, 2004). Worldwide, the Muslim faith, too, is growing as it hasn't in a long time, but it's also suffering from an inaccurate image as wholly intolerant of other religions (Küng, 2003). Now the younger generation comes along and learns that the organized extermination of a religious people, as in the Holocaust, is the stuff of ancient history. But at the same time, they've read about the systematic rape of Muslim women by Christians in Bosnia-Herzegovina and the Rwandan massacres between Christianized cultures, not to mention the phenomenal 9/11 terrorist attack by religious extremists. And as I write this chapter, we're still embroiled in the conflict in Iraq where the different Muslim sects vie for power.

The struggle for religion's trustworthiness defies easy explanation; it kind of has the flavor of the nineteenth and twentieth centuries' science/religion debates when religion denounced "Godless science" and science refuted "the illusionary dogma of religion." But there's a funny twist to the struggle: today science is actually being used to "prove" the importance of religion. As Wayne shared in chapter 1, there's more and more evidence that religious belief (like belief in god or a friendly power bigger than us) helps protect us from getting ill — or helps us heal. In spite of some fraudulent claims about the power of intercessory prayer (Masters, Spielmans, & Goodson, 2006), the link between belief and health appears pretty strong when you check into the health of those who believe in a caring god — or something similar (Sperry, 2001; Wulff, 1997). It's as if there is "something else" going on alongside the religious practices that brings the noted benefits. I contend that this "something" is what people are calling "spirituality." And they call it that precisely to distinguish that "whatever else" from religion.

There are lots of ways to tell spirituality apart from religion. Religion, for example, contains clear faith statements that support doctrine. It's often considered "content oriented." Spirituality, on the other hand, is kind of a pathway leading somewhere — a pathway to anywhere you might find answers. It's often considered "process oriented." Another indicator is that religion tends to involve organized public church communities, whereas spirituality prefers individualized, private practices.

But as much as we compare and contrast the two, there is something at the heart of spirituality that isn't necessarily tied to religion at all. The mystics of many religions for a long time have proposed it's this: where religion focuses on answering, spirituality encourages questioning. Yes, spiritual questioning *can* be responded to by religious answering, but it can be answered in other ways as well — by science and philosophy and art, for example. But the questioning itself stands on its own, apart from religion. On our way into the labyrinth, let's take a look at spirituality again in this original, "questioning" way.

Spirituality and the Big Questions

There are Big Questions that — everywhere and at all times — have expressed human wonder about how things work:

- Why am I here?
- Does it matter at all that I am here?
- Why is there something instead of nothing?
- How does it all work?

This isn't an official list, but the really Big Questions can be summed up as "What's it all about?" or "What's the meaning of life?" People are always looking for the answer to that one. Today both believers and nonbelievers are thinking about it. The Big Questions reveal a deep concern about humanity in spite of all the religious fights and horror stories and in spite of all sorts of scary religious enthusiasm that results from people fighting over which religious answers are more correct.

Religiously oriented people are aware of the growth of spirituality, and many suspect something's up — like the conversion of the world or something. But other people who feel pushed aside by organized religion *also* claim that spirituality is important to them. I call them the "refuse-to-leavers." They flat out refuse to let go of their higher values — like honesty, trustworthiness, kindness, and the like — even if they learned them in churches whose leaders

- encourage intolerance toward those of a different sexual orientation;
- treat women as if they are not equal in dignity to men;
- claim god wants the followers to pay hard-earned money for the pastors' comfort; or
- make a joke of their values by sexually abusing the refuse-to-leavers' young.

It's safe to say that believers and nonbelievers, the doubters and refuse-to-leavers, are *all* concerned about finding answers to the Big Question: "What's the meaning of life?"

I don't mean to "just" make sense out of life. This challenge isn't the same as trying to make sense out of skills we've learned in school or on the job, for example, where we make sense out of things without much actual thinking. For example, the mathematic equations learned in class can be applied in the auditor's books without having to see how they fit into the way the world works; and office Internet technology is developed one day and learned the next without a second thought about discarding it when newer information arrives. No worries here about permanent, unchanging conditions of the universe. Here's the point: although job and book knowledge are important in their own right, they just don't address the Big Questions.

But sometimes, even in the middle of everyday happenings, we run up against "limit" or "barrier events." These are often tragic events that limit our usual understanding, or they impose a barrier to understanding so that life is "hard to get." These events can push us to our limits and stop us dead in our tracks, as if we've hit a barrier, for example, when a loved one dies, or when a large natural disaster occurs, or when men (right, usually males) declare war on others. It's at these times that the Big Questions force their way into our awareness as we ask: "What does it all mean?"

When faced with tragedy, we can feel frustration and anger toward the unknowable. It's all quite understandable. At these times prepackaged, churchy responses "to not doubt" or "to trust god's mysterious will" aren't very likely to be helpful. At these times we don't want stopgap answers like "You can't understand it now, but will later." Such answers put us off and keep us from thinking the matter through, rather than helping us make sense of it.

Nor do we want patchwork answers that mix up different religious beliefs and symbols. Someone who doesn't know the differences between reading tarot cards and praying the Rosary, yet recommends we do one or the other, doesn't help the matter much. No, we want heartfelt answers that come only from a deep understanding of who we are and that we have a relationship to the greater world we live in.

My point is this: when we run up against the "unanswerable" issues in our lives, we don't look for *tentative* suggestions; we look for *final* solutions — however they might come to us. And right then and there, when you find you're looking for Big Answers, you've entered the realm of spirituality: the search for ultimate answers that supply deep meaning to our personal lives.

It's this process of creating a Big Answer to our Big Questions that guides our lives in the small, day-to-day aspects of life, too. The value we give the process helps guide us through the many minute-by-minute decisions we face. By helping form a Big Answer or "ultimate meaning" in our lives, we find guidance all along the way of life.

A good example of this is Tariq Khamisa's father, Azim. Tariq was a responsible high school student who was thoughtlessly gunned down while working his pizza delivery job. Azim Khamisa could have been bitter and resentful when he encountered this barrier event. But the senseless death of his son that stopped Azim in his tracks didn't stop him permanently. Instead, he took to heart the importance of understanding the gangland violence that victimized innocent people. Over the years, he met with his son's killer in prison and eventually formed a movement that reaches out to others touched by such tragedies. It's Azim Khamisa's everyday actions toward people of different cultures that make a difference in the lives of so many and that are the substance of his national presentations to curb gangland violence (Tariq Khamisa Foundation, 2000).

Azim illustrates how we can't believe just *anything* and get the same positive results. In fact, the more people-friendly the quality of our belief is, the more direct the relationship with "peace of mind." Think about it: believing in a way that is good for ourselves and others (such as the Golden Rule) vs. believing that we must get it *over* others (as competitive sports sometime teach) affects our overall quality of living. We worry less about missing the big opportunities and are more willing to share in the benefits we receive. Research indicates this benefit is the rule no matter what your standing in society (Sperry, 2001).

Science and faith *can* go together, and they provide a different and reasonable way of thinking about spirituality. Here's what is important about the *process* of questioning: it can move us from a "minus" feeling to a "plus" feeling.

- Our "not knowing" everything we want to know feels like a minus (–) and "believing I can know" feels like a plus (+).
- Our "not seeing" the way the world fits together as a whole (–) but "wanting to see the Big Picture" (+) is part of the path to wellness.
- The minus (–) pushes us to strive for the plus (+).
- Moving from negative (–) to positive (+) is part and parcel of spirituality.

Imagine this movement as a process involved in taking "what I do know" and comparing it to "what I don't know," "what I am learning," and "what I want to learn." The result of the comparison is "I still *don't* know it all."

Can you see that there's a real *risk* that we won't learn enough if we only hold onto what we know? At the same time, the fear of not knowing enough provides the opportunity to learn more — to ask more questions — whether through personal reading, more education, or seeking wise counsel. What a great starting point! Why? Risk and opportunity don't simply cancel one another out. Whether we face the risk or take the opportunity, we increase our ability to know more about the world!

Now, let's go into the center of this asking opportunity, of "knowing our world," and look closely at how we make sense of our place in that world.

Second Movement — into the Sacred Center

The experience of creativity is really the entry into the sphere of mystery.... The key is to abandon the self to the energy that generates the birth of all phenomena.

— OSHO RAJNEESH

I invite the second movement into the center of the labyrinth by showing first how we actually construct and come to know that world we want to make sense of. I emphasize that this is done quite distinctively given our unique families, geographies, physical imperfections, and the like. This draws together the individual and community aspects of knowing the world — it's one essential aspect of the "sacred center."

The second part of this movement within the center explores knowing the world on a spiritual level. You're invited to understand soul and spirit in ways that are sacred *and* holistic. This movement presents soul and spirit in a way that expands on the metaphor I used in the introduction: the inward movement of authenticity, of being rooted to our deepest convictions; and the outward movement of being connected to something greater than ourselves.

Coming to Know the World

How do we come to know about our world? Not just how we acquire the facts, now, but how we become *aware* of the world — what is around us, how it fits together, what our place in the Big Picture is. We had this sense of wonder, once-upon-a-time. How'd we lose it? Is there a way back? Here in the center of the labyrinth, I invite you to explore with me the different ways we gather knowledge about the world — via our unique family setting, our physical imperfections, our particular geographic experiences, and the way we were taught spiritual matters.

Starting out as children, we are all small and dependent. Yet, too often in spiritual matters — as well as in physical and psychological matters — we speak of ourselves as if we sprang full grown onto the scene. We say that "god made us that way." But "made" doesn't mean — for believer or unbeliever — that we sprang complete on the scene with our current intellect, outlook, prejudices, preferences, wisdom, superstitions, and cultural awareness.

These personal aspects all came from *somewhere*. Our physical imperfections, our personal and family histories, our geographic setting, our culture, and our religious outlook all played a part in how we came to understand the world. With so many things influencing how we came to know, it's no wonder we all see things a bit differently.

Physical influences. Physicians contend (Stone, 1995) that due to the genetic contributions from our parents, every human body has as many as nine physical anomalies — "imperfections," things that don't work in us quite like they do in most other bodies — some of us have flat feet, others a curved spine; a few experience a tipped uterus or an undescended testicle; and still others have one leg shorter than the other or need glasses.

We all have combinations of such things. The anomalies in each of us — although they don't dramatically affect our well-being — result in our receiving different information and developing different ways of understanding our world and ourselves in it. Your way of processing is absolutely unique.

Family influences. Then there's the family. We assume that parents raise all their children the same. They *are* the same parents that did it, after all. But do they really? Surely parents learn from experience to experience, and the parent of a firstborn is far different from the same parent three, two, or even one child later.

If you're a firstborn (and even twins know which one is older), you only need to ask yourself whether you're like any of your siblings. How did your brother or sister become so different from you? How could they not?! Having an older, more practiced person modeling the way for them? And although firstborns may have much in common with other firstborns (and on through the sibling lineup) in other families, the uniqueness of each person's body and family couldn't possibly be identical.

Are you the second? Can you imagine what it would be like not having your older sibling cutting the waves in front of you, and blocking your view? However pleasant or frightening that is to consider, you get the idea: the world is perceived differently by each child — necessarily and understandably so. The same goes for the broader concept of "extended family," which is more prominent elsewhere in the world where families differ by the number of those counted as part of it: grandparents, aunts and uncles, and even the deceased family ancestors

Geographic influences. The same principle of individual outlook on the world can be applied to geographic location. How different are the experiences of the children raised in Seattle, Washington, from the children in Grand Forks, North Dakota? Though nearly the same global latitude, the climatic and cultural differences are profound — starting with a sixty-degree difference in average winter temperature! Then add the differing senses of history and culture (and whether you are native to the area or not), agricultural vs. maritime awareness, and on and on.

Religious traditions influences. But here's the important point: don't forget that this individualized "coming to know the world" that we do through absolutely unique bodies, families, geographies, and the like *also* applies to the religious and spiritual ways we come to know our world. The "Faith of our Fathers" (and mothers) may indeed be a holy faith, but it's not transmitted free of light and dark from one person to another, let alone from one generation to another. It simply isn't accurate that stories were told from one generation to the next — for centuries — without changes in the story.

No, the study of ancient texts supports a different conclusion. Variations of sacred stories are found clashing in the same texts. For example, the stories we're so familiar with in the book of Genesis actually include two different versions of human creation. The first one, in chapter 1, states that humans are created in the procession of the other creatures, and the second one, in chapter 2, has humans made at the beginning and the rest of the creatures afterward.

The very things that provide knowledge of our world (our bodies, families, geography, religion) also ensure that how we tell the stories about our world (or write about, read about, or listen to them) is absolutely unique to each person. So even when we think we're holding to a "sure faith" as given by our elders, our personal understanding of it is different, to some degree, from that of others who share that faith. How could it be otherwise?

You get the picture. The world may or may not be as simple as the way we see it. But, at least now we know that the *way* we come to know it isn't at all simple! The world is about as complex as all the variations we bring to our way of knowing it.

Whoa! With so many people seeing everything so differently, how do we ever agree on anything?

Social influences. Well don't forget we are, after all, social animals. For millennia we've known that humans are most likely to survive the elements and one another by banding together into a community (Sawyer et. al, 2007). And communal living demands setting aside differences in order to ensure the survival of the individual and the group. That's how we developed our social sense; it's something we come by honestly enough. The social sense, taught imperfectly from parent to child, guides us to transcend our own needs and to care for the larger group. So, although some would say individualism (caring mainly about *me*) has been developed to an unhealthy degree in Western culture, caring about the *other* (as individuals and as a larger group) is the reason community involvement has evolved so richly into various cultures.

Again, concern for the group and the individual is at the root of society in general as well as of our individual cultures. And it's only by a sense of general agreement, some kind of consensus, that we come to agree on the rules used to govern society, the social aspects of our world, that is. I don't mean just our governmental system, but also the cooperative, consensus-focused way that we respond to disaster as well — natural or human.

This is how I would say we come to know the world: by agreeing on the information we gather by means of our unique bodies, our unique minds, and (this is where we go next) our unique souls or spirits. It's something like this: if a fingerprint represents our physical uniqueness and our personality represents our psychological uniqueness, then our soul or spirit represents our spiritual uniqueness.

Spiritual and soulful influences. And so the question arises: What do "soul" and "spirit" mean anyway? It's easy enough to understand for those of us with a parochial school education. On the blackboard Sister Mary Elias would draw the outline of a human body — in my mind's eye it's similar to the ones you see at crime scenes on TV; she emphasized that this was the physical body. Then she would turn the chalk on its side and fill the inner space with softer, thicker, richer strokes: that was your soul.

It made perfect sense then. It makes different sense now. Then, it seemed as if I were made of two parts: inner and outer. Now I see the wholeness of what she was drawing. Both turns of the chalk defined perceptions of a whole person — a boundary for sure (something that could distinguish me from others) but also a fullness that was drawn from the same chalk (things that I had in common with others) with shaded strokes (something that showed my uniqueness).

Most religious and spiritual people today are still comfortable with the idea of a soul considered separate from the body, as "a part of us" that will outlive the body. But a growing number are less comfortable with the idea of the soul being separate from the body. Because of their familiarity with the science that eases their daily lives (like vibrator chairs, soothing music, or telephone calls to friends), they can't quite imagine how a soul principle could exist apart from the body. They're not opposed to the idea of a life force or something as part and parcel of the *living* body; but in our era of scientific discovery, souls surviving death sounds to them like too much science fiction — or worse, like a ghost story.

There are still others who reject the idea of the soul altogether. Some of them feel that humans aren't different from other animals — alive and important now, dead and gone later. Some of these people, too, are saddened to think that this life is all there is yet conclude that this is all we have. So, although most go along with the "bodily" and "mental" ways of knowing, when it comes to knowing beyond what we see, feel, and touch, fewer and fewer people agree. I think reconsidering spirituality, as I'm doing in this chapter, will remedy this.

Perhaps there is a way of imagining soul and spirit that accommodates theists and nontheists alike. Maybe we can find a way to think about soul and spirit that would offer common ground for spiritually oriented believers and nonbelievers alike. It's sure important enough to try, because it's at these deeper levels — at the levels of making sense out of our other ways of knowing — that we become truly *aware*. We become aware not only of our world and our place in it but also of life itself. *Awareness*, the positive essence of spirituality, is the realm of fully experiencing — and thereby making meaning — of life.

Knowing the Soul and Spirit

In the midst of our childhood "coming to know" about the world, people present us with models about how they believe the world works. We learn lots in formal educational settings, but not just in this way. For example, even before going to preschool we experience examples of how *they* see the world: adults, that is, "big people" — parents, grandparents, aunts, and uncles.

Again, because of your unique body, family, and geography, you don't adopt any of these views wholly as your own. That much is clear from the discussion above. Rather, you make your own unique hodgepodge of how you think the world works. Of course you don't use adult logic but a kind of hit-and-miss approach to figuring life out.

Nonetheless, there is always doubt that comes with your discovery: "It might be different" or "There's got to be more." And so for the years of your childhood you keep on learning and learning, always escorted by the nonverbal, emotion-laden, inexpressible doubt: "I might not have it quite right." It's expressed in the child's natural inquisitive: "How come it's that way?" The great "why."

Soulful feeling. Surely at a level that defies words, this amounts to feeling "I'm not done yet." In many it takes on a tougher edge: "The world is so big and I'm so small!" This is both a statement of fact and a first taste of what we know as anxiety. It's the "inward movement" I mentioned in the introduction. It's here that we get a sense of *soul*. This is all about our littleness, our incompleteness, our defenselessness (Hillman, 1994).

Much of this will stay with us a lifetime. It will be reawakened in our experiences of vulnerability on the job, among our friends, and especially in the throes of love. We're likely to believe: "I'm not good enough this way; I must do more." That belief has stimulated much of our culture as story, poetry, music, and even comfort food. Its coloring is somewhat "blue," we might say (and is expressed well in the blues music scene); it's a lack, sometimes felt as a "longing for." This is the felt negative (–) aspect of the spiritual movement I spoke of as we were moving into the labyrinth.

Whatever the tone and hue, the purpose of "feeling little" is experienced in how you respond to it. Your littleness is experienced as manageable when you strive to overcome what is in front you — to truly know and understand, to master the unknown, to become wholly *aware*. Even the pleasure of pausing to console yourself with comfort food or soul music serves the purpose of gathering your strength in order to move on, to move forward, and to continue striving for completion of whatever task is before you.

This is a different way of looking at the "blind drive" theory that some imagine our survival instincts to be, as if they come from nowhere and go to nowhere. From the spiritual point of view, our instincts aren't so much "drives" as they are "strivings" — effort that moves us *away from* a feeling of littleness and *along to* a sense of being competent.

Spirited movement. This sense of movement (striving) away from littleness to bigness; away from ignorance to knowing; away from inability to mastery has been called *esprit*. Long before commercial advertising took it over for a line of designer clothes or a compact car, this French word was in use to express a certain spiritedness, even "spunkiness." It's the "outward movement" I mentioned in the introduction. I'm speaking of the *indomitable human spirit*: a can-do, will-do, must-do attitude that animates human striving, movement, life. It's more than a word; it's action — *movement* forward (Hillman, 1994).

Step by step, we actually do learn more and more. But this information comes in fragments because it depends on those parts of the greater world that we have the good fortune to encounter and on how we put together the information about those parts. This is something we do both accurately and inaccurately. It's how we create such an endless number of inspired motley assortments about how the world works and how we fit into it. This would be the felt positive (+) aspect of the spiritual movement I spoke of as we moved into the labyrinth.

Some spiritually oriented psychotherapists such as Bob Powers (2003) of Port Townsend, Washington, identify soulful and spirited feelings as the two lenses of our "binocular vision." Similar to the way our eyes are spaced just far enough apart that we perceive what is before us in a three-dimensional manner, our spiritual movement is "binocular," allowing our meaning-making perceptions of the world.

A soulful feeling of littleness ("I'm so vulnerable!") is one of the lenses and the other is a feeling of competence or sense of connectedness, spirited direction ("I'm a part of it all!"). However we conceive this double movement (as vision, walking, breathing, the heart beating, or the like), we sense the interactive movement stimulated by a feeling of not knowing (soul, "minus" or lack) and *at the same time* a moving toward knowing (spirit, "plus" or abundance).

Then — lo and behold! — by around age five or six we settle on "a view of the world and our place in it" that makes some kind of sense, a view that we can live with. This is the fruit of years of keen observation. But at the same time it's an instance of poor calculation. I say this because from here on out, instead of asking: "Now, *HOW* is it that the world works?" we tend to see examples of: "Yes, that *IS* how the world works!" Based on what knowledge we've gathered through our bodies, families, geographies, etc., we tend to look for, and therefore *find*, confirmation for our answers rather than continue to *look* and to formulate new questions.

This is when we set aside our first naiveté, of wide-eyed childhood wonder. What remains of the really scary (–) but exciting (+) phenomenon is a sense of insecurity. There we go, thinking we "know it all" all the while having either a vague feeling or strong conviction that we're at risk of harm or ridicule or death or something else dire if we don't know it all. We act as if we know the truth about how to be happy by behaving and pleasing others or by getting whatever we want in spite of others, and on and on and on.

By this time in your growth you look at the world pretty much the way you're going to look at it the rest of your life. This isn't fate; it's the fact that we don't think we need to work on it anymore. Some spiritual writers look at what happens in this stage as if an internal computer has been programmed that we mistakenly, but mindlessly, believe we must obey (DeMello, 1992). Others see this as the point when we begin wrapping ourselves in a cocoon that's meant to protect us from danger and death but that also, unfortunately, shields us from fully living (Trungpa,

2002). However we conceptualize it, this phase of "knowing" obscures the larger truth: we will never understand it all; in fact, by thinking we get it — when we "know it all" — we really miss the Big Picture altogether.

Before heading out of this centered "knowing that we don't know," I'd like to suggest that you stop and breathe in this very important possibility of not knowing.

Third Movement — into a Sacred World

Serenity, plenitude and ecstasy should not stay latent within you like a simple possibility. They need to flower and spread their perfume into the environment, reaching your friends and also strangers.

— OSHO RAJNEESH

Leaving the sacred center, the third labyrinth movement is used for reintegrating into the potential chaos of our workaday world. First by understanding how we come to fuller "awareness" as the healthy result of walking a spiritual pathway, and second by distinguishing healthy spiritualities from unhealthy varieties found in the marketplace.

Becoming "Aware" in the World
As we turn now to leave the sacred center and the insights gathered there, let's consolidate them. Within our earliest understanding of the way the world "out there" works is our earliest formulations of spirituality: along with believing we've worked it all out, we figure we have it right about god as well. It's as if we've already placed god in his heaven so that all is right with the world. Here is our first formal movement into *answers* and away from *questioning*. Never mind that we've forgotten (or ignored) that there is much more to be known and much, much more that simply *can't* be known. We do our best to obliterate the thoughts and reminders that provoke our sense of littleness! Instead we act as if we always feel secure. It's this somewhat mistaken understanding that we project onto the world around us.

But don't despair. There's a beautiful irony in it all. The irrepressibility of life is not in its strength but in its weakness. Remember the two-way movement of spirituality: a soulful sense of inadequacy spurs a spirited response; risk begets opportunity; without the low spot, there's no sense of movement to the higher ground; strength arises from weakness. The generated activity never ends. It leaves us wanting to overcome our littleness and make sense of our place in the world — once and for all, now and forever. We really do want to finally get it.

You can see that any bad news here is quite possibly good news. The hushed whisper of our childhood littleness persists. Part of our animal nature or an aspect of human nature hasn't been clarified, but no matter how we try to quiet it, it persists: "Is there more to know?" "Do I have it right?" And if we listen to it with gentleness and acceptance, the littleness leads us to question anew, to seek the wonder of the world. That is, *awareness* awaits us.

And there's still better news. Not only do we retain this motivating sense of littleness from our childhood but we also get to respond to it as the talented, experienced adults we've become! Now, as "big people," we're able to apply the experiences and talents we've developed over the years to keep on searching. Here's how it works: we move *from* the exciting and scary place of childhood wonder *through* the adult world of thinking we know it all *into* a place of wanting again to know. But this time our wanting to know includes "knowing that we don't know" and being okay with that. This is what some call "being aware." This is what we can bring with us as we journey back through the labyrinth and into a newly perceived world.

Incorporating this wonder, this spiritual way of knowing into the Big Picture of physical and mental knowing might look like this:

- The way we tend to interact with the world physically is known as our "physiology." Wayne showed in chapter 1 how by coming to know your body and its interactions and reactions you can adjust your responses to your everyday world in a way that helps you act and experience it anew.
- The way we tend to interact with our world mentally is called our psychology or, nowadays, our "personality." Gary showed in chapter 2 how by coming to know your likes and dislikes, your fears and joys, you could watch for your typical reactions and practice reacting differently.
- And the way we tend to interact in regard to the Big Picture — how we make sense out of all of it — is our "spirituality." This chapter shows how the dual movement of your soul and spirit can be used to experience things very differently.

There you have it: a way of understanding spirituality from a holistic perspective. It can make sense for the believer, who sees god as the author of the marvelous way we are made, as well as the unbeliever, who can also see the unfolding of life in a wondrous way.

Wellness and Spirituality

Still, this doesn't yet say anything about spiritual health or illness. Surely not all spiritual pathways — ways of making meaning out of the Big Picture — are equally healthy any more than all uses of the body and mind are healthy. No, not all spirituality leads to awareness. No way! We've seen how our early childhood spiritual movement, after a few years of processing questions, is intent on providing partial answers. Because of the incompleteness of the answers, they tend to obscure the reality around us. How, then, do we come to understand or get a sense of spiritual wellness? And what type of "vitamins" might we take to ensure a robust, hearty spirituality?

To explore this, let's continue along the lines already established here: we want to know how the world works and how we fit in:

- We do this by striving to move from not knowing (–) to knowing (+).
- We have varied experiences (physical, familial, geographic, etc.), and we integrate them into our original (mis)understanding of life.
- We realize that striving to master life is not dependent on ourselves but occurs among others with some sense of communal agreement.

Whether seeking "deep within myself" or "far beyond myself," we can speak of this spiritual movement as a transcendence of the self. That is, when speaking of spirituality we aim to discover and understand the Big Picture. Such Big Picture arrangements are what some understand as god or higher power or, as theologians of spirituality call it, the person's "ultimate value" (Schneiders, 1989).

Here "ultimate" stands for the sense of "once and for all, now and forever" that's part of spiritual movement, and "value" stands for how we come to define the importance of things in our lives. At the same time, the notion of ultimate value avoids the power orientation of "higher power" and the historical negativities of "God." More and more spirituality scholars put it this way: Spirituality is a striving to integrate our lives in a self-transcending way in the direction of whatever value we hold as ultimate in our lives.

Each of the significant aspects — striving, integration, self-transcendence, and ultimate value — are separate facets of a single wellness continuum leading to a full awareness of life. The two ends of the wellness continuum extend infinitely in either direction with health, wellness, or heartiness represented as a broad area of balance between the extremes.

Healthy Balance

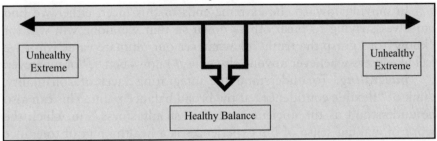

Illness occurs when we go too far in one direction or the other, whereas wellness is a healthy balance in the middle of the continuum. Mostly, we find ourselves somewhere in between. The near perfect balance of the facets is awareness. In the following, I draw out each aspect of the continuum as separate balance beams, showing the healthy center and the unhealthy extremes.

Striving. The striving facet of the wellness continuum is constructed with "cooperation with others" as the broad area of balance. Healthy striving has the tone of collaboration, "me in relationship to others." Even if others aren't present, the striving is team oriented because we work with others in mind. "What I'm doing will help me and the others." Such striving has the feel of actively accomplishing something for ourselves and others. It's vastly different from expending effort alone and only for oneself.

In striving to accomplish a task involving our spiritual awareness, we can imagine a benefit for others. As we see, it shares with healthy

Team Orientation

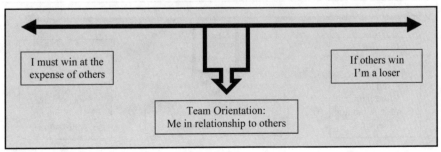

self-transcendence an intimate connection with others; but in this case rather than being focused out toward the larger group, we find ourselves "in the mix" of real human interaction and not so much "at the center" of things.

In moving toward the extreme ends of this facet, either we find ourselves striving to push others down so that we alone will win (or "know" or "grasp the truth" or whatever our ultimate value is) or we feel like losers whenever anyone else wins, "knows better," or whatever.

Integrating. To understand the integrating facet of spirituality, think of "flexible confidence" at the broad balance point. This can also be understood as the ancient virtue of "steadfastness," in which the work of making sense of life experiences is a healthy mix of tolerance and firmly held principles. You hold on to what you believe is true for yourself and willingly hear and appreciate what others believe. In other words: "Your way is *your* way and my way is *my* way, but neither is *the only* way." You might even hold quite tenaciously to what you believe and expect others to hold just as tenaciously to what they believe.

Integration also involves accessing a certain ability to discern between rigid beliefs, fixed ideas, and blind faith, on the one hand, and gullibility, magic, or superstition, on the other. Still, it involves a certain childlikeness that allows one to ponder the mysteries by asking anew: "HOW is the world?" This has been called a "second naïveté" by philosophers of religion: realizing that our childhood words aren't any more accurate or harmful than the explanations we use today (Ricoeur, 1978), one that replaces the abandonment of our first naïveté (thinking that our understandings were perfectly accurate) that we developed in our earliest years. We remember the importance of a critical open-mindedness while using our values to help grasp the Big Picture.

Steadfastness

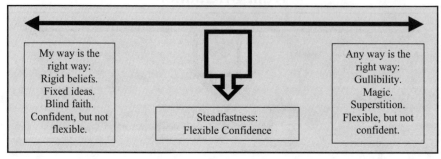

If we moved toward the extremes of integrating, we would find ourselves supporting a narrow view of the world, one defined solely by our quite personal religious or spiritual doctrine. Our beliefs would point approvingly to condemning others for their disbelief, questioning, or infidelity. We'd certainly have confidence but with no flexibility. At the other extreme of the continuum, we'd find it nearly impossible to commit ourselves to any set of beliefs. We'd end up accepting all sorts of values or the most varied doctrinal interpretations. Although we might have favorite interpretations, we'd demonstrate no governing principle for our acceptance or rejection of them. We'd have flexibility but no confidence.

Self-transcendence. Self-transcendence, when in its area of balance on the wellness continuum, inspires a very real concern for "others in relationship to me." It manifests this concern perhaps more on the community level than on the individual level. Going beyond oneself — whether in an external or internal way — brings one into contact with the larger community, where the possibility of well-being awaits. You transcend the self by moving more intentionally toward community and by living consciously engaged with it while distancing yourself from enmeshed, dependent relationships. You can also transcend the self via an internal exploration: by meditating about what is most authentically of value to you.

Community Focus

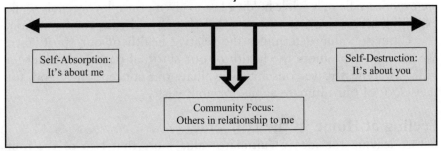

Moving toward the extreme ends of this balance beam, we'd show a tendency toward self-absorption at one end and self-destruction at the other. Self-absorption, positioning oneself as most important in all interactions, is the exact opposite of the inward focus just described. When self-absorbed, we feel: "It's all about me." Similarly, self-destruction, denying one's own goodness and place in the world, is the opposite of a focus on community. Self-destruction embodies submissively agreeing to do whatever you're told to do.

Ultimate value. Finally, our ultimate value is also a facet on a wellness continuum but has a different type of balance point. We find our striving, integration, and self-transcendence perfectly reflected in our ultimate value. It's an embodiment of what we hold most important about our spiritual path. In the traditional sense then, our conception of god reflects our personal style of striving, self-transcendence, and integration.

Ultimate Value

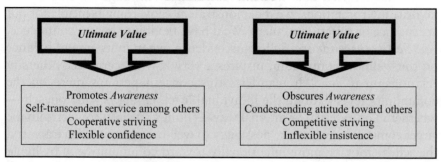

Ultimate Value	Ultimate Value
Promotes *Awareness* Self-transcendent service among others Cooperative striving Flexible confidence	Obscures *Awareness* Condescending attitude toward others Competitive striving Inflexible insistence

As the diagram shows, your ultimate value (a) promotes a fuller awareness of life or obscures such awareness; (b) endorses a self-transcendence that includes others and service among them or a condescending attitude toward them; (c) fosters cooperation or competition; and (d) integrates life-experience flexibly while holding fast to given principles or rigidly while expecting others to agree with your beliefs to avoid your condemnation.

Ultimate value determines the relative health of our spirituality. We restore or promote the health of our spiritual path and achieve a fuller awareness if we consciously evaluate our conception of god, for theists, or of our ultimate value, for nontheists.

Feeling at Home in the Universe

Before leaving the idea of ultimate value, note that two of the four facets are especially intertwined with social sense. One facet, striving, points the way to cooperative (immediate or long-term) interaction with specific others. The second facet, self-transcendence, goes beyond the self to others and the world at large.

Seeing the striving and self-transcendence facets as balanced activities in spiritual movement raises the issue of service as an aspect of spirituality. In all cultures the measure of well-balanced spirituality has always included caring for those in our world who aren't well cared for. That is, spiritual concern "for the group and the individual" truly means all others — in fact, the whole universe. In today's world this includes service among believers and unbelievers alike.

Wellness is not only an issue of doing for others but also one of understanding the others as included in "us" (Levinas, 1996). This encompasses the awareness that we help ourselves by helping others and that we help others in caring well for ourselves. At the balance point of wellness is concern and actual involvement with others. Neither losing oneself in service to others nor, at the other extreme, altogether ignoring those in need, it endorses Hillel's admonition: If not us, who? If not now, when? (Goldin, 1957).

Spiritual writings that use our social sense to promote awareness support wellness in many ways. They speak of a mutual respect that encourages us to help others to truly help themselves and to develop ourselves as a gift to the other. Spiritual writings in this area also encourage wellness as neutral nonattachment (rather than a judgmental, negative detachment) from the world, that is, a balanced appreciation for the world without either overly depending on or altogether disconnecting from the community. The slogan "Live simply so that others may simply live" embodies the healthy form of our social sense.

We've completed the labyrinth walk and developed our understanding of spirituality. We can see clearly the potential for exercising a healthy spirituality and perceiving the universe as a whole as our home. This spirituality strengthens the relationship between the other and me and bolsters a healthy view of the world. Remember, the healthy spiritual path can dwell within religion but it need not.

Nurturing the Soul, Nourishing the Spirit

Perhaps you feel like a flowering garden, receiving benedictions from everywhere, spreading your contentment in order to share it with everyone. . . . Thus comes forth unification, integration, crystallization.

— OSHO RAJNEESH

Having journeyed into, paused within, and journeyed out of the spirituality subject, we are ready to review the fruits of our exploration. What follows is a proposed regimen to keep our spirituality vibrant and healthy.

I've suggested thinking of spirituality as our unique way of making sense of the Big Picture, of making ultimate meaning. Throughout this chapter, I've urged becoming *aware* as the healthier path. After all that has been said, it's possible to think of spiritually healthy behaviors as the vitamins that promote vigorous spirituality — a spirituality that's cooperative, other-focused, and yet assures us that we are part of the movement along with others, a spirituality that's steadfast and guided by an ultimate value.

Vitamins for the spirit can be grouped into five general areas. I identify the vitamin by name, explain what practices it encompasses, and then offer a figurative posture that embodies the practice.

Vitamin A = Ask

Ask anew: "What is it all about?" Step outside the realm of what you know and be okay with not knowing again. Sure it can be uncomfortable, but it's a discomfort that opens us to the wonder and mystery of the wider world, the mystery of the unknown that we've sealed ourselves off from so effectively.

As practice, ask others how they make sense out of life. In your readings ask how things work. In your observations of nature, ask about its harmony. Ask the universe and yourself how it all fits together. Ask whether and why it all matters.

Prayers of petition or intercession from the Christian tradition may be a part of asking, but not in the sense of asking for things — not even answers. Instead ask to be open once again to the wonder of life all around you — whether you believe in god or not. For believers this is "God's wonder," and they should be confident in praying to be in tune with the Big Picture — even if you don't get it just now. To everyone, this is the wonder of our ultimate values, and we all can feel free to ask anew.

The posture of asking is one of opening our eyes wide to wonder.

Vitamin W = Wait

Then: wait, quietly. This is content-free activity. You're not waiting for answers; you're waiting for those important questions to arise. Or if an answer comes, continue your patient vigil and let it dawn on you that this is only one of *many* answers. It makes sense to you and maybe to a few others. But wait with your answer; you can be sure that because the answer comes from your unique perspective on the situation, it probably *won't* make sense to a lot of other people just now.

As practice, consider making room for quiet time in your life. This can include meditation, which has variations in most spiritual traditions. Sitting quietly in some fashion is a very important practice at this point. It has its own rewards and helps open the mind to reality-perceived-differently. Minimally, quiet time models the dual aspects of our spiritual movement — a half hour in the morning and the evening, one to reflect upon the inward path and the other to reflect upon the outward path.

The posture is one of a softly fixed gaze not too far in front of you, attentive and focused.

Vitamin A¹ = Apply

Only after asking and waiting — only after being still — will the application of creative approaches make sense to you. And by then, the success or failure of your action will be less important than understanding that you're striving in a manner that's cooperative and harmonious with others.

As practice, apply new spiritual activities, including service among others and communal involvement with other religious congregations or spiritual seekers. This awakens new interactions with others and the world around us. It's a sure way to awaken new insights and a new understanding of reality.

The posture of applying is one of bending low to work. This posture is simultaneously bowing in service of others.

Vitamin R = Reflect

This is meant as a re-viewing (seeing again) and re-membering (bringing back together), the asking and waiting in light of your applying action. It isn't a re-dredging of the past but a re-assessment of yourself, here-and-now, in the midst of all that is around you. This vitamin feeds your capacity to change and grow as you engage in the practice. It is a continual reappraisal of life lived fully. In essence, you're remembering to ask and wait.

As practice, quiet time is again called for; but now periodically focus on your activities, rather than solely on emptying yourself. This allows you to reintegrate knowledge flexibly and steadfastly, to make meaning from acquired knowledge. This can occur only after seeing the effects of our actions in the world.

The posture is a graceful *glance upward*, in expectation of what is presenting itself at this new moment.

Vitamin E = Experience

Strive to integrate your experiences in a self-transcendent way in light of your ultimate value. Experience the grace of harmonious interaction all around you. Here is only forward movement and awareness of the integrating process of life. Let your integration be a oneness with all that you're learning, let yourself be connected and caring toward all others.

As practice, "Be here, now!"

The posture is a smile.

In this chapter I used a labyrinth exercise to distinguish spirituality from religion and show that spirituality — with or without religion — makes sense out of our experience and makes meaning in our lives. I've encouraged certain practices focused on bringing about a fuller awareness of life. The next chapter addresses the importance of humor for our health — whether recovering from an illness or searching for fuller life. You'll discover ways to create humor in your life.

Vitamins for the Spirit

- Some people think of spirituality as part of religion because it can embrace one's approach to life and closeness with creation. Others make clearer distinctions between the two. For example, religion tends to focus on a set of beliefs, moral codes, and observances, whereas spirituality deemphasizes these and emphasizes an inner sense of direction, or the pathway. Both religion and spirituality can be thought of as leading to answers. But whereas religion tends to emphasize right answers, spirituality aims to encourage further questioning.

- The Big Questions can be summed up as "What's the meaning of life?" By helping form a Big Answer, or "ultimate meaning" in our lives, we find guidance all along the way of life.

- There's a risk if we hold on only to what we know. At the same time, the fear of not knowing stimulates the opportunity to learn more.

- Our physical imperfections, our personal and family histories, our geographic setting, and our culture and religious outlook played a part in how we came to understand the world.

- Awareness, the positive essence of spirituality, is the realm of fully experiencing life.

- To strive, to integrate, to self-transcend, and to have an ultimate value are separate facets of a single wellness continuum leading to a full awareness of life.

- Vitamins for the spirit involve the AWARE process: vitamin A = ask, vitamin W = wait, vitamin A^1 = apply, vitamin R = reflect, vitamin E = experience.

"YOU'LL LIVE LONGER
IF YOU DIE LAUGHING":
THE VALUE OF HUMOR

*Imagination was given to man to compensate him for what he
is not; a sense of humor to console him for what he is.*

— FRANCIS BACON

We're sure you've noticed as you've been reading this book that we value humor. Most of the proceeding chapters have some humor in them, and humor is in the following chapters as well. Why? — Because humor heals. It has benefits for the body, mind, and spirit, as you'll discover as you read this chapter.

Laughter is medicine: it improves immunity, lowers blood pressure, aids in recovery from surgery, and helps in coping with chronic pain. The late humorist Erma Bombeck said: "Humor is great in health care. I still can't figure out why Blue Cross doesn't pay for it!" Humor helps you improve your mind, handle your discouraging beliefs, and improve your social relationships. Bob Hope reported: "I have seen what a laugh can do. It can transform almost unbearable tears into something bearable, even hopeful." Humor is good for the soul. "God is a comedian playing to an audience that's afraid to laugh," said Voltaire. Humor is a recurring theme throughout the Hebrew Scriptures and the Diaspora. As Tevye in the musical *Fiddler on the Roof* says: "God, I know we are the chosen people, but couldn't you choose someone else once in a while?" Even if you're not a god believer, humor can lift your spirit.

Let's begin our study of the benefits of humor by looking at the psychological aspects of humor. Do you mind?

Taking Humor Seriously

Gary D. McKay

> *Through humor, you can soften some of the worst blows that life delivers. And once you find laughter, no matter how painful your situation might be, you can survive it.*
>
> — BILL COSBY

Humor and laughter can lift your mood, increase your creativity, help you see options, and assist you in solving problems. As said in my book (written with the late Don Dinkmeyer, Sr., 2002) *How You Feel Is Up to You:*

> Humor is the ability to make a perceptual switch, for example, from pain to pleasure — or at least to tolerance. . . . Humor is more than jokes. It's a state of mind that frees you from . . . a discouraged outlook on life.

Find the Funny in the Frustrating

In chapter 2, I discussed the concept of reframing. Instead of dwelling on the negative and thinking DUMB thoughts — "It should or must be different." "I can't stand this." "It's awful." "You are (I am, or life is) rotten." — and increasing your PsyDNA (Discouraged Negative Attitude), you look for what's positive in the situation. Humor can help you see the positive — help you create REAL thoughts.

For example, I was getting a blood test and there was an older woman ahead of me who had trouble giving blood — she had deep veins and very little blood was coming out, so it was taking a long time. I was feeling frustrated and angry, I had a lot to do that day, and I felt I didn't have time to keep waiting. Yet I'd fasted during the night and had no breakfast, and I didn't want to go through that again.

So, deciding to wait, I chose to work on my anger by finding something funny in the situation. I said to myself: "Well, if she gets shot, at least she won't bleed to death!" As the woman was leaving, she commented, by way of apology for taking so long, that this always happened so I shared my little joke with her. She laughed. When it came to my turn, as the nurse brought me to the drawing station she apologized for taking so long with the older woman. I told her: "That's okay; I came here to get stuck." She roared.

Through reframing with humor, I was able to defuse my anger. Did the situation change? Did I get more prompt service? No. But when one's stressed out, angry, or depressed, it's impossible to remain so when one focuses on the humor in a situation. The situation probably won't change, but you have. It's like cleaning up doggie doo-doo in the backyard: sure it'll be there later, but for now the yard's clean!

When you encounter people who are quite annoying, you can reframe and keep yourself from being angry and causing problems by imagining them as a cartoon character or some other funny image. Don't laugh out loud of course, but this can help you laugh inside and survive the encounter. And be sure to monitor your nonverbal behavior, so that you don't broadcast that you're laughing at the person.

You can also be prepared for unexpected events by having a funny line available. One that I use is "S . . . happens, carry toilet paper!"

Humor helps in very painful situations, too. When my father died, we held a memorial service for him. In the memorial talk I gave to honor him, I recalled funny times with Dad from my childhood and into adulthood. Doing this helped me handle my grief.

Think about situations you find upsetting. Search for the humor in the situation. There's always some. If you dig deep enough, you'll find it.

Use Humor to Combat Discouraging Beliefs

Although there are a vast number of things people believe that can be discouraging, there are five common ones: "I must be in control." "I must win." "I must be perfect." "I must be superior." "I must please others." These irrational (DUMB) beliefs can be combated by humor. Many of the humorous lines I'm going to give you under my description of each of these beliefs come from a good friend of mine in Scotland — Mac Logan. I'm sure you'll agree Mac has one great sense of humor.

As you read about each belief, see which one (or ones) applies to you. In addition to the humorous lines given, see if you can create your own. (By the way, I'm sure you'll see that these beliefs are just NUTS — Negative Unrealistic Thoughts; McKay & Dinkmeyer, 2002).

I must be in control. Oh yeah? Well, lots of luck! We discuss controlling in chapter 5 on anger and aggression. Trying to control others can get you in big trouble, as nobody likes to be controlled — unless they want you to take the fall for making decisions that go wrong: "See, you made me do it!" or "Well, it was your idea!"

But you can refocus your control on controlling your thoughts and behavior. You can also control the situation by stating your own limits, without telling others what they must do (For example, if someone asks you to do something right away and this isn't convenient for you,

you could say: "No, I won't be doing that today. I'll be happy to do that when my other obligations are finished.").

The next time you think you must control what others do, realize that you're exaggerating your importance. So when you're upset because someone doesn't obey your orders, you could say to yourself: "Move over god, it's my turn!"

Also, you can remind yourself of the futility of trying to control others by getting a cat! Most dogs (except some terriers) act as if they're saying: "What can I do for you, master?" Cats on the other hand say: "You want me to do *what*? You've gotta be kidding!"

I must be perfect. The late professor and author Leo Buscaglia would tell people who think they have to be perfect: "You don't have to be perfect until I am, and you have a very long wait!" By trying to be perfect, you deny your humanness — a mistake is not just a mistake — it's a "catastrophe!"

You demand perfection in others too and "can't" tolerate their mistakes. (But you may not want them to be too perfect, lest they surpass you!) Making mistakes makes you and others human. Mistakes provide an opportunity to learn and grow. Rudolf Dreikurs told people: "Have the courage to be imperfect." Be satisfied with your best effort or the efforts of others — you'll be less stressed out.

So if you think you have to be perfect, imagine yourself wearing a cape and a pair of tights with a big "S" on it! Or you could decide to accept yourself despite the mistake and follow Mac Logan's advice: "Don't take yourself seriously; nobody else does!"

I must be superior. To be superior, you don't have to be perfect — just better. Mac would tell us that superiority seekers say: "Those of you who think you know everything are particularly irritating to those of us who do!"

These folks discourage others as well, because to be better, someone else has to be worse. And of course they discourage themselves because even coming in second isn't good enough. Like perfectionists, those who seek superiority are often creative, competent, and helpful. They can use these talents to contribute. But by overdoing it, they can stress themselves — and others — out by always trying to be on top. Also, remember, if you're on top, you're always in danger of being toppled!

I must be right. If you believe you have to be right, then you can't see any compromise — everything is black and white or right and wrong. "Righters" fear being wrong and may frequently argue, trying to prove their point. If people don't agree with them, those who disagree don't just have a different opinion, they're wrong! As Mac would say, those who have to be right will tell you: "I always listen to both sides of the argument, mine and the wrong one!"

If you've ever been in a discussion with one of these folks at a party, for you the party may be over. Or if this is you at the party, you're a party pooper! On the other hand, they often have good ideas. So, share your ideas, people may appreciate them, as long as you don't try to force them down their throat — this could put a hiccup in the relationship!

I must please others. Pleasers believe they must gain others' approval at all costs. They strive to be liked. They believe: I was placed on this earth to please others. What the others were placed on this earth for, I have no idea!

Pleasers can be pleasant to be around and that's great, as long as you don't overdo it. If you seek to please, regardless of the consequences for you, you're disrespecting yourself. Others may take advantage of you. In the long run, what does this do to your self-esteem? Not only that, but you'll resent them for it.

If you feel you must please others, Mac would tell you to be sure to "keep a civil tongue on the boss's shoes."

If you have difficulty identifying that any of the above apply to you, then examine your thoughts when you're upset. For example, if you tell yourself: "He must do what I say." Then guess what? You're probably into control. If you say: "I made a mistake, that's awful," or "Look what she did, she's an idiot!" you may be seeking perfection. Superiority seekers may tell themselves something like: "I'm the best person to do this. They should know that!" Those who have to be right may say: "She's wrong, and she just won't admit it. How stupid of her!"

If you believe you have to please and fail, you may think: "This is terrible. He didn't like it. I should have known better!"

Develop Your Humor Muscles

Some folks find humor quite easy; others find they have to work on it to build up their "strength of humor." Exercising your humor muscles can be done in a variety of ways. Here are some ways I find very helpful. Do whatever "suits your hoot!"

Build humor in your daily life. Be a humor observer: watch for the ludicrous, the silly, and the bizarre. Watch sitcoms and stand-ups on TV. Watch young children play — this will probably bring a smile to your lips. Collect cartoons. Go to a comedy club or a funny movie.

Read a joke book. Associate with people who enjoy humor and a good laugh. Tell jokes and encourage others to tell you some. Have fun with your family and friends. Check out "Humor and Laughter" on http://www.HelpGuide.org for more ideas.

Sharing a laugh helps bind relationships. Spend time with your family sharing humor. You can laugh together by watching sitcoms, renting a funny movie, sharing cartoons, telling jokes, or doing whatever brings a laugh. Another way is by having a conversation at the dinner table each day in which you share funny things that happened that day.

Make light of yourself. Some of my favorite comedians are those who include making light of themselves in their acts. The late Rodney Dangerfield was a good example. One of Rodney's classic lines was: "I don't get no respect." For example, he said: "I tell ya, I get no respect from anyone. I bought a cemetery plot. The guy said, 'There goes the neighborhood'" (Rodney Dangerfield, The Health Clock: When Will You Die?).

Another comedian who laughs at himself is Jay London. Jay wears his hair long and dresses roughly. He tells his audience: "You might recognize me; I'm the fourth guy from the left on the evolutionary chart."

There are several such "one-liners" you can use on yourself, for example: "I don't collect antiques because I have my own antique. I see him every time I look in the mirror!" Some other ways to make light of yourself are comically telling the story of your life or making light of your profession. Here's how I comically tell the story of my life:

Until a couple of years ago, I used to tell people that I'm at an awkward age: "Too young to be a hippie, and too old to be a dirty old man." But now, I just say: "I'm too old to be a hippie."

I started life as a wonder child — people would see me and wonder why my mother ever had a child. As a young child I was so unpopular that even my imaginary friends wouldn't talk to me. But as I got older, I became the talk of the town. When people in the town saw me, they'd say: "Watch out, here he comes!"

As a teenager, I had all the girls — running in the opposite direction! In school, the teachers referred to me as a pain in the class. Despite that, I decided to be a teacher.

I went to the university to earn my degree, a B.S., which means Bachelor of Science, not what you think it means — though some could argue it could be that too!

As a teacher I ran a democratic classroom. This worked okay until the kids voted me out!

Then I decided to become a psychologist. We psychologists help people stand on their own two feet by lying on the couch (Sigmund Freud). I went back to the university for my M.S. — which means "more of the same" and then my Ph.D., which means "piled higher and deeper" (Jorge Cham).

When I started my practice, office space was hard to find so I shared office with a proctologist. We called our practice "odds and ends" (Mosak, 1987).

We would interview patients together to decide which end needed to be cleaned out first. Dr. Upyourbutt had quite a sense of humor. He would laugh while examining a patient. The patient would ask, "What's so funny?" The doctor would reply: "Sorry, it's an inside joke" (Rodney Dangerfield).

I decided to specialize in differential diagnoses. One time I was walking down the street with some friends. All of us were doctors, me a psychologist, George a neurologist, and Sam an orthopedic surgeon. In the distance, we saw a man walking toward us. His legs were pressed together and he was struggling to walk. I said to my friends, "Let's bet five bucks on what causes his condition. I say it's psychosomatic." George said, "No, it's neurological." Sam said, "You're both wrong, it's definitely a problem with his spine." So, I said, "Okay, how are we going to decide who's right?" "Well," Sam said, "let's ask him."

When we reached the man, Sam said, "Pardon me, sir, but we're three doctors and we're wondering about your condition." Pointing to me, Sam said, "He's a psychologist and he says it's psychosomatic. He is a neurologist and he thinks it's neurological. I'm an orthopedic surgeon and I say it's a problem with your spine." The man replied, "Well, gentlemen, I'm sorry to say, but you've all got it wrong. I'm also a doctor, and if I don't find a restroom soon..." (Mosak, 1987).

Finally, I decided to be a writer. You know — those who can, do; those who can't, write about what others should do. (Well, you're reading this aren't you?)

Okay. That's me — what about you? Give it a shot. Write about your life. It doesn't have to mirror who you are, it's meant to be funny, so make up whatever tickles your trachea. You may have some funny lines you've read or heard, so borrow them if they fit for you. I did.

Make light of professions. Making light of professions can bring you a laugh. For example, lawyer jokes. These poor people have been the butt of so many jokes that they probably want to kick us in ours! So, I won't tell any lawyer jokes here. Instead, I'll make light of my profession (Erik's too): psychology. Here we go:

- How many psychologists does it take to change a light bulb? Just one, but the light bulb has to want to change! (Mosak, 1987)
- Two psychologists meet in the street; they great each other. One says: "You're fine, how am I?" (Mosak, 1987)
- I'm a retired psychologist, which means now I get to lie on the couch!
- Anyone who goes to see a psychologist ought to have his head examined! (Sam Goldwyn)
- Everyone knows that when seeing half a glass of water the optimist will say the glass is half full and the pessimist will see it as half empty. But, half a glass of water can help in a more specific diagnosis. For example, antisocial personalities will look at the glass and say: "Who the hell's been drinking my water?" Those with a paranoid personality disorder will say: "Oh my god, someone's been drinking my water!" People with obsessive compulsive disorder will ponder: "Now, let's see, is it 49.99 percent full or 50.01 percent empty?"

Whatever your profession is (even if you're a lawyer), how can you make fun of it and bring yourself a laugh?

Sing funny songs. Do you have any favorite songs that you find funny? One of my favorites is by Vince Gill and the Notorious Cherry Bombs: "It's Hard to Kiss the Lips at Night that Chew Your Ass Out All Day Long." All by itself, the title is funny and so are some of the lines of the song. There are other singers who include funny songs in their collection, for example, the late Johnny Cash: "Boy Named Sue" and "Understand Your Man." You may have a favorite comical singer as well. Dr. Albert Ellis had many humorous "rational" songs that spell out people's "DUMB" thinking. Here's an example from one he wrote in 1977. It's sung to the tune of the Yale "Whiffenpoof Song"("We're poor little lambs who have lost our way...").

Whine, Whine, Whine

I cannot have all of my wishes filled —
Whine, whine, whine!
I cannot have every frustration stilled —
Whine, whine, whine!

Life really owes me the things that I miss!
Fate has to grant me eternal bliss!
And if I settle for less than this —
Whine, whine, whine!

(ELLIS & BECKER, 1982)

You may have some other ways to exercise your humor muscles. As long as they're healthy ways, great, use them. My final section talks about healthy humor vs. sick humor.

Healthy Humor vs. Sick Humor

The techniques and examples I listed above are all forms of healthy humor. They help you laugh at yourself and situations. Healthy humor can bring people together. Sick humor involves using humor to attack others — individuals or groups. Although some teasing may be appropriate with good friends, sometimes teasing will be seen as insulting. So be careful with this. Being sarcastic or telling jokes or making humorous comments that insult or offend individuals or ethnic groups, genders, nationalities, religious groups, etc. can create resentment. Besides, they say more about the teller than the told-on.

Next, Wayne tells you how humor and laughter can help with your physical health. And then Erik shows you how your spirit can grow through a humorous perspective.

Is Laughter Truly the Best Medicine?

Wayne F. Peate

A good laugh and a long sleep are the best cures in the doctor's book.

— IRISH PROVERB

Humor is a part of our daily lives even from an early age. The fact that children laugh without lessons indicates there is something innate about humor in our species. Adults teach kids all kinds of things about daily living, but few offer "home school" on humor.

There is almost universal recognition that humor is a positive. One of the best compliments to pay someone is: "You have a good sense of humor." I've never had a person disagree with that assessment. I did a small experiment and tried that line on the gloomiest people I know. The closest I came to a disagreement was from an acquaintance who replied with: "You're funnier than I am."

Humor comes in many flavors. Sometimes it's slapstick (known as broad humor), and other times it's more intellectual. A wide-ranging spectrum exists between both these poles of humor. There even appears to be a genetic predisposition to either type, though one's environment seems to be more important than inheritance (Cherkas et al., 2000). A relative of mine roared with delight at the late British comedian Benny Hill's broad humor; much of it I found to be ridiculous and repetitive. Professional comedians survive on their ability to make others laugh and are especially challenged because not everyone finds the same thing funny.

Ever listen to a world-class comic before an audience? It appears everyone is laughing. Bob Hope, one of the top comedians of all time, videotaped his best performances. To everyone's surprise, if 70 percent laughed the perception was that everyone was laughing. If Hope's percentage went below that, he "died' on stage — lacked a critical mass of laughers. An explanation for this phenomenon in a group setting is there is a laughter contagion between people in an audience who don't even know each other. (I tried this on all of my daughters before they could speak. I started to laugh, and then they did.) But why do we need humor and how can we benefit from it?

In *Reader's Digest*, author Richard Reeves told the story of the late president Ronald Reagan who, after he was shot in the chest and while being taken to the operating room for emergency surgery, relieved the tension with a spontaneous comment. As the surgeons prepared for the surgery, the President said: "I hope you're a Republican." Everyone laughed. Suddenly the nervous tension in the room about operating on the most powerful man on the planet changed for the better. The patient survived (Reeves, 2005). No wonder *Reader's Digest* has a section called "Laughter Is the Best Medicine."

Most of us haven't had as dramatic an example in our life, yet everyone can recall a moment when humor helped relieve a tense situation and things started to improve. Recently, while I was kayaking with a group in Antarctica I experienced a similar event. Another kayaker fell into the frigid water. The temperature was so low that we had been warned that two minutes of immersion could kill. Fortunately, he was pulled out in the nick of time onto a larger boat.

Later while we were huddled together in that vessel the impact of what nearly happened — a fatality — struck hard. I said to him: "We would have got you out of the water sooner except that all of us were reaching for our cameras to take a photo of you in the drink." All the passengers in that boat broke out in laughter, including the near victim! It was the levity we all needed to cope with the aftermath of what could have been a tragedy.

The more rational person would rightly condemn my comment. How dare I make light of someone else's misfortune. On the other hand, based on the favorable response of the others on the boat, there is clearly a benefit to humanity in our humor. Perhaps the ability to laugh at yourself defines what it means to be human. To laugh requires self-awareness, a characteristic of higher intelligence.

What is the science behind humor and is *Homo sapiens* the only species that laughs? Some primate specialists have suggested apes laugh. Others believe it's only monkey business; what appears to be a laugh is just ordinary communication spoken at a more raucous, higher volume. So if we're the only ones in the universe that can laugh, why do we? Is humor as essential to our well-being as finding food, water, and shelter?

How Does Humor Heal?

Let's think about the physiology of humor as an explanation for its existence. Think of the last time you laughed so hard your tummy hurt. Maybe your eyes watered. It's obvious even to the nonscientist that humor can have an intense effect on the human body, psyche, and spirit. Humor has been shown to have positive physical effects, including improving immunity and lowering blood pressure (Sultanoff et al., 1999).

Can laughter prevent a heart attack? Dr. Michael Miller and co-researchers (2005) at the University of Maryland School of Medicine think so. Their study found that laughter is linked to healthier blood vessels. Heart disease patients laugh 40 percent less than others. The cause of this finding is still unclear. Prior work had shown that stress negatively impacts the endothelium, the inner lining of blood vessels that plays an important role in circulation, response to infections, and trauma. Dr. Miller and colleagues were concerned that heart disease patients might laugh less because they're ill. So, he checked blood flow on healthy volunteers. One group was shown serious movies like *Saving Private Ryan*. Another group watched funny movies. Those watching humorous shows had improved blood flow.

The reasons for these fascinating findings requires further investigation in the scientific community. But one conclusion that's already clear is that the mind and body are connected, and the body can be enhanced by mental activity. Of course the reverse is also true. Lowered physical activity can lead to lowered mental activity. I've had many patients who were inactive and overweight and complained of fatigue. A simple increase in physical activity and decrease in calorie intake were all it took to restore their energy.

As pointed out in chapter 2, laughter is like jogging in place. One could conclude that because humor has so many benefits, it likely has been passed on as a genetic advantage. The advantages of humor extend from our ancestors right up into our own time. I knew a young man whose face was disfigured by a fire and who married a wonderful woman. She told me that she had never been with someone before who made her laugh so hard that she forgot all her troubles. Humor can thus help you overcome a bad break and still pass on your healthy DNA.

You read about Norman Cousins in chapter 2. He isn't the only one to use healthy humor to overcome disease. Several doctors practice laugh therapy, including Hunter Campbell "Patch" Adams, whose clinic was featured in a 1998 movie starring Robin Williams.

Nobody has done a head-to-head study comparing the various nonmedical approaches to each other (such as laugh therapy, meditation, or positive imagery) for various illnesses. Stay tuned. Someday soon we docs may prescribe time in a humor gym.

Humorizing Your Life

"But I can't tell a joke, what can I do?" As Gary said, make light of yourself. The late Mo Udall, congressional representative and noted political humorist (author of *Too Funny to be President*), agreed. He insisted the best humor is when you poke fun at yourself. No one else gets their feelings hurt, and listeners will think you're the better person for being able to point out your own flaws or a stereotype about your group. Udall once said: "Lord, give us the wisdom to utter words that are gentle and tender, for tomorrow we may have to eat them." About a political caucus he once said: "I have learned the difference between a caucus and a cactus. On a cactus the pricks are on the outside" (Morris K. Udall Quotes).

Senator John McCain told about his experience in losing his bid for the presidency in 2008 on NBC's "The Tonight Show": "That night I slept like a baby. Got up every two hours and cried."

A masterful example of someone making fun by stereotyping his group is former Massachusetts governor Mitt Romney. When asked what he thought about gay marriage, he responded: "As a Mormon, I believe marriage should be between a man and a woman, and a woman, and a woman" (Mehren, 2006). Here is your laugh therapy. Think of a ridiculous or funny time in your life and replay the tape. I heard Bishop Gerald Kicanas of the Roman Catholic Diocese of Tucson, then in his sixties, relate one of his favorites.

> One day while reading a book to young children, one asked me how old I was.
> I asked back: "How old do you think I am?"
> Without a moment's hesitation, the little girl said: "102."

Think of the healing power of humor and how much we are in charge of our own lives because of its benefits. Down and out? Think you need a highball or a drag on a cigarette to feel better? Try humor. It's cheap, has no known negative side effects according to the Surgeon General, and it's always available.

I have a patient I'll call Eeyore. Like that character in the Winnie the Pooh stories, he always saw the bad side. If asked if he was a "glass half empty or glass half full kind of guy," he would say: "Half-empty and what's in the glass is poison." I asked him to write down the ten funniest things that had happened to him or others he had known. I instructed him to keep the list in his wallet, and whenever he felt bad or discouraged to pull it out and read it. Creating the list was a struggle for him, but he succeeded.

After three months he reported definite progress in his view of life events. Most of the humorous events on his list coincided with difficult times in the past. When he hit a new rough spot, he told me he expected that there would be another laugh to add to his list. He also said he became less critical of others as a result of this exercise.

Try it yourself. List your ten humorous life events. They can be something you saw or did; there are no limits. If you don't have ten, that's okay, just list as many as you can. Notice how you feel when you complete your list. A colleague named Paul tried this and got stuck at the first one! "I'm not a jokester." By coincidence we had a funny miscommunication in the clinic that involved Paul one day when he came for a social visit. I was talking about Dennis, a physical therapist helping with a case. Paul, my humor-impaired co-worker, thought I said "dentist" instead of Dennis. Here's how it went that morning:

"Who is that?" asked Paul.

"That's Dennis, he does physical therapy."

Paul, thinking I said "dentist" seemed surprised: "I didn't know they did physical therapy."

"He does it all the time; he even helps us with some of our burn patients," I responded. I treat 1,200 firefighters and burns are a common injury.

"That doesn't seem right. How does he have the training to do that?"

"He worked at a hospital burn center for eleven years."

"I don't care if he did. He doesn't have the education for that kind of work. Next thing, he'll be doing rehab on someone's injured knees."

"That's his specialty," I said with puzzlement.

"The dental board needs to hear about this."

"Why would the dental board be interested in Dennis?" I asked.

"That's their job, to supervise dentists."

A light came on. "Paul, I said 'Dennis' not 'dentist.'"

We both had a good laugh, and now Paul had a funny circumstance for his list. You might think that a couple of chuckles aren't going to change a life, but I'm a great believer in incremental change. Want to be a millionaire? Invest two dollars a day. Hope to lose weight? Drink one less soda a day (or substitute a diet soda) and you'll weigh twelve pounds less next year (unless you replace the calories with something else). Like to be more physically active but don't have the time? Park the car farther away and walk ten minutes more.

I admit when I first tried this "think of ten funny events" exercise, I felt frustrated. Surely I could easily think of ten. I couldn't at first. Then it got easier. I did have ten; I wasn't in need of a remedial humor course. As weeks passed, I revised my list. It got longer and funnier as my recall improved. Even better, I realized how much humor involves others: friends, family, those we admire and love.

I made a few overdue phone calls and sent several emails to people who were part of my list. Some hadn't heard from me in such a long time that they were fearful something terrible had happened. I have a cousin who calls me only when a relative has died. Then again, I have behaved the same toward him. This time I called him and before he could inquire who had expired, I brought up the time we played a practical joke as kids. Best of all, he added details I had forgotten. What a laugh we enjoyed together! I felt renewed for days after. He now calls me when he has a good joke to share. I also get a steady stream of humor from the Internet from others. Some of it's good, plenty isn't, but I appreciate that someone is thinking of me.

Another way to develop your sense of humor is to think of one thing that was funny each day. If you really search, you'll probably find something.

Next Erik talks about humor and your spiritual life. For those of you who believe in God, God must have a good sense of humor. After all, God made us, right?

Ain't Nothin' Sacred?!

Erik Mansager

All you need in the world is love and laughter. That's all anybody needs. To have love in one hand and laughter in the other.

— August Wilson

The Danish newspaper *Jyllands-Posten* is being protected by security guards and several cartoonists have gone into hiding after the newspaper published a series of twelve cartoons about the prophet Muhammad. According to Islam it's blasphemous to make images of the prophet. Consequently, Muslim fundamentalists have threatened to bomb the paper's offices and kill the cartoonists. The newspaper published the cartoons when a Danish author complained that he could find no one to illustrate his book about Muhammad. *Jyllands-Posten* wondered whether there were more cases of self-censorship regarding Islam in Denmark, and asked twelve illustrators to draw the prophet for them. Carsten Juste, the paper's editor, said the cartoons were a test of whether the threat of Islamic terrorism had limited the freedom of expression in Denmark (Malkin, 2005).

So ran the blog statement of syndicated columnist Michelle Malkin, written a full year after the furor of this now infamous case of humor vs. religion. Maybe we'd best think again before going about the business of hee-hawing at religion.

"Laughter? Well and good," say some. "Just don't forget that some things are sacred and off limits." What they mean by this is: "Don't be making fun of *my* faith." Gary is surely right in what he said about sick humor in the opening section of the chapter. And Wayne shared how Mitt Romney lightheartedly poked fun at his own religion. But there's nothing healthy about ridiculing other peoples' faith, family, culture, or gender *in order to* demean them. The humorist Cliff Thomas (2003) once said: "When someone blushes with embarrassment, when someone carries away an ache, when something sacred is made to appear common, when someone's weakness provides the laughter, when profanity is required to make it funny, when a child is brought to tears, or when everyone can't join in the laugher, it's a poor joke."

Such humor is a cheap attempt at self-esteem building. Healthy esteem can be measured in the feeling of solidarity — sharing the same fate among those we love and honor. With true self-esteem, we have the sense that we're actually doing our part or that we're doing something useful for others and thereby earning another's appreciation and respect, as they have ours.

On the other hand, those who *don't* feel up to the tasks of doing their fair share are too often content to gain the *feeling* of being better by making others appear worse. They feel "below" and artificially seek a position "above." They strive desperately to be "up" by putting others "down." So, did the Danish publication intend only to test the freedom of speech implications, or was it a psychological ploy intended to elevate one culture by pushing down another?

We know this much: the overt issue of the Danes poking fun at the Prophet Muhammad incensed the Islamic world. So we can legitimately ask in regard to the Danish cartoons and the emphatic Islamic response: "To what degree does humor and spirituality maintain or undermine mental health?" I explore the healthy aspects of spiritually oriented humor, the heart of which I believe is the ability to laugh *with* others, not *at* them — to make fun of our own limping faith, not that of other. I illustrate this with a good deal of "humble humor" that aims to demonstrate that we can be serious about our spirituality without being somber.

I return to the Islamic issue in closing.

Lifting Our Spirits

Even the weightier matters of faith can be more easily borne and more thoroughly grasped with a lighter grip. There's no question that by looking for humor in the sometimes dire situations we face, we can gain a wholly (holy!) new perspective on the situation. This means that potentially new solutions also abound. As Wayne points out, just as the oxygen intake and internal jostling of a hearty laugh is healthful for the whole body, so too is the "lifting of our spirits" good for the soul. It can reposition us in the atmosphere of hope where we actually experience what ancient wisdom has maintained: "A joyful heart is the health of the body" (Proverbs 17:22).

As with humor generally, along our spiritual path the first step is to not take ourselves too seriously. If we can see the humor in our own lives, we're far less likely to be offended by outside attempts to deprecate us or our faith. This isn't to say we become insensitive to defamation. But we're clearly more able to distinguish the inconsequential accusations of troubled individuals from the individual troubles every faith does well to acknowledge.

Gary and Wayne both reference making light of ourselves. Some call it "self-deprecating humor." I prefer to think of it as "humble humor"—something very different from putting ourselves down from lack of self-confidence. In fact, it can be a sign of real confidence. For example, when a critic of U.S. president Abraham Lincoln called him two-faced, old Honest Abe denied this accusation with the reply: "If I had two faces surely I wouldn't wear this one."

As Gary pointed out above, we function better when we "have the courage to be imperfect." We must never relinquish the right to screw up. In fact, I advise others to do as I do and keep track of personal bloopers. It's a healthy, mindfully aware decision to remind people that we make no claim to divinity. ("My name's Erik," I used to remind my kids: "I never said I was God.") We all have our share of errors, and some days we feel like we're going to make *more* than our share. But if we learn from our mistakes, let's give ourselves permission to be really smart, by being great mistake-making people.

Sharing our mistakes in a light-hearted way shows others we're at ease in our humanity and allows them to feel the same. For example, next time you err, try this one: "I didn't do it, and I'll never do it again!" A light-hearted approach can give others the confidence to learn from their own errors. Terry Paulson (1989), who wrote on the use of humor in the workplace, says self-deprecating humor means we can take things seriously enough to joke about them. The same goes for our faith lives.

I spent my college undergraduate days in a Roman Catholic seminary. During that time, I learned to appreciate the healthy aspects of religious humor. We were a sincere lot, young men studying for the priesthood. Our regular attendance at Mass and telling of our Rosaries kept us focused on a mission that we hoped would prepare us for parish life and all its ups and downs. Still, in seeking the depth of the mysteries, we never shied away from adding our own to the Rosary such as "the five culinary mysteries." These told of the wonders of great food and a Jewish mother putting up with a less than appreciative male household back in tiny Nazareth. It was inside humor that simultaneously made our faith real and kept us from taking ourselves too seriously.

Such "spirit lifting" placed us back in an atmosphere of hope. We had plenty of help from others. Back then Charles Schultz, famous for his comic strip, *Peanuts*, had observed that "No one would have been invited to dinner as often as Jesus was unless he was interesting and had a sense of humor" — an insightful theological observation I've come to appreciate more and more. It made me wonder if Jesus himself might not have originated a joke about his mom that goes like this: "Inquiring minds wanted to know her response to the interview by a Nazarene tabloid. 'What it was really like, after all, being the Mother of the Son of God?' The Virgin Mary was said to have replied: 'Well, I really would have preferred a girl.'"

Humble humor is only one aspect of spirited wittiness. For example, here's a down-to-earth list of glossary terms that a Catholic buddy sent me. It may bring a smile if you have any experience with religious ritual:

Amen: The only part of a prayer that everyone knows.

Bulletin: Your receipt for attending Mass.

Choir: A group of people whose singing allows the rest of the congregation to lip-sync.

Holy water: A liquid whose chemical formula is H2O-ly.

Hymn: A song of praise usually sung in a key three octaves higher than that of the congregation's range.

Procession: The ceremonial formation at the beginning of Mass consisting of altar servers, the celebrant, and late parishioners looking for seats.

Recessional hymn: The last song at Mass often sung a little more quietly, because most of the people have already left.

Incense: Holy smoke!

Jesuits: An order of priests known for their ability to find colleges with great basketball teams.

Justice: When kids have kids of their own.

Kyrie Eleison: The only Greek words that most Catholics can recognize besides *gyros* and *baklava*.

Magi: The most famous trio to attend a baby shower.

Pew: A medieval torture device still found in Catholic churches.

Relics: People who have been going to Mass for so long, they actually know when to sit, kneel, and stand.

Ushers: The only people in the parish who don't know the seating capacity of a pew. (Catholic Dictionary)

Catholics, by no means, have a lock on humble humor. So you won't want to miss the *Beliefnet* humor page at http://www.beliefnet.com. It's full of wonderful ever-changing religious jokes and follow-up comments. I haven't drawn from them here, but you'll enjoy exploring them, I'm sure.

Garrison Keillor, of *Prairie Home Companion* fame, is surely the guru of Lutheran wisdom. He suggests that the Ten Commandments are the most important top ten list not given by late-night talk show host David Letterman. Here's a rephrasing a friend sent me that's fitting of the strong, good-looking, above average folks from Lake Wobegon:

1. Der's only one god, ya know.
2. Don't make that fish on your mantle an idol.
3. Cussing ain't Minnesota nice.
4. Go to church even when you're up north.
5. Honor your folks.
6. Don't kill. Catch and release.
7. There is only one Lena for every Ole. No cheatin'.
8. If it ain't your lutefisk, don't take it.
9. Don't be braggin' about how much snow ya shoveled.
10. Keep your mind off your neighbor's hot dish.

Holy Humor!

This brand of humble humor is a healthy way of showing we don't have to take ourselves so seriously that we forget our humanity. It helps us get over ourselves and at the same time remain appreciative of the challenges we struggle with. Humor is a bridge-building project — it keeps us linked with both our human foibles and our ultimate concerns. Laughing not only builds personal morale but also has been shown to be just as effective as crying when it comes to the bonding process, people coming together for common endeavors.

In my work with college-aged students who have undergone life-changing conversion experiences, I look for healthy indicators of their new faith lives. These experiences are often formative for them as young adults. I'm most assured of the wellness of their movements if they haven't been robbed of their humor and, if they retain it, it's not used mockingly against other faiths. In a recent email exchange with some students, we howled — well, in a cyber kind of way :-) — as they shared Internet insights about the typical collegian's outlook on Christianity.

For example, I learned that if college students had written the Holy Bible, the Ten Commandments would actually be only five —

double-spaced and written in a large font. And get this: they would be published every two years as a new edition in order to limit reselling! The forbidden fruit, an email said, would indeed have been eaten — not due to temptation but due to the simple fact that it *wasn't* cafeteria food! And the Last Supper would have been eaten the next morning — cold! I learned that the reason Cain killed Abel would have been because they were roommates.

Still more intriguing, the reason Moses and his followers walked in the desert for forty years would have been because they didn't want to look like freshmen by asking for directions. The most endearing insight, however, was learning that instead of God creating the world in six days and resting on the seventh, he would have put it off "until the night before it's due!"

Holy humor can come in many varieties. A colleague of mine who has long practiced Tibetan Buddhism shared an Internet list of "Zen sarcasms" that had us both holding our sides. Some of the insights were aphorisms about the nature of things:

> "The journey of a thousand miles begins with a broken fan belt and a leaky tire."

> "Some days you're the bug; some days you're the windshield."

Others were direct commentary on moral precepts:

> "Give a man a fish and he will eat for a day. Teach him how to fish, and he will sit in a boat and drink beer all day."

> "Before you criticize someone, you should walk a mile in the person's shoes. That way, when you criticize you're a mile away and you have more shoes."

> "If you lend someone twenty dollars and never see that person again, it was probably worth it."

Still others are closer to recognizable koans ("unsolvable" questions or comments):

> "No matter what happens, somebody will find a way to take it too seriously."

> "Generally speaking, you aren't learning much when your lips are moving."

This one has a sequel that is a bit more directive:

> "Never miss a good chance to shut up."

As you can see from this list, there's nothing sacrilegious about smiling to yourself about religion. Furthermore, there's nothing wrong with smiling in the face of adversity. It can sometimes be just the thing that strengthens us for life's long journey. So give it a try, think about any traditionally morbid or revered issues and spin them in the direction of health and wellness. For example, when I ponder long what my own workaholic tendencies will get me, I keep in mind that once I was told that ruts in life were coffins with the ends kicked out. Nope, there were to be no such ruts for me as I capitalized on the internalized rule: "Keep planning, keep moving, and keep doing!" On the other hand, my dear life partner soothes me when I stress about my over-commitments by reassuring me that death is nature's way of telling us to slow down.

Lest we think that some faiths are devoid of humor, remember the observation that "One deserves Paradise who makes one's companions laugh." This quip, I'd like to remind you, is by none other than the Prophet Muhammad, who recorded it in the Holy Koran (Qur'an). So, in closing, I can't help but wonder if, in the face of the quagmire created by the Iraqi War, the last religious laugh might be on those who view that war-torn land as altogether godforsaken. Don't forget that the stories of the tower of Babel, the fiery furnace, and the Garden of Eden, all took place in Iraq. That's where Daniel faced the lions, where Jacob found Rachel, and where Nineveh was located. (Remember Jonah preaching there after living through an original version of the *Jaws* screenplay?)

And as the ravages of war are still being experienced in Iraq, we do well to listen to humorist Jim Boren, who reminds us that "even though a humorist may bomb occasionally, it's still better to exchange humorists than bombs. You can't fight when you're laughing."

Humor is just good stuff. Good for the mind, body, and spirit. Gary reminds us of the importance of taking ourselves lightly and even developing a stand-up routine about our lives. Wayne, the doc among us, reminds us of the cardiovascular benefits of laughing. Practicing what he preaches, he prescribes laughter for his patients by having them watch for ten funny events in their lives. The spirit, too, is strengthened by good laughter. Take your own faith lightly and let humor show you the way to a deeper knowledge of yourself and those you love. The following chapters discuss a range of very specific issues and views from the interrelated perspectives of body, mind, and spirit.

Vitamin H: Humor

- Humor and laughter can lift our mood and increase our creativity.
- Although there are a vast number of things people believe that can be discouraging, these irrational (DUMB) beliefs can be combated by humor.
- Build up your "strength of humor, " and avoid sick humor.
- Perhaps the ability to laugh at yourself defines what it means to be human.
- Humor has been shown to have positive physical effects. A study found that laughter is linked to healthier blood vessels. Laughter has health benefits similar to jogging in place.
- One way to develop your sense of humor is to think of one thing that was funny each day.
- By looking for humor in the sometimes dire situations we face, we can gain a wholly (holy!) new perspective on the situation.
- As with humor generally, along our spiritual path the first step is to not take ourselves too seriously.
- Holy humor can come in many varieties. There's nothing sacrilegious about smiling to yourself about religion.

Part II

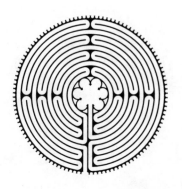

APPLICATION TO THE
CHALLENGES OF LIVING

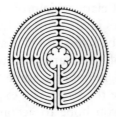

CHAPTER 4

DE-STRESSING YOURSELF

There cannot be a stressful crisis next week. My schedule is already full.

— HENRY KISSINGER

What if we had arrived sooner or tried another medication?" Paul asked me, his eyes holding back tears. The thirty-year-old firefighter paramedic was extremely stressed and experiencing depression and self-anger as the result of a double tragedy.

One evening, Paul and his paramedic partner were dispatched on a 911 call to a familiar address, the home of his favorite uncle. They found Paul's uncle collapsed on his living room floor from a massive heart attack. In spite of their best efforts, they were unable to resuscitate the victim.

Though the emergency care offered was faultless, Paul became immobilized by self-torture. His work performance declined, as did his relationship with friends, family, and co-workers. Someone else's worst day of his life had become Paul's worst day, only that day stretched into weeks of self-recrimination.

Stress arises from normal, everyday life events such as changes in relationships, your financial situation, the death of a loved one, changes or demands on the job, and threats to your safety or that of your loved ones — violent crime, fears of terrorism, and school shootings. The list of stressful life events goes on and on. Weather, noise, pollution, and other chemical and environmental factors also bring on stress. Anxiety, fear, rigid beliefs, demanding schedules, and other lifestyle or emotional factors trigger the feeling of stress. Relationship problems such as communication conflict and power struggles invite distress. Even positive events such as holidays or weddings can be stressful (McKay & Dinkmeyer, 2002).

The physical effects of stress are profound and can include heart attacks and compromised immunity. Some are able to handle stress better than others. Because the stress you experience is related to your beliefs and the purposes you hope to accomplish, in this chapter we discuss how to change your thinking, prioritize your life, avoid situations that invite distress when possible, and reduce your stress through deep breathing, relaxation, imagery, healthy habits, exercise (physical and spiritual), and humor. You'll discover various ways to become involved in spiritual activities and the effects of prayer and meditation on stress.

Stress Is Part of Daily Life

Wayne F. Peate

Why do people in industrial societies, who have so many material things in contrast to the rest of the world, suffer so much? Why hasn't the technology that has reduced the physical requirements of making a living decreased our stress? Our recent ancestors' lives were brief and brutal. They worked twelve-hour days six days a week, and they frequently died from malnutrition and disease. If they had a time machine to let them see our lives, they would ask: "What do you have to be stressed about?" The answer is "a great deal," and you can diminish much of this stress by following the suggestions in this chapter.

In the introduction, I discussed a condition I called "modernitis" — the physical effects of stress that are so frequently encountered in today's demanding society. Many of us have high-speed Internet services and cell phones that do everything from fax to broadcast the television stock reports. We expect instant results, and this expectation contributes to our stress.

Stress doesn't come only from a bad day on the job or grinding traffic. Stress arises from both the *known* tensions in your life, like a missed deadline, and the *unknown* tensions. You can feel stressed because you think your boss might fire you. It hasn't happened, and maybe it never will, but the uncertainty can affect your health.

Smoking and other unhealthy behaviors that lead to physical disease affect your level of stress. Isolation from others causes stress; it increases stress hormones, weakens immunity, and elevates blood pressure.

Stress Effects

Stress can make you sick. Like running your car engine past the red line, leaving your toaster stuck in the on position, or running a nuclear reactor past maximum permissible power, sooner or later, something will break, burn up, or melt down.

Stress aggravates many physical conditions, such as asthma. My daughter and many of my students report that their asthma gets worse before exams. Conditions caused by stress are wide ranging, and they're more common than you might imagine. Stress triggers your basic "fight-or-flight" response, which causes your heart rate and blood pressure to rise.

Chronic stress aggravates heart disease, anxiety disorders, and depression, and it leads to reduced sex drive, high blood pressure, diabetes, digestive disorders, gum disease, and back pain. High levels of stress for prolonged periods can weaken your immune system, making you more vulnerable to illnesses and minor infections.

Everyone experiences stress a little differently, but there are some common signs of too much stress — muscle tension, fatigue, headaches, back pain, anxiety, irritability, depression, changes in appetite, sleep problems, and loss of concentration. Some experience numbness in their lips and fingertips from breathing too fast. Others experience excessive sweating or frequent urination.

What's a Body to Do?

Part of the challenge is to recognize that your reaction to stress is something that you can change for the better. Paying more attention to when you're stressed helps decrease stress-related effects. Doing something about stress now can help for many weeks.

Stress Busters

For fast acting relief, try slowing down.

— LILY TOMLIN

It's never too late to start doing stress busters — activities that reduce stress. Edward McAuley at the University of Illinois found that physically active seniors have less stress and higher self-esteem and confidence. Those benefits occurred even in those who didn't start the program until their seventies and eighties (McAuley et al., 2007). Yes, even old dogs can learn new tricks!

Several stress busters are available for all ages. Here are some you may find helpful:

Try insight meditation. With this technique you focus on whatever is present, such as a noise or body sensation, and *not* your thoughts about the sensation. Don't analyze it, just focus on it. You can chant a mantra or you can repeat "ohm," but neither of these is necessary. Doing this twenty to forty minutes a day will help you feel less stressed.

Minibreaks help too. The late Eddie Rickenbacker, CEO from 1938 to 1959 of the now defunct Eastern Airlines, could be found several times a day silently meditating. He found the few moments of not working allowed him to refocus and become more productive.

Breathe. Several times a day, take four or more deep breaths. You'll find yourself more relaxed. By the way, it's best to do this in private, not during a conversation with others lest they misinterpret. It also helps before a stressful event to take four deep breaths, and as you exhale rehearse in your mind: "I am relaxed." (Look again at chapter 2 for more breathing exercises.)

Use humor. Bob Hope said: "Laughter is the best medicine." Besides taking your mind off what's stressing you out, laughing actually relieves stress. You can use laughter exercises to help you with your stress. Here's one website that gives instructions for laughter exercises, jokes, funny videos, and more: http://www.laughteryoga.org. Cartoons, watching a good comedian on TV, and reading a funny book also help. Learning to laugh at yourself takes the sting out of stressful events as well.

Exercise. Walking, running, biking, and swimming all help drain stress away as well as maintain physical health. Work out for at least twenty minutes three times a week. Some like to work out alone, others like to form exercise partnerships or belong to a club. (Refer to chapter 1 for more on exercising.)

Get a massage. "Ah, that feels good — getting the kinks out." Massage relaxes the muscles and relieves stress. A professional massage practitioner costs money, it's true, but can be worth it. Also, you may be able to get free massages from students who are learning to be massage practitioners. Stretching also helps relax your muscles and relieves stress.

Anticipate. Sometimes simply planning to do something about stress is beneficial. A fascinating finding from Stanford professor Brian Knutson's (2007) brain image research is that the anticipation or preparation for an event such as shopping, a wedding, or a stress-relieving work break provides greater happiness than the occasion itself. Intuitively this makes sense. "Anticipation is totally underestimated," says Knutson.

Eat a balanced diet. Experts believe that complex carbohydrates and proteins enhance mental performance in stressful situations. Sugar- and caffeine-rich foods, on the other hand, though they give you a quick burst of energy, leave you feeling even more worn out. So go easy on the sweets and caffeine-laden stuff and eat healthy. (See chapter 1 and the websites listed in the appendix for dietary recommendations.)

Relax. Breathe deeply, meditate, take a shower, pet the dog, and do relaxation exercises (see chapter 2). If you're at work, get up and stretch and take a walk or short run if you can.

Sleep. Insufficient sleep makes you frazzled and unfocused — leading to performance issues at work and home (as if you weren't already stressed). If you're unable to get the amount of sleep every night that is optimal for you, take naps when you can. Even a short nap can leave you feeling refreshed.

Socialize. Part of the reason for the amount of modern stress and our inability to deal with it is we have fewer friends than we did twenty years ago, according to a recent study done at Duke University and the University of Arizona (McPherson, Smith-Lovin, & Cook, 2001). Half of the participants reported they had no one to confide in; this represents a loss of a significant stress-coping safety net. The support of friends and family and counseling through work-based employee assistance programs, by clergy, and by mental health professionals can be invaluable.

So, you see there are many, many stress busters that help reduce the amount of stress in your life and keep it from developing into distress. Gary will take the next step and address the psychological aspects of this everyday issue.

Minding Your Stress

Gary D. McKay

> *The greatest weapon against stress is our ability to choose one thought over another.*
>
> — WILLIAM JAMES

Yes, we're surrounded by stress, and that stress — as Wayne pointed out — can cause us physical problems, and he's given some great ideas on how to relieve stress. But, do we have to *feel* stressed? As you learned in chapter 2, we choose our emotions based on our thoughts and our purposes. Some people are energized by stress — they love it! They use it to get them going. Others are stopped dead in their tracks and seek to avoid it at all costs: they get anxious, angry, depressed. They even view otherwise positive events as too stressful and avoid having fun! Most of us are somewhere in between — certain stresses we like; others we try to avoid.

How to Stress Yourself Out

We do many things in our head that increase our stress. Below are some popular ones.

Procrastinating. Many procrastinate, putting off things they know they must get done — but don't want to do! Procrastination can stimulate anxiety — the longer you put it off, the more anxious you may get. So what's the cure? Plan a time to do it, and then do it! As comedian Larry the Cable Guy says: "Git-R-done." Think about how much better you'll feel when it's done.

Focusing on past failures. The Bible tells the story of the destruction of Sodom and Gomorrah. As Lot and his wife were fleeing Sodom, angels told them not to look back. But Lot's wife disobeyed, looked back, and was turned into a pillar of salt. Well, at least her stress was over!

Although you probably won't be turned into a pillar of salt if you look back at your failures, you'll certainly discourage yourself by worrying about how you didn't handle a problem in the past. But, if you look back in another way, you may learn a way to handle the current stressor. If you focus on your past *successes*, you may just find a way to handle what's going on now. So *do* look back, but *don't* look for mistakes. Instead, look for a success in the same or similar event. Ask yourself: "How can I apply my past success to this current situation?"

Worrying about what can go wrong. When facing a stressful challenge, you may worry about all the things that could go wrong or that you will screw up. True, you could screw up some things — it happens — but you almost guarantee screwing up if you concentrate on what can go wrong. Instead, look at what could go right — *find something positive* in the stressful situation.

For example, suppose you have trouble at work. Your boss wants to see you to discuss the situation. You're scared to death: "Will the boss fire me?" That's a possibility, but is it a guarantee? Why not focus on some ideas you could share with your boss on how to solve the problem? You may still experience some fear — that's normal — but you'll also experience feelings of confidence. And, if the bottom line is that you are fired, what are some other positions you could go after?

Sometimes when I'm going to give a talk, I get nervous and stressed out, worrying whether or not I'll do a good job. First of all, I prepare my talk carefully. If that doesn't do it and I'm worried the day of the talk, I use a technique I learned from one of my mentors, Dr. Harold Mosak, who when facing a stressful situation told himself: "Unless I get hit by a truck, I will survive." So I tell myself as often as I need to in order to calm myself down: "I will survive." (That's certainly positive!) When I do this, I feel more relaxed. And so far, so good — no trucks! Think how you can use this "survival" technique.

Okay, these are some ways we stress ourselves out and some ideas for counteracting the tendency to procrastinate, focus on past failures, and worrying about the bad things that can happen. But there are other ways as well, such as taking on too much and thinking DUMB thoughts. Let's take a look at how we can analyze and manage our stress.

Don't Let Stressful Events Pile Up: Organize and Prioritize

You can begin to manage your stress by looking at all the things in your life that invite you to feel stressed as well as the physical and emotional symptoms you experience. Then organize and prioritize stressful events using your journal. List the activities that stimulate your stress. Arrange the events you find stressful into three columns: "Must Do," "Maybe Do," and "Forget It." In your "Must Do" and "Maybe Do" columns, prioritize: list the events in order of importance. Now, really scrutinize the items in your "Must Do" column. Decide which ones are essential, such as earning a living and caring for your family. Are you sure there aren't some in the "Must Do" column that can be moved to the "Maybe Do" column and some in that column that can be moved to the "Forget It" column?

For items you believe you must do, decide what can be delegated to others and who you can recruit. One working mom lamented how little time she had at home to relax because of household chores. She asked for a family meeting. She explained her plight to her husband and daughter and then asked for help. Her daughter said she wanted to learn to cook, and if she had some guidance she could do three dinners a week. Her husband took over the laundry. Sometimes the stress from others is "contagious." You might notice the distress of others and call a meeting yourself. Be prepared with an open mind and possible ideas.

If you have children, think about all the extracurricular activities they're involved in. If they are participating in too many activities, providing transportation, supervision, etc. will invite stress. Or, if you're stressed out from driving your children to and from school every day, for example, consider a carpool.

Too many activities invite stress for your children too. So, in your journal, don't forget to list your kids' activities, too. Which ones can you eliminate? Don't make this decision yourself, talk it over with your kids, and let them choose which ones to eliminate. Try this: "Kids, I've decided that you and I are involved in too many activities, and I'm really feeling stressed out. Maybe you're feeling that way too. So, I'll tell you what, I'm willing to be involved in (___ number of) activities. Let's list your activities and see which ones you want to be involved in most and which ones you're willing to drop" (McKay and Maybell, 2004).

As you work to relieve your stress, choose some of the stress busters listed above as well as working on your thoughts and purposes as discussed next.

Identify Your Thoughts and Purposes

Sometimes when people are under stress, they hate to think, and it's the time when they most need to think.

— BILL CLINTON

If you're feeling stressed out, identify your thoughts and purposes. Remember in chapter 2, I said that we could think of our negative thoughts as DUMB thoughts. Let's review DUMB thoughts.

Demanding. You make demands on life, others, and yourself. You proclaim things should, must, have to, or always happen or shouldn't, mustn't, or never happen. So when things don't go your way, you get very upset.

Underestimating. You discount your ability to accept what's happening. You tell yourself that you just can't stand it, handle it, or take it. In this way you excuse yourself from functioning.

Maximizing. You maximize the situation by judging it to be a catastrophe. You tell yourself that the event is awful, or terrible, or horrible. In other words, your world is coming to an end.

Blaming. You blame life, the other person, or yourself for the problem. You judge life, others, or yourself as totally bad.

Let's apply this concept to stress. Suppose you told yourself:

"I can't stand this [underestimating]. Everyone expects too much of me — this is awful [maximizing]. Don't I have a life? People shouldn't expect so much of me [demanding]. If they'd get on with their own damn lives and stop expecting me to take care of everything, I'd be a lot better off! [blaming]"

If you tell yourself these things, you're likely to feel stressed, angry, and maybe even depressed. The purpose of your stressed and angry feelings could be to punish those who expect so much of you. If you're depressed, your purpose could be to back out of all expectations.

To change these feelings, prioritizing is your first step: what expectations can you eliminate, what responsibilities can you shift to others? Next, rethink and create REAL thoughts. As I said in chapter 2, REAL thoughts involve the following:

Reevaluate your demands. Just because you wish something was the way you want it to be, as psychologist Albert Ellis (1998) said: "What universal law says it should or must be your way?" When you place demands on others, life, or even yourself, you set yourself up for strong disappointment.

Eliminate excuses. "I can't stand it," is just an excuse for wallowing in your upset feelings. Where is the evidence that you can't stand something that has happened? You've probably stood many unpleasant things in your life. What makes the current situation any different?

Accept disappointments. Few things in life are catastrophes. What happens to us may be frustrating, unfortunate, inconvenient, or disappointing; but it is seldom awful.

Let go of blame. We can't judge a person by his or her behavior. Each of us behaves in positive or negative ways. When we try to place blame, we end up judging the whole person. So, judge behavior, not personhood. When you think someone has done you wrong, focus on the behavior — separate the deed from the doer.

So, using REAL thinking, you could tell yourself:

"I don't like this; it's unpleasant, but I can stand it [eliminating excuses]. Although it's true that people expect too much of me, it's not awful; it's just very frustrating and inconvenient [accepting disappointments]. I do have a life and I don't have to succumb to everyone's expectations [reevaluating demands]. Although I don't like people dumping things on me, they're not bad people; they're probably just as frustrated as I am. I'll evaluate what I'm willing to take on and let others handle their own responsibilities [letting go of blame as well as making a positive plan]."

If you tell yourself these things, you'll probably still feel frustrated, but you'll most likely feel determined as well — determined not to be dumped on. Your purpose would now be to manage your own life despite others' expectations.

Additional Ways to Manage Your Stress

I mentioned in chapter 2 several ways to manage emotions, such as reframing, laughter and humor, deep breathing, relaxation, imagery, exercise, talking about your feelings, and seeking meaning. In this chapter, Wayne also mentioned some of these activities and how they can help.

How could you reframe the situation in the above example? Instead of telling yourself it's awful that people expect so much of you, you could tell yourself that it's very flattering — people trust and have faith in you. What's funny about the situation? Well maybe you could see yourself as a superhero, donning your cape and tights! Deep breaths can help you relax. We presented breathing exercises above and in chapter 2. Relaxation takes many forms — from a warm bath to listening to relaxation tapes. Do whatever helps you feel relaxed.

Create positive images such as lying on the beach (or maybe everyone serving you rather than you trying to serve them). And, as I said in chapter 2, you can use imaging to rehearse how you'll tell people to handle their own responsibilities. Exercise. As we've said, physical activity can drain away stress. Tell your spouse or a friend how you're feeling; seek their counsel. If things are pretty bad, consult a professional therapist.

And remember, trying to make sense of life is what it's all about. As Erik pointed out in chapter 3, seeking meaning underlies your sense of spirituality. In the next section of this chapter, Erik discusses how to manage stress with spirituality.

De-stressing Spiritually

Erik Mansager

> *A knower of God (Jnani) and a lover of God (Premika) were once passing through a forest. On the way they saw a tiger at a distance. The Jnani said, "There is no reason why we should flee; the Almighty God will certainly protect us." At this the Premika said, "No, brother, come, let us run away. Why should we trouble the Lord for what can be accomplished by our own exertions?"*
>
> — RAMAKRISHNA

Wayne helped us understand what we can do physically about the stress we encounter in our busy days. He suggests being conscious of the stressful events and practicing stress busters. Developing healthy life patterns is very helpful, indeed. Gary took us to the mental level and suggested practical ways of replacing DUMB thinking with REAL thinking. I especially like the idea of being an example to our children and helping them de-stress their lives as well.

You can see the holistic effects of good health. Wayne, from the physician's viewpoint, reminds us of the benefits of meditation. Both Wayne and Gary, from the physical and psychological viewpoints, suggest humorous imaginings and enjoying a good belly laugh. And from the spiritual viewpoint, I remind you of what you read in chapter 3, that spirituality isn't just a whole "otherworldly" enterprise. You can effectively incorporate spiritual stress busters in your everyday life as well.

We encounter spiritual stress on many levels, to be sure. We get most in touch with it when we experience guilt and "vexations of the spirit." Let me start with vexations, then I'll get back to guilt — the preeminent spiritual stressor — and I'll close with comments about how prayer and mindfulness can impact them both.

Are You Vexed?

After distress, solace.
— SWAHILI PROVERB

Feeling vexed or "ticked off" is an internal irritation we sense as if it's related to outside events.

You've run into it before — probably lots of times. You're going along fine in your day, getting things accomplished on your long list of activities, when all of a sudden an annoyance jumps out of nowhere and really (really!) ticks you off. Truth be told, the vexing incident probably has been there for a while at a lower level (for example, your boss's constant, low-level criticism or the repeated difficulty finding that telephone number you need).

Then you catch yourself snapping at somebody — sometimes not even the one at the root of the annoyance. Since the snapping almost feels good, you feel a bit guilty about it. Still, you're so surprised and embarrassed that you try to ignore it, "compose yourself," and move on rather than deal with what's plaguing you. By now, though, every little thing the other person does or says bugs the heck out of you. (Or as Gary would say, you bug yourself about what's going on.) As usually happens, the irritation comes to the surface at the least opportune time — you have many hours to go before the day ends and you dread that it's just going to be one long annoyance.

Such annoyance comes in any number of ways, actually. We might feel ill at ease, as if something is going to happen that we can't control.

Maybe we're afraid our temper will rise and we'll pop off at someone. Or we dread facing that other person who seems about to pop! You know the feeling: "If just one more thing comes along, I'm going to scream!" (See chapter 5 for suggestions on dealing with your and others' anger.)

The difference between physical and psychological stressors and the spiritual ones might best be understood by getting in touch with this low-level, but persistent dread: "Something not so good is about to happen!" What can we do about such vexations of the spirit?

Rest assured, there is a lot that you can do. I'm writing third in this chapter because you can go a long way toward relieving vexations of the spirit by following Wayne's and Gary's suggestions first. Calming ourselves and thinking differently are essential to such vexations to keep them from escalating. But as you read in chapter 3, our spiritual aspect really focuses more on the long-term outlook. At the spiritual level, it's more a matter of thinking in terms of replacing the low-level sense of dread with a higher-level sense of joy.

No, it isn't automatic. Sure, it takes practice. Yes, you can do it.

Pema Chödrön (2000), a Buddhist nun, and the late Anthony DeMello (1995), a Catholic priest steeped in the Hindu traditions, suggest complementary ways of moving from vexation to awareness. I'll share tips from both of them and show how their schemas fit in with the spiritual vitamins I shared in chapter 3: asking, waiting, applying, reflecting, and experiencing.

Chödrön's approach comes in three parts: getting in touch with the irritation, changing one thing about how you deal with it, and continuing to practice the change until it's a habit. Here's how it works:

- In the course of a daily quieting-time, we can get in touch with our agitations. By setting aside time on a regular basis — remember I suggested twice a day in chapter 3 in acknowledgement of the give and take of life — we can compare how we're doing from "then" until "now." The routine helps us better focus on our feelings of agitation and, even if we have difficulty identifying the belief that underlies the feeling, we become more and more conscious of it.

- You see, it doesn't take complete clarity to resolve the vexation. Increasing our consciousness of the vexation itself — rather than trying harder and harder to avoid it — provides enough for us to act on. In being quiet with it, we better see the pattern we're involved in that brings the agitation with it. It's from here, in seeing the pattern, that we can choose one aspect of that pattern to do differently.

- Strategically chosen and regularly applied, the minor change allows a vexation to become less an annoyance, less a sense of dread, and more an exercise in self-awareness. DeMello goes about it somewhat differently.

Where Chödrön's threefold movement — consciousness-change-practice — focuses on moving from conscious to immediate action, DeMello goes the route of interior understanding of how we perpetuate our own irritations:

- Upon experiencing the annoyance, our task is to ask whether we're in charge of the annoyance or it's in charge of us.
- This leads to the realization that there are likely innumerable people who could be in an identical situation and not be negatively affected.
- So we arrive at the understanding that it isn't the person or situation that vexes us so, but the way we have learned to deal with such things.

Sounds familiar, doesn't it? Yet at the spiritual level, we're invited to think deeply about our overall situation — the Bigger Picture — to realize again that the world may not be at all as we perceive it. Getting in touch with stressors at this level is the precondition for deep resolution and fundamental shifting of our outlook.

Imagine such a switch. It allows us to see again, to see differently, that the upsetting situation is not to blame — no matter the person or circumstance. Especially regarding people who vex us, we can see that they too have been conditioned by the way they come to see the world. Never mind how the irritations got there, though; you've come to understand at a very practical level what you can do about it: *let it be.* Here is the path to joy through gratitude: the irritation itself becomes the opportunity to remember that life is bigger than those irritations. Here is the gift, given again and again, that reminds us how we limit our own joy.

In a case of being late to dinner, a trail of toys left about, or the uncertainty of your job, it would be a matter of reframing like this: Think how happy a great number of people in the world would be to have the benefit of the meals you eat, a home with more than enough toys to leave around, or any kind of a paying job. Moving *into* gratitude, crowds *out* the irritation. Letting it be as it is, even in this small matter — especially in this small matter — leads the way to greater inner peace.

Reframing may not be all you'll want to do. Elsewhere in the book you'll find ways of interacting respectfully, showing others what they can do, and positively expecting them to do their part. Still, the effort to reframe an "unmanageable vexation" as something wholly manageable will enhance those techniques.

Spiritual Guilt Tripping

Either do wrong or feel guilty but don't do both; it's too much work!

— RUDOLF DREIKURS

The other common spiritual stressor, guilt, doesn't come from the outside. Rather it's an inward self-evaluation that we aim back toward others, guilting ourselves with: "What will people think?"

Remember, spirituality is concerned with how we make meaning out of it all when we look at the Big Picture. In that context, an inward sense of having gone against a value we openly proclaim as essential to who we are brings about guilt. It could be anything we're vocal about that helps us identify our "true selves" to others, for example,

- the importance of being frugal
- being available to others
- caring for the environment
- voting one's conscience rather than a straight political ticket

Acting *against* such values can lead to a deep sense of guilt.

All is well and good with us spiritually when we perceive the Big Picture in such a way that follows our stated values, since our values help us make sense out of it all. But now and again, it's a serious inconvenience to follow our own values. At such times, we may temporarily suspend our values and totally disregard them. To follow the example values mentioned here, perhaps we

- go on a shopping spree in spite of a rising credit card debt
- don't visit a friend we know is in need because we have other pressing matters
- leave our picnic garbage behind because there are no garbage cans available
- vote a straight party ticket because we haven't taken the time to explore the individual candidates

Isolated incidents like these may, in fact, not disrupt our making meaning of the Big Picture even though they go against our proclaimed values. We nonetheless "feel bad" about them. We probably do so to keep ourselves in line with our temporarily suspended value. It's as if we act to punish ourselves by the guilt, the "feeling bad," and in that way we try to assure ourselves that we're not going to do that particular behavior again.

There's a funny thing about guilt, though. In certain matters or in certain circumstances, we get stuck in feeling guilty *instead* of "not doing it again." Any time we say one thing and consistently do something differently, guilt will act as a stressor and debilitate us spiritually, mentally, and even physically. At such times we do well to ask ourselves: "Why do I espouse one thing and do the other?" Well, psychiatrist Rudolf Dreikurs has suggested: "Guilt expresses good intentions we really don't have."

Quiet-time examination can reveal a dynamic that regularly follows this pattern: you want people to think one thing about you, and you want to do another thing. The guilt feeling in such a case is only window dressing. By punishing yourself with guilt — perhaps as you were punished with a spanking or scolding as a child — you give yourself an odd sense of "permission" to continue the behavior rather than change it. After all: "I've taken my licks for it." It's similar to the old joke about the father disciplining his son in the woodshed. Since he had to travel for business the following week, he swatted his boy for last week's misbehavior as well as the coming week's, and since the boy had taken his licks he was free to misbehave. That's kind of what we do to ourselves. The stress is a powerful tension as we pull ourselves between "what we think we should do" and "what we want to do" — stretched like a rubber band. How do you alleviate this type of stress?

First, in the quiet moments when you're aware of contributing to others' lives and receiving care from them, you can try on this new understanding of guilt. It's obvious that you "want to do" something other than what you believe you "should do." During quiet time, work to ask clearly: "Who is responsible here?" Then you quiet the voice that says anything other than: "I am responsible." No blaming Mom and Dad, no blaming "fallen nature," no blaming "a weak moment," and no blaming yourself. Indeed, there's no room for blaming at all. Blame is part of the old reward-punishment approach. Instead, you simply accept responsibility.

Breathe, calmly and deliberately. Wait, and ask again. Ponder who benefits from the "should" behavior and who benefits from the "desired" behavior, who is harmed by the "should" behavior and who is harmed by the "desired" behavior. We can imagine a four-way matrix of benefits and harm that conveys these options:

1. I benefit and others are harmed.
2. I benefit and others benefit.
3. I am harmed and others benefit.
4. I am harmed and others are harmed.

From this perspective, only the personal costs of option 3 need deeper consideration, as options 1 and 4 likely eliminate themselves.

But the actual point of the exercise is that in examining option 2, we find a resolution to the self-imposed guilt. You do well to admit clearly that others may believe one thing and you can choose your own path. With such personal congruence, the stress is alleviated, the punishment lifted, free choice restored, and calm and joy have the chance to return.

If we were to take one of the example values above — say visiting a friend in need — we could run it through the matrix:

1. I will do my shopping rather than visit my sick friend.
2. I will do my shopping sometime after visiting my sick friend.
3. I will forget my shopping and simply visit my sick friend.
4. I will neither do my shopping nor visit my sick friend.

You can see in this simple example that options 1 and 4 are easy to eliminate. Option 3 is doable, but I'm likely to feel resentful about it. Option 2 will take some thought as to the details, but it's clearly the option of choice.

What about Prayer?

Pray as if all depended on God. Act as if all depended on you.

— St. Alphonsus Liguori

In instances of the spiritual stressors discussed — vexations and guilt trips — there are spiritual activities that reduce and eventually eliminate the stressors. But I'd be remiss if I didn't mention that the most effective means for many is simply prayer. Admittedly, there is nothing really simplistic about communing with god — but it can be a simple, gentle movement. For the believer in god, it can take many shapes. Conversation, petition, gratefulness, and rejoicing are all ways of reframing one's thinking about spiritual annoyances.

Speaking to god as if to a trusted friend has shown its effectiveness in many Judeo-Christian traditions. A good way to begin is by sitting quietly and putting forward your concern while thinking of god as a beloved parent or sibling advisor who can provide an answer.

Petitions, or requests for change, often closely follow a heartfelt conversation. It's natural to entrust to a loved one your hope for things to be different. Don't hesitate to do so with your god. Petitions are different from bartering. Bartering is about you doing "this" so that god will do "that." This approach itself leads to further vexations of the spirit if what you bartered for doesn't happen. The prayer of petition isn't like that. Rather, it's recognizing your desire for the annoying event to change. In petitioning, you realize that it may well be your heart that needs changing, and you open yourself to that possibility first and foremost.

Gratefulness often follows from the petition. This is a prayer of remembering, one that aims to get you back in touch with how things were before the stressor ever occurred. Long before the sense of dread began rearing its head or you began feeling guilty, there was a moment or space in your life that you experienced real peace of heart. It's the contrast with that peace that you're likely experiencing as stress.

So, for example, if the pending dread or guilt has a monetary tinge to it — "How am I going to make it to the end of the month with the regular bills and the kids' unexpected doctor bill to cover?" or "I shouldn't have spent that on myself." — recollect an earlier time. In the very face of your concern, think back on a time, for example, when all the bills were met, when the kids weren't sick, or when you were experiencing really solid trust that it would all work out. Pause. Yes, pause there in your recollection and experience the calm; connect with your gratitude. Give yourself a full five minutes here. That's all. Pause, and move on. You'll find yourself dramatically less stressed even after this brief exercise. And that is when the prayer of joy will be most effective.

Stressors are, after all, the texture of life. Don't avoid them, but recognize and work through them. The scriptures of all major religions address the importance and the promise of working through hardships rather than avoiding them. And all those textures represent divine lessons for you to learn.

Step by step, we find our way through difficulties and on to a better way of dealing with the world. Here, within the joyful moment, we can casually converse, we can ask for assistance to change our minds and hearts, we can pause to recollect and be thankful. All such prayer is a reframing of a world that only temporarily feels unbearable. "Rejoice, always!" said Paul the apostle. He reminded us again: "Rejoice!"

Stress is a debilitating matter — whether immediate physical stress, self-imposed DUMB thinking, or Big Picture spiritual stress. By investing a little time to control stress, you keep yourself healthier — and a whole lot happier. We hope the benefits of these stress-busting procedures are of help. To sum up this chapter, Wayne tells the story of how he used vitamins for the three dimensions to help a patient manage his stress.

Paul's Story: "The Worst Day of Your Life"

Wayne F. Peate

Firefighters help people on the worst day of their lives: heart attacks, devastation of a family home, loss of loved ones and favorite pets.... Paul, the firefighter paramedic whose story opened this chapter, confessed to me that: "I just can't get that image of my uncle out of my head. What if we had arrived sooner or tried another medication?"

"Paul, nothing I could say would ever erase the grief you must feel," I offered. He nodded in agreement. "I am certain there are many good memories of your uncle that you have."

"Yes, he taught me how to ride a bike, to catch a ball; he was always there for me." Paul put his head in his hands. "Do you think I'll ever be right again?"

Stress is multifaceted. For some the time pressures of daily life are consuming, for others it's financial or family factors that stress us. For Paul, his stress was self-created. He had done the best anyone could for his uncle, but that wasn't enough.

What to do? Reassurance is often helpful; but it wasn't in this case. A senior co-worker reviewed the case. His assessment was Paul and his partner had followed state-of-the-art procedures. For Paul that was insufficient. "I've gone over the case a hundred times in my head. I realize that I followed correct procedure. I just keep seeing my uncle's face — dead."

Taking Vitamins for the Three Dimensions

My experience has been that intervention from one dimension may work for someone who is stressed, but that the synergy of techniques that incorporate the mind, body, and spirit hold greater promise. Here's how I applied the mind, spirit, and body integrated approach to help Paul.

Mind. I've found substitution can be effective in such cases. I asked him: "Paul, that image of your deceased uncle is a negative. What is the most positive image you can have now?"

He thought and then his face brightened: "My daughter was born before my uncle died. I was there for the delivery. It was a miracle."

"Can I see a picture?" Paul, the proud father showed her photo to me. "What if every time you have a negative image of your uncle, you substitute it with a positive one — take the picture of your daughter out of your wallet and focus on it."

I also provided Paul with a simple breathing exercise to use. I advised him to take four deep breaths in and then out. As he exhaled, I urged him to think of a reassuring word. He chose "peace."

Spirit. Since I know that spirituality plays an important healing role in the lives of many, I asked Paul about his sense of spirituality. It turned out that he was affiliated with a local congregation. With his wife's assistance, we scheduled a session with his pastor.

However, there Paul expressed his anguish that he had let his uncle down: "He was always there for me, and when he needed me most I let him down."

The pastor reframed Paul's conclusion: "Paul, you've told me your uncle was extremely proud that you were a paramedic and that your life's mission was to help others."

Paul agreed and added: "He always said if he was ever in trouble he wanted me by his side. If only it had worked out differently."

"Paul, perhaps God had other plans for your uncle the day he died. He is with God now. But your uncle got his wish. You were at his side when he passed to the other side, from this life to the next. Imagine how alone he might have felt if there was only a stranger with him. Instead he had the presence of a loved one — you."

Paul and his pastor continued to talk over the next weeks. Paul not only said the word "peace" during his relaxation breathing, he also began to feel more at peace inside.

Body. Paul couldn't eat or sleep and his energy level plummeted in the days after the death. Previously he had been physically active in a regular workout program and described feeling unwell if he missed a gym session. He had what I call a "positive addiction" — a health-promoting behavior that compels one (for others it might be yoga or Tai Chi). I told him he would feel better if he restarted his physical activity program.

He declined: "I just don't have it in me to lift weights or do sprints."

"You seem to be okay with walking; you walked from your car to my office." He admitted that wasn't a problem. I asked him to just walk, with his wife or a friend or one of his older children. The company and the distance didn't matter. But the activity did make a difference. Later that week, he reported that his stress seemed to melt when he was walking. Getting out of the house and exercising his body helped his mind and spirit.

Paul worked on his grief for many months, visualizing positive images, practicing relaxation and deep breathing, acknowledging that he really had "been there for" his uncle with caring attention at the end, and slowly increasing his physical activity. He gradually began to find himself experiencing less stress, fewer bouts of depression, and a more positive outlook on life. He never forgot his uncle or the tragedy of that worst day, but he eventually regained full confidence in his work and became his "old self" again.

The topics of the following chapters are all related to stress. For example, chapter 5 discusses aggression that involves anger, and anger is often related to stress. Some stressed out people get angry, and some get depressed — the topic of chapter 6. Chapter 7 discusses addiction. Severe stress can lead to a chemical addiction, such as alcoholism. Chapter 8 discusses chronic illness, which, of course, can be very stressful. As people get older, the topic of chapter 9, they may experience stress as their lives change.

Vitamins for Stress

- Chronic stress can aggravate heart disease, anxiety disorders, depression, and a host of other problems and can weaken your immune system.
- Stress busters include insight meditation, deep breathing, humor, physical activity, massage, eating a balanced diet, relaxation, socializing, and adequate sleep.
- There are many things we do in our head that increase our stress, such as procrastinating, focusing on past failures, and worrying.
- If you're feeling stressed out look for your DUMB thoughts. To change these feelings, prioritizing is your first step. Next, rethink and create REAL thoughts and positive purposes.
- Spiritual stress is best understood by the sense of persistent dread: "Something not so good is about to happen!" Calming ourselves and thinking differently are essential to such vexations to keep them from escalating.
- A common spiritual stressor, guilt, is an inward self-evaluation. We get stuck in feeling guilty instead of "not doing it again." By punishing ourselves with guilt, we give ourselves "permission" to continue the stress-causing behavior rather than change it.

CHAPTER 5

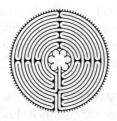

"WHO'S ON TOP?": AGGRESSION AND ANGER

Aggression only moves in one direction — it creates more aggression.

— MARGARET J. WHEATLEY

Jake was a much beloved neighborhood baker who started a food bank that fed hundreds every day and made generous donations of his time and funds to that cause. But Jake's cheerful demeanor and community service hid a dark past. On his arm were tattooed numbers from a German concentration camp. "As a boy I lost all my family. When I was released from the camp, I swore revenge against their killers. I could think of nothing else. Then I realized I was still a prisoner of the Nazis because I was allowing them, through my anger, to take over my mind."

Jake's anger was also affecting his physical and spiritual well-being. He developed severe headaches; the angrier he got, the more his head ached. He also felt detached from the faith of his fathers, whose core value was "Love your enemy as yourself." Jake came to a startling realization. The commandment's first admonition was to "love . . . yourself." His deep anger had turned into a destructive self-hatred as he had tormented himself with his failure to inflict revenge. Worse, he felt he had become estranged from what God wanted from him. "I didn't survive Hell just to continue to live in it by my own choices and actions."

With that spiritual inspiration and the recognition that his mind was wrecking his body, Jake was able to make productive plans. "The Nazis never gave us enough to eat, so I swore to make sure others got enough." Jake's anger didn't vanish; he transformed it for a better purpose. Jake could have spent the rest of his days hunting down a few murderers. Instead, he reformed that aggression into a positive — a life vocation that nourished thousands.

Aggression Is Everywhere . . .

. . . And it takes many forms: war, school shootings, violent crimes, and family violence are far more prevalent than we realize. Emotional aggression is another problem, from attacking and discouraging remarks in political campaigns to family accusations and arguments. Daily irritants such as being put on hold for what seems like forever; traffic and road rage; bratty kids; noisy neighbors; computers that malfunction; problems with relatives; hubristic religious claims — you name it! — they get to us. With all the irritation and aggression in this world, it's a wonder we manage to exist — why didn't early *Homo sapiens* kill each other off — why do we survive?

But still, just as aggression is everywhere, so is cooperation. And guess what, we live and advance more through cooperation than through aggression. Humans have the capacity for both cooperation and aggression. It's a matter of choice, like all human behaviors — and emotions. As Benjamin Franklin said: "We must, indeed, all hang together, or most assuredly we shall all hang separately."

Anger accompanies aggression, but is not the cause of it. Aggression — no matter what form — elevates the aggressive person, puts him or her "on top." Aggression and anger are created and controlled by your mind; they result from what you choose to think and the purpose of your behavior and emotion. Deciding to let go of anger and controlling your aggression will improve your relationships and life in general. Spirituality (not religiosity, which is obtrusive religiousness) helpfully addresses aggression as well. When is anger right and when is it best to let it go? Becoming aware of the physical effects of hostility, such as increased blood pressure and cardiac problems, as well as deciding to make positive changes will improve your physical health. We'll begin our examination of aggression and anger by looking at what goes on in our heads.

Aggression, Anger, and Attitude

Gary D. McKay

Remember in chapter 2 I talked about PsyDNA — your Discouraged Negative Attitude? Well, it certainly comes into play with aggression and anger. Aggression comes from your belief that you have to be superior, you must be in charge, you must win at all costs, or only you know what's right. Sometimes aggression comes from the desire to get even if you think your rights have been violated or you don't get what you want. Aggressive people are concerned only with their rights and ignore the rights of others.

Although aggression causes multitudinous problems when it leads to war between nations, terrorism, violent crime, and other forms of violence, it's especially sad when it occurs in families. How do you "cure" it? If you're the aggressor, if you're frequently angry, consider the consequences for you in your relationships. When you get what you want at the expense of others, what does that do to your relationship?

If you're the target of aggression, you can protect yourself; and if you have kids who are also the target, you can protect them too. If you, or your kids, are being abused, it's time to seek help. Call your local abuse hotline — check the phone book. In an emergency, dial 911 (911 in all of North America and 112 in the European Union).

Anger, like all emotions, is the energy behind the behavior. It's difficult, if not impossible, to act without some emotional input, be it anger or calmness. In the case of anger, the emotion serves as the "fuel" to carry out aggressive acts. Even if you are angry, you don't have to be aggressive. Learning to manage your anger helps you avoid aggressive acts. You begin by accepting responsibility for your aggression and anger.

How You Make Yourself Angry

You don't lose your temper, you throw it away.

— RUDOLF DREIKURS

From previous chapters in this book, you've learned that no other person or event causes you to feel anything — your emotions are based on your purposes and beliefs. When it comes to anger, your purpose can be to control, win (as in an argument), get even, or protect your rights or someone else's (McKay & Maybell, 2004).

No one likes to be controlled — do you? When you try to control another person, that person is likely to resist your efforts, give in, and blame you when things go wrong, or get even with you. You can turn around your desire to control instead of trying to control others — you can control your anger. Or you can focus on controlling the situation by setting limits.

Those who believe they have to win create losers, and it's often themselves when the first loser gets even. Instead, you can work for the win-win — seeking cooperation.

If your anger is generated to help you seek revenge — another form of aggression — consider this Irish saying: "If you want to get revenge, dig two graves: one for your enemy and one for yourself." Instead, concentrate on your "opponent" — what's she or he feeling that would lead to the actions that you find hurtful? The person must be hurting too, or she or he wouldn't be behaving this way toward you. When you consider this, your desire for getting even may turn into compassion.

Anger can be useful in protecting rights, but it can also turn into a fight. Consider other ways you can protect your rights or others'. Be firm, but calm and state your limits: what you'll accept and what you will not.

Now, what about your beliefs — what thoughts do you have when you're angry? Angry thoughts are often DUMB thoughts.

Demanding. You believe this situation or person should or must be different or do what you say or shouldn't have done what she or he did.

Underestimating. You give yourself an excuse for being angry because you just "can't" stand what happened.

Maximizing. You truly believe this event is the most awful thing in the world.

Blaming. You cast blame on the person or situation (or yourself if you're mad at you).

Do these thoughts help you? Do they solve the problem? If you acted on the thoughts and expressed your anger, did things get better or worse? If we act when we're angry, things often get worse — creating more anger, stress, and guilt. In other words: "You got mad, are you glad?" If you are and somehow won the battle, watch out! It's the loser's turn to get mad!

Sometimes we don't act aggressively on our anger but are passively aggressive. We keep quiet about it and smolder. Does this help? No. Carrying around a bag of irritation can get heavy. And, often, we punish with our silence. "Something wrong, honey?" "No, I'm just fine!"

So, how do you get REAL?

Revaluate. "Okay, I'll admit I really want this to be different, but what logical reason says it should?"

Eliminate your excuses. "I really don't like this, but I *can* stand it, I'm *not* helpless."

Accept disappointments. "This is very frustrating, but it's not awful — nobody's dying."

Let go of blame. "Yeah, he's being a prick about this, but he's not a total one. He's got his good points."

Now, if you tell yourself these things you'll be annoyed and frustrated, but you won't be full-blown angry. And once you have yourself in control, your chances of solving the problem increase. You can approach it more rationally. (See below for ideas on how to communicate your feelings and seek resolution.)

Vincent's mother, an elderly widow, had fallen in her apartment and ended up in the hospital. She had a subdural hematoma (bleeding beneath the skull). The doctors said she could no longer live by herself; she needed to be in an assisted-living facility. Vincent had a demanding job, making it very challenging for him alone to spend the time locating a home and moving his mother. He called his younger sister Tanya, who lived on the other side of town, and asked for her help. Tanya complained that she had too much to do already and that Vincent would have to take care of it. Vincent got very angry and accused Tanya of being selfish and lazy. Tanya hung up on him.

Vincent smoldered, telling himself that his sister never helped out and had expected Vincent to do everything since they were kids. This was just one more example. He saw Tanya, who was five years his junior, as the "little princess" of the family, seated on her throne, expecting everyone else to serve her. How could he have expected her to help? Vincent admonished himself: "How stupid of me!"

Although one can understand why Vincent would be so angry, what good did it do? Did it gain Tanya's cooperation? Obviously not — it just strained the relationship further.

First Aid: Stop, Think, and Act

To reduce your anger, you need to get in touch with what you're telling yourself and discover the purpose of your anger. This takes time and practice. It helps to journal your thoughts, look for your purpose, and rethink the incident so that you're prepared for similar incidents in the future.

But what do you do in the heat of the moment? When you feel your hackles rise, how can you interrupt your anger and calm yourself down so you can approach the situation productively? There's a technique called *Stop, Think*, and *Act* (Barrish and Barrish, 1989; Horton, 1996). In my book *Calming the Family Storm* (McKay & Maybell, 2004), I tell readers how to use this technique:

> In this approach, you first Stop — preventing the escalation of angry feelings by avoiding your first impulse, telling yourself to stop, inserting calm phrases or using imagery, counting to ten, taking a time-out — whatever it takes to calm yourself. Then you Think about what is going on for you and what an appropriate action might be. Finally, Act on that thought — replace reaction with action.

Telling yourself to stop, repeating to yourself soothing phrases like "calm down," conjuring peaceful visualizations of a lake or a mountain, and counting to ten are all done in your head, of course. If you find it necessary to take a physical time-out, tell the person that you are too upset to talk now and that you'd like to take some time and discuss it later when you've calmed down. In your time-out, you can think about what's going on and how you can approach the problem differently.

While in their time-out, some folks find a mantra or a prayer for patience and guidance helps them take charge of their feelings. Some find humor — laughing at themselves — helpful. "Lord, grant me patience, and I want it right now!"

What Lies Beneath Your Anger?

Annoyance, frustration, fear, disappointment, fatigue, stress, pressure, hurt, embarrassment, rejection, guilt, feeling cheated or threatened — a host of feelings — can lead to anger. So, besides anger, what else are you feeling in this incident? Consider whether you'd be more effective at getting the problem solved if you concentrated on the accompanying feelings rather than your anger?

Your significant other agrees to go out for dinner, then comes home from work, complains he's too tired to go out, and says he's just going to fix himself a bowl of soup and go to bed early. You're angry — you were really counting on getting out, but what else are you feeling? Are you disappointed? Hurt? Feeling cheated?

Suppose you concentrated on those feelings and told yourself something like this: "This is disappointing, but it hardly qualifies as awful. I don't like this, but I can take it. I'll resist what I really want to do — get even. I've had a tough day too, and I really wish we'd go out. But from his point of view, there's no reason he should suck it up and go — even though I really want to. I'll talk it over with him later and see if we can come to an agreement about future plans that's satisfactory to both of us."

Sometimes it helps to talk with the other party about the situation that invited your anger; sometimes it's best to let it go. How do you decide? The basic question is, do you think it'll do any good to talk it over — is there a possibility of gaining understanding and cooperation? If so, the following suggestions will help.

Say What You Mean, Mean What You Say

Approach the other person during a peaceful time with nonaggressive, yet assertive statements and manner. When you're assertive, your intent is to gain your rights while also respecting the rights of the other person. When you're aggressive, you're unconcerned with the other's rights. Being assertive involves gaining the person's cooperation. Begin by saying something like: "I'd like to talk with you about what happened . . . , is this a good time?" If it is, proceed. If not, set up a mutually convenient appointment.

Use "I-messages" to communicate your feelings (Gordon, 2000). An I-message is a statement in which you take responsibility for your feelings instead of blaming the other person. Most people send "you-messages" when there's a problem (Gordon, 2000). You-messages attack and blame the other person and create resentment with little possibility of cooperation. I-messages tell the person how his or her behavior is affecting you. A simple "formula" will help (McKay & Dinkmeyer, 2002).

Tell the person the behavior you find objectionable: "*When . . .*"
Then state how you feel: "*I feel . . .*"
Then state the consequences the person's behavior has for you: "*Because . . .*"

Let's apply this formula to the examples above. Suppose, at a later time, Vincent decided to express his feelings to Tanya regarding her refusal to help with their mother. He'd be better off identifying the feelings that accompanied his anger than expressing anger. Besides, he already did that, and she knows he's angry. Perhaps he also felt let down and frustrated. He could express one of those feelings: "When I heard you were too busy to help me with Mom, I felt let down because I have so much to do too and I really need some help." No guarantee that his sister will pitch in, but it's worth a try to gain her cooperation. It at least doesn't worsen their relationship, and perhaps Tanya will reconsider or have some suggestions on how to obtain help.

What about the situation where your partner broke the going out to dinner date? You might say: "When I learned you were too tired to go out to dinner, I felt angry (or disappointed) because I was really looking forward to it — I could use a break."

As you can sense here, it's usually best to leave the word "you" out of the sentence even though the person knows you're talking about him or her. Why? Because sometimes the "you" seems like an accusation even if it isn't. Let's see some more examples of how you could rephrase these two conversations without saying "you."

"When I need some help and it's not available, I feel really frustrated because I'm at a loss as to what to do."

"When we have dinner plans and don't follow through, I feel disappointed because I really enjoy it when we go out together."

When you decide to express either your anger or the feelings that accompany your anger, you'll have to decide the best way to form your I-message and which feelings to express based on your knowledge of the receiver. You don't have to follow the formula. There are other ways to express your feelings in an I-message. For example, you might want to begin your message with "I feel" rather than "when."

"I'm feeling let down because I really need some help on this; I can't do it by myself."

"I really wanted to go out to dinner; it's been so hectic lately, and I could've used the break. I'm dealing with it, but I'm really disappointed."

When you state your feelings, be prepared to listen. The person will probably have something to say. The following section gives you ideas on listening.

Be Prepared to Listen

In any conversation, the first one to draw a breath is declared the listener.

— MARK TWAIN

A skill that's very helpful for hearing another's feelings is "reflective listening." This involves reflecting what you hear and see regarding the person's feelings as well as stating the circumstances related to the feeling. A simple formula is "You feel . . . because . . ."

EXAMPLES:

"You feel angry because your boss embarrassed you in front of your coworkers."
"You feel sad because your best friend is moving."
"You feel excited because of all the prospects of the new job."

As with I-messages, you don't have to follow a formula. Other ways to phrase a reflective listening response are "I'm sensing that you're feeling . . ."; "It seems to me you feel . . ."; "Sounds like you feel . . ."; "Could it be you feel . . . ?" The important thing is to catch the feeling and reflect it in your own words. Don't just parrot or repeat what the person said; she or he won't feel understood.

When you make the effort to listen to others' feelings, they are more willing to listen to yours. Reflective listening is especially important when you send an I-message about your feelings. Let's look at the example of Vincent and Tanya. Vincent went to visit his sister at her house.

Vincent: When I learned you were too busy to help me with Mom, I felt let down because I have so much to do too, and I really need some help.
Tanya: I'm sorry you felt that way, but I don't see what I can do.
Vincent: I appreciate that you are overwhelmed with your job and the kids and all.
Tanya: Yeah, well I'm glad you see that.

Vincent's effort to let his sister know how he felt and to listen to her feelings has a chance of improving the relationship and gaining some cooperation. In the next section we discuss "exploring alternatives," a way to negotiate.

What about when your partner breaks the dinner date? How can reflective listening help here?

You: When we have dinner plans and don't follow through, I feel angry (or disappointed) because I really enjoy it when we go out together.
Partner: I'm sorry, Honey, it was just that it was such a bad day.
You: Sounds like you are really down about it.
Partner: Yeah, but I'll get over it.
You: You're feeling confident that you can handle it.
Partner: Yeah, well you know me, always rise to the challenge.

If your partner wanted to talk about the bad day, you could continue to reflect your partner's feelings. Then bring up your concern again about the broken date and how to handle this kind of situation in the future.

Exploring Alternatives

Once you have sorted out your feelings, you may want to negotiate. Exploring alternatives helps. When you explore alternatives, follow these steps (McKay & Maybell, 2004):

1. Connect and clarify. Using I-messages and reflective listening, you make sure the problem is clear to both of you.
2. Brainstorm solutions. Each of you gives ideas. Agree to withhold judgment of the ideas until you've both finished making suggestions. Rejecting ideas immediately shuts down creativity and discourages problem solving. However, sometimes an acceptable idea just "jumps up" and you both agree.
3. Evaluate solutions. If several ideas come up and you're both through giving suggestions, evaluate each one. Some things you or the other person will find acceptable, others not.
4. Choose and use a solution. Once you've evaluated each idea, pick one that you can agree on and make a commitment to use the solution. If appropriate, agree to experiment with the solution for a certain period of time and then evaluate. Commit to actually doing the suggestion, not just trying it. As I said in chapter 2, trying and doing aren't the same. Trying is like buying insurance for failure.

Let's look at how Vincent could use exploring alternatives with Tanya. After stating his feelings and listening to hers, as illustrated above, Vincent could say...

Vincent: Because we've both got so much on our plates, would you be willing to look at the list of tasks and see if there's anything you think you'd have time to do?

Tanya: Well, I don't know what I can do, but sure, what's on the list?

(Vincent showed Tanya the list.)

Tanya: I think I can call these different assisted-living places and see what they have to offer and how much they cost.

Oh, and you left one thing off — helping her unpack and get things arranged in her room. I could probably do that too.

Vincent: That would be great! As things progress, if you manage to free up some time, do you think you might be able to help with some of the other tasks?

Tanya: Maybe. We'll see. Why don't you email me the list?

Vincent: Okay, will do. Thanks so much, Sis, for your help.

With improvement in their relationship, Tanya may decide to do more down the road. But what if Tanya decided not to do anything, complaining she just didn't have the time? The ball is in Vincent's court on this one. It's his problem; he can't force his sister to help out. So what could Vincent do? Obviously getting angry with his sister doesn't work, nor does anything else he did. He may just have to "bite the bullet" and do what he can. Life's like that sometimes.

Concerning the issue with your partner and the broken dinner date, following the discussion of feelings — connecting and clarifying, you could initiate a discussion on what to do in the future.

You: Could we talk about what to do in the future when we have plans and something like this happens?

Partner: Sure, what do you have in mind?

You: I thought we could brainstorm some ideas. What do you think we should do?

Partner: Well, maybe we could reschedule?

You: I have an idea too. Maybe you could call me from the office so that I don't have to get all dressed?

Partner: Sounds like an idea.

You: Any other ideas?

Partner: Well, maybe we could plan to go on Saturday nights, no work that day, so no problem.

You: Okay, I'll put that on the list. Any more ideas?

Partner: No, that's all I can think of.

As you discussed the list, suppose you rejected the Saturday night idea because the restaurants are so crowded and you'd like a more quiet time. That leaves two ideas. Suppose you and your partner decided to combine these ideas: your partner would call you if it was a bad day and he wasn't up to going out. Then, when he got home, you'd both look at your calendars and pick another date.

Now, what happens if you don't reach agreement? In this case, you can table the issue to give each of you more time to think. Or, if it looks like it's just not going to work out, do whatever you have to do to take care of yourself, keeping in mind that things will get worse if you ignore or violate the other person's rights in favor of your own. Look for ways to maintain mutual respect and still take care of yourself.

Okay, you've got some ideas on how to "mind" your anger and communicate: how to be assertive rather than aggressive. Next, Erik will discuss the spiritual aspects of aggression and anger.

Spiritual Aggression?

Erik Mansager

I think when there's enough will and aggression, there's no shortage of talent either.

— JURGEN KLINSMANN

To understand anger and aggression from a spiritual perspective, we'll have to take a broad perspective. Anger is one of a very few "root emotions" that all humans share. To consider the full range of emotions is an endless task. It seems as if we're able to experience an infinite variety of feelings: alarm, annoyance, apprehension, delight, dread, ecstasy, elation, fright, fury, grief, happiness, irritation, mourning, panic, pleasure, rage, regret, sadness, and terror.

This is hardly an exhaustive list! Think about the feelings that you experience on a clear, sunny day in winter or the feelings generated by a quick, cooling rain shower in summer. What about the feelings you have when your child sounds out a difficult word for the first time? Or what you feel when you hear a racist or sexist remark? The range of our emotions is incredibly varied.

The few emotions I mentioned above are arranged alphabetically; but there are other ways of arranging them. Here's another: by most accounts there are four emotions all of us humans share, and so we can consider them universal emotions. Some even say that we can find the whole spectrum of emotions among these or in combinations of them. They are anger, sorrow, joy, and fear. An easy way to remember is to use the rhyming scheme: Mad, Sad, Glad, and Egad! Again, each of these emotions has a wide range of variations.

Of the quick list I provided, for example,

- mad (anger) incorporates annoyance and irritation as well as rage and fury;
- sad (sorrow) includes sadness and regret as well as mourning and grief;
- glad (joy) includes delight, pleasure, and happiness as well as elation and ecstasy;
- egad! (fear) includes apprehension, alarm, and fright, all the way to dread, panic, and outright terror.

There are many other ways of conceptualizing them, too. In grouping the broad range into the four universal or root emotions above, I placed them from relatively low key to very strong in each category.

Still another way to arrange them is in the typical response that each emotion generates. As we've discussed in prior chapters, the action that follows emotion doesn't happen for no reason. Our evolution as human beings has equipped us with such emotions for good reason. For example, we learn early in our education about the "fight/flight responses." These are the typical responses generated by the root emotions of anger and fear. When angered we're ready to fight; when scared we're ready to run. The two other root emotions can be seen in this evolutionary schema as well and are called the "face/freeze responses." When we're joyful, we tend to be open to experiences and willingly face the world around us to join its activities more fully. When some loss saddens us, we tend to slow down — sometimes even "freeze." That is, we stop to reconsider what our world is like in light of the saddening situation.

So this is the larger context in which anger and aggression belong. Anger, like all of our emotions, has a reason for being part of our makeup as humans. If we're readied for a fight when we get angry, it's also the case that we get angry in order to fight. This is what Dreikurs meant in Gary's earlier quote: "You don't lose your temper, you throw it away." And this is the aspect that brings us to considering spirituality. Is there a spiritual use for anger? Does anger have an aspect that impacts our Big Picture view of things? Does it add meaning to our lives? Given all the physical and mental downsides of anger, is there any possibility of applying it for good?

The answer to these questions depends on the "quality" of the fight over which we have gotten angry. Whom is the anger directed against, and for what purpose? The rest of this section will explore these "fighting with" issues as well as the "fighting for" or "fighting about" issues.

Fighting with Whom? Fighting for What?

When you clench your fist, no one can put anything in your hand.

— ALEX HALEY

Anger, itself, comes in many shapes and sizes. It's most often thought of as being directed at another person; but, it can also be self-directed or aimed at a negative situation.

As we learned from Gary, anger arises from believing something cherished — whether our life or a value — is being threatened. Imagine the case of Sam:

Sam, just out of high school, literally believes that his eternal life depends on adhering to a strict set of beliefs and behaviors. When he arrived on the college scene and took his first psychology and philosophy courses, Sam found that not only did his professors not share his theistic beliefs, but also many of his classmates downright disdained his seemingly prudish, no-partying behavior. Sam understandably felt angry about the situation. He felt he had to fight to defend his beliefs in class, and he felt threatened and aggressive toward his classmates as they continued to harass him about his attitude toward their party life.

This is an example of anger aimed at fighting with others. In such a case, Sam felt threatened by those who didn't agree with him and used the energy of anger to defend his cherished opinion.

Now, imagine how such a situation might also lead a person to fight inwardly, as in the case of Jessica.

Jessica arrived at college and faced similar first-time academic challenges to think critically. She, however, felt very different from Sam. Rather than feel her beliefs were threatened, Jessica felt ill prepared. That is, she wanted to understand, but found herself unable to reason through all the new challenging thoughts of her coursework. Perhaps her girlfriends and mentors saw things differently. Their easy ability to respond and their freedom from her seemingly prudish hang-ups angered Jessica in a different way. She thought to herself: "How could I have gone along with such narrow-minded thinking? I was naïve and gullible to accept it all. I need to get on board with the others."

This is an example of fighting with one's self. Here, Jessica felt threatened — even embarrassed by her lack of preparation and used the consequent anger to do all she could to fit in with those she found different and compelling from what she experienced growing up.

And there is yet another type of anger-based outcome. This is aggression acted out against a negative situation. Of course, it occurs with people of all ages, but the cases of two more young adults, James and Amy, serve to illustrate this third alternative.

James went to college on an athletic scholarship and found from the time of his "initiation" to the freshman team all the way through to the victory celebrations after their considerable wins that sexual exploitation of the women students was the norm. Being the middle child between an older and younger sister he found his teammates' behavior and attitude literally revolting.

Similarly, Amy entrenched herself in her college classes and was introduced to a number of feminist scholars. She initially felt quite ill equipped to grasp problems and had difficulty accepting the radical solutions she heard being espoused. She thought: "If I am to survive here, my old understandings just won't protect me!" So she directed her anger toward the poor preparation for college she experienced in her high school education.

Both James and Amy could have felt angry and directed it toward others or focused it inward and personally. However, instead of defending their positions or behavior, they assertively set out to broaden their outlook over a range of issues, authors, and settings, and used the energy of anger to prepare themselves with richer "survival" skills than they had developed previously. James' protests resulted in an inquiry into the sexually exploitive aspects of the team's activities, and Amy became the chair of a campus political party that supported expanding women's roles at the school. They directly and effectively impacted their Big Picture and found greater meaning in their lives by utilizing their anger effectively.

Just as anger is only one of a range of emotions that we have available to move us into action, so, too, are the experiences of these young adults only a couple of the thousands of ways that threats to our values or very selves lead us into action. We can feel angry about our inner relationship with ourselves, our interpersonal relations with others, or our transactional relations in the world. I shared briefly how some people responded to these movements. More specifically now, I'll share what we can do about angry emotions from the spiritual perspective.

When Is Anger Right On?

If there is no struggle, there is no progress.

— FREDERICK DOUGLASS

Anger is a frequent theme in the Judeo-Christian scriptures. In spite of common expectation, it isn't accurate to characterize the Hebrew Bible as portraying a primarily angry God and the Christian Testament as portraying a primarily merciful God. There are examples of a tenderhearted God in even the most relentless of the prophetic books. For example, Isaiah reminded his people "with enduring love your redeemer takes you back" (Isaiah 54:7). And he insisted that God would not forget the Israelites any more than a mother could forget her child. Indeed, it's as if Zion were carved on the palm of God's hand (Isaiah 49:15).

Just as tenderness is found in the prophets, anger is found in the Gospels. The most popular example of Jesus' anger is his "cleansing of the temple." This was well known enough to be recorded in all four accounts of Jesus' ministry (Mathew 21, Mark 11, Luke 19, and John 2). A less popular, but just as important account of Jesus' anger is his indictment of the religious leaders of his day. In charge after charge, Jesus criticizes the leaders for laying "impossible burdens" on the people without lifting a finger to lighten them (Luke 11). Whereas the Temple cleansing incident seems to lament the misappropriation of sacred space for nonspiritual purposes, the critique of authority is an attack on the so-called leaders' efforts to limit spiritual growth.

Whatever else the stories mean within the different Christian doctrines, in cleansing the Temple and in criticizing the Jewish leaders, Jesus, as every good Jew would, insisted on being aware of something beyond the material. He railed against the self-satisfied security found in rituals and called for experiencing a trust that transcended place (Temple) and time (seasonal rituals) and emphasized openness to trust as more important than one's personal security.

Jesus' right to be angry, his "righteous anger," represents well the effectiveness of anger with a positive purpose. He was quite willing to fight for the betterment of others, to fight against those who would oppress others, to fight for the greater good. His anger wasn't an anger that sought to get even by means of revenge. As a practicing Jew, he left vengeance to God (Leviticus). Rather he seemed bent on a real justice acted on in the here and now. He certainly isn't the only spiritual person who stood for justice, but coming from the prophetic tradition, he serves as a prototype of such a person. Other traditions address anger differently.

When Can We Leave Anger Behind?

If you are patient in one moment of anger, you will escape a hundred days of sorrow.

— CHINESE PROVERB

We find a contemporary presentation of another ancient practice in the practices of Tibetan monk Chögyam Trungpa (2004). He promotes the practice of tonglen. This is the meditative practice of conscious breathing, with a twist. Rather than the frequent practice of being aware of each act of inhaling and exhaling, practitioners of tonglen specifically focus on negative encounters with life. He adapts the Buddhist belief that the consequences of disharmony in the world are diminished by an individual's acceptance of them — rather than vengefully retaliating. Specifically, the tonglen practitioner breathes inward deeply while aware of and accepting the negative aspects of a situation. Then, as if one's body-mind-spirit acts as a cleansing agent, the person breathes outward only thoughts of loving kindness.

Chögyam especially commends this practice for matters of anger that run to the extent of rage. He advises sitting quietly and then intentionally bringing forward the very thought about which you're angry or the image of the person at whom you're angry. Breathe, he advises. Breathe in deeply as you think of the pain and the hurt and the anger and the rage. Let the feelings well up. Be with them. Breathe.

Next, exhale deeply as you disengage the thought or person from the anger; and yet maintain the full feeling of outrage. Let go of the person or thought along with your breath, he writes. And exhale.

Inhale again and feel the disengaged anger. Know its dimensions by the pace of your racing heart or the forced shallowness of breathing. Inhale feeling the freed, yet intense anger. Breathe.

Now exhale in loving kindness, knowing you can still feel angry upon the in-breath. Inhale. Exhale in compassion, free of the anger itself.

Inhale and exhale; inhale the rage, feel the purging take place, exhale kindness and compassion.

With practice we learn that we can leave anger, even to the degree of rage, behind. This is especially helpful when we have been unable to find a useful purpose for the energy of the anger we experience. It need not damage us, as it surely will if we continue to generate the thoughts by which we so agitate ourselves. Discerning between the right to be angry and the time for it to be left behind is itself a practice that brings us to awareness.

So that's a way to work through anger to awareness. Next Wayne will discuss the physical aspects of anger.

Aggression, Anger, and the Body

Wayne F. Peate

What's the matter, you dissentious rogues? That, rubbing the poor itch of your opinion, makes yourselves scabs?

— WILLIAM SHAKESPEARE, CORIOLANUS

Bill slammed the chart on Sally's desk with such force that her coffee spilled. "You blew it. Get it right or get out," he growled as he stormed out of the clinic on the way to his hospital rounds. Leave she did, the fourth medical records clerk to resign from Dr. Bill's practice in as many months.

William "Bill" Hardwood had always been hotheaded. In grade school his temper had earned him his share of black eyes and bad grades, until a teacher-coach directed his aggression into sports, a course that earned him a college scholarship. At college, Bill thought he had discovered both a label and an excuse for his tempestuous behavior. "I'm a Type A Personality," he would offer as an excuse when he blew his top at classmates and dates.

A Type A Personality is a way of describing a person who is competitive, goal oriented and often stressed when the world doesn't conform to his or her time lines. Bill used to say he suffered from a "tyranny of unmet deadlines." *Dead*line seemed appropriate, because he later endured a debilitating heart attack that almost killed him while rushing to work. What's the most common day of the week and time of day to experience an adverse cardiac event? Monday morning. The psychological stress of heading to work after the weekend appears to harm the heart.

Bill was half right about Type As. There are two Type As according to a recent study in *Circulation* (Kawachi et al., 1998). Men who explode in anger damage not only their relationships with others, but their health. Hostile men who speak in anger have a 30 percent higher risk of an irregular heart rhythm that leads to stroke than do nonhostile men, and a 20 percent greater risk of death from all causes. Interestingly, angry women are the stronger sex in this regard. They are less likely to suffer the ill effects of hostility to others.

From a body-mind-spirit standpoint, it's evident that your state of mind affects your heart. Although you may have heard that it's better to act out your anger, to "let it all hang out" or to "blow off steam" this study's evaluation of 1,769 men and 1,913 women suggests we need other strategies.

In the example of Bill, what could he have done instead of exploding? He could have used the Stop, Think, and Act technique Gary mentioned above — counting to ten, using imagery, whatever it took to calm himself down. He could have taken four breaths and put things in perspective. A year from now, how much will it matter what someone just said or did (McKay & Dinkmeyer, 2002)? If he felt expressing his feelings would help, he could use an I-message as Gary talked about above. He might have said to the clerk: "When all the parts of the physical are not organized for me to review, I get frustrated because it takes me longer to find everything I need; and this just keeps the patient waiting." This has less chance of putting the clerk on defensive and may encourage her to improve her performance in the future. He could also, in considering the Bigger Picture, breathe tonglen as Erik suggested — with the result of establishing a sense of loving kindness in the practice.

Medical Mystery Solved?

Up to half of heart attacks occur in individuals who exhibit no risk factors whatsoever. It's been a mystery why until now. Research at Duke Medical School has shown that C-reactive protein (CRP), a marker of heart inflammation that's associated with stroke and cardiac disease, increases with anger, hostility, and depression symptoms in those who are otherwise in good health. CRP has been detected in the plaque that blocks heart arteries. The study at Duke was the first to uncover a connection between the mind and elevated CRP in those without risk factors for heart attack (Suarez, September 2004).

High CRP is typically found in people with known cardiovascular risk factors such as smoking, obesity, diabetes, hypertension, high cholesterol, and an inactive lifestyle. But many without any risk factors have an unaccountably high CRP. The Duke study shows that anger and hostile behavior, as well as symptoms of depression, may account for why those persons who lack risk factors have higher amounts of CRP and a greater risk of heart conditions and stroke.

For many years, scientists have known that those with mild to moderate depression have an elevated risk of death from a heart condition. Now the study's lead investigator, Dr. Suarez, and his colleagues have also demonstrated that those prone to anger, hostility, and depression respond to stress with an increased output of norepinephrine.

A spike in this stress hormone puts the immune system into overdrive and activates inflammation. Inflammation is correlated with a bump in CRP. Increases in CRP have been shown in fever, infection, and trauma; but higher levels (such as those in this investigation) are associated with cardiovascular disease. The following diagram outlines the process.

CRP Elevation Process

Mind: Experiences anger, hostility, aggression, depression

↓

Body: Adrenal glands respond by releasing

↓

Norepinephrine, a stress hormone
Stress hormones foster production of high levels of CRP

↓

CRP is found in artery plaques (plugs in blood vessels), and is associated with inflammation

↓

Heart attack/stroke occurs

Psychologically, those inclined to burst out in anger are also likely to suffer low-grade depression. "The world doesn't work the way I want it to, damn it" kind of attitude leads to feeling down — and a heart condition. Suarez, in earlier work, found that hostile individuals with depression had elevated interleukin 6. Like CRP, this is a marker of inflammation that's a predictor of heart problems in those who are currently healthy. Although this study found that a tendency toward anger was sufficient to effect CRP levels adversely, one didn't have to have an overt clinically evident psychological diagnosis to have higher CRP.

The above-mentioned studies provide further evidence for the powerful influence of the mind-body interaction. If emotions in healthy individuals lead to heart attacks, imagine the impact of feelings on those with risk factors like high cholesterol. Obtaining a psychological evaluation or getting help with anger management may be just as important as a blood pressure check for predicting and addressing future cardiac disease.

Roads to Rage

In Viktor Frankl's seminal book *Man's Search for Meaning* (2000), he describes three challenges of modern living: depression, addiction, and aggression. Drive our streets and you confront the latter. Road rage, discourteous driving, and tailgating are daily events. The emergency rooms and cemeteries are filled with the sad consequences of that aggressiveness. So are our headlines. Bombings, assassinations, and terrorism are parts of our daily vocabulary. Sadly, many practitioners of aggression such as terrorism misuse spiritual language as a justification for their attacks. Every religion has its "black sheep" who hijack the peaceful words of their prophets for their own evil purposes. Christians have the Ku Klux Klan, Jews the Jewish Defense League (referring to the plot to blow up the mosque in Los Angeles), and Muslims suffer bin Laden.

The physical effects of aggression are often more subtle than the headlines. While serving in a refugee camp in Somalia amid a daily onslaught of civil warfare, I observed the less obvious signs and symptoms of the struggle to survive in an aggressive environment among my co-workers. Those in less dramatic circumstances can also experience any of the following.

Numbness. When dozens are dying all around you, you can become indifferent to death and inattentive to the schedule of daily activities. You miss meals, your sleep is irregular, your relationships become shallow. (You may be dead tomorrow; what's the point of a relationship?) The move to counter this numbness is to avoid isolation. No matter where you work, plan on a regular time of reflection and sharing with a friend, relative, or colleague. Doing this helps you restore balance and a sense of meaning and purpose even in a disorderly and aggression-filled world.

Flashbacks. The child you could have saved may haunt you. The mistake you made at work may have cost you that promotion. The anchors of the past that can't be changed can prevent you from succeeding in the future. Learn to learn from the past, but don't be tortured by it. The spiritual approach of "Let go and let god" helps. Let go of the past, and let your god guide your path to a better tomorrow. Many believe we are all god's children, and like any youngster we make mistakes and then can learn to do better. In Aramaic (the language of Jesus) sin means "misfire." When an archer shoots, there are many misfires — shots that don't hit the bull's-eye. So it is with some people's sense of sinfulness — with effort we will get closer to god's purpose for us.

Loss of effectiveness. A week's vacation for refugee camp workers was mandatory every three months. At first I thought this rule was frivolous, after all people were dying all around me. What was the point of a holiday? After a month I had changed my tune and was counting the days until the break. Everyone needs a Sabbath, a time for regeneration. So important is this concept that it's the Fourth Commandment in the Judeo-Christian spiritual world. The Sabbath is more than a time of loafing. It's a time of connection with the creation, a "re-creation," a time to recognize the bounty all around us. Friends, family, fellowship, sunsets . . . you choose what gives you joy. Within that joy is the catalyst of regeneration that will help you overcome the difficulties of the workweek.

Aggression, Competition, and Cooperation

What is the origin of human aggression, and how does our understanding of our history improve our present? Erik mentioned the "fight/flight" and "face/freeze" experiences that describe human reaction to threats. Anger triggers the fight/flight reaction. Fear, excitement, and anxiety also elicit this reaction. When you feel threatened, your body feels a sudden rush of adrenaline and your mind becomes intensely focused. The adrenal glands barrage the body with stress hormones. The brain diverts blood from other organs to the muscles to prep them for attack or escape. You might notice the hair stand up on the back of your neck and a tingling in your extremities. Vital signs like breathing rate, blood pressure, and body temperature rise. Dry things turn wet (armpit) and wet things turn dry (mouth). The mind is under alert.

Our predecessors used to show their teeth as a warning to strangers to beware. The human smile is thought to be a friendly version of this teeth baring — the corners of the mouth are turned up to show lack of intended aggression. Early humans were once thought to have survived in a win-lose world. If your tribe improved your lot by taking my water hole or grazing area, I lost. "Winners" who conquered others' territory were obviously resented by "losers." Your gain becomes my loss. This cycle was thought to be the root of today's aggression. But current anthropology (Sawyer et al., 2007), less male dominated than in the past, suggests a different outlook — one that says cooperation is at least as old as competition. It seems our prehistoric ancestral tribes learned cooperation to get enough food for all and to ward off dangers common to all.

All this led to the possibilities we have today of living in a win-win world. If I do better economically, I have more cash to dispose of to buy from my neighbor. If he's doing well, he can reciprocate. Your gain is now my gain. "I've got mine, to heck with you" is no more viable in a modern economy than it was as our ancestors faced common death threats. One of the reasons Europe has had over sixty years of peace, the longest in the history of that blood-soaked continent, is the Common Market or European Union. It makes little sense to bomb the hell out of your neighbor when you're economically interdependent. An exception has been the persistent conflicts in the Balkans, an area not in the European Union.

There are exceptions. After 9/11, a colleague of mine countered the win-win position I'm talking about with: "Why did the Saudis fly planes into our buildings if we are such good customers?" My response was that oil in Saudi Arabia isn't owned by a profit-making company within a democracy. The Saud family owns the oil and lives precariously between fundamentalist clergy who condemn the "Western" excesses of this royal family and a growing populist movement that wants to remove the monarchy. Hitler demonized the Jews so that the German public would turn a blind eye to the barbaric Nazis all around them. In the same way, the royal Saudi families allow extremists to demonize "The West" so that the Saudi public will ignore the need for their government to reform.

There is a profound spiritual component to aggression. Few human institutions are as aggressive as the enslavement of others. John Newton, a slave-ship operator, had an epiphany during a vicious storm while crossing the Atlantic with a hold full of slaves. He wrote the song "Amazing Grace" and became a pastor and an advocate for the abolition of slavery. He inspired William Wilberforce, one of his parishioners, to become the "conscience of Parliament" and inspire the elimination of slavery in the British Empire. Unfortunately, today 27 million people, mostly women and children, are still enslaved in the sex trade worldwide or as contract laborers without hope of release (Salt of the Earth).

The Mind-Body-Spirit Connection

You might ask: "What do mind, body, and spirit have to do with economics, international politics, and child slavery?" The answer? A great deal. Experts now have a new understanding of aggression, and its solution has much to do with our three themes.

Mind. If we create a new awareness of the benefits of the win-win approach, we curb aggression. Go it alone, independent, "I got mine, to heck with you" attitudes are destructive. Fortunately, people don't attack friends or customers, usually. That's why the benefits of international exchanges and fellowships are so powerful at creating friendships. Examples include the People-to-People, Rotary, Fulbright, and Marshall programs.

Body. As explained above, anger increases heart rate and blood pressure. So does physical exertion. The difference is that a person running can stop and heart function rapidly returns to normal. In the angry individual the recovery may be delayed. In addition, physically active people who maintain a regular exercise program develop healthy heart muscle that's "trained" to handle stressors on the body. People who work out infrequently feel the pain in their muscles the next day. Similarly, angry people don't have the protection of a conditioned heart, so they are more likely to experience pain, even a heart attack or stroke.

Spirit. Religious groups too often practice a "theology of contempt" according to Bishop Gerald Kicanas, Diocese of Tucson. Christian leaders routinely proclaim their superiority over Jews during weekly worship sermons by emphasizing Jewish "legalism." Most Christians are surprised to learn the contrary is true. For example, if asked, they would say that the origin of the saying "Love your neighbor as yourself" is Jesus. Jesus' source was actually Leviticus 19:18 of the Hebrew Scriptures. The Golden Rule is also found in each of the world religions! (See the recommended websites in the appendix.) The spiritual solution is this: My faith works for me. The faith of others works for them. This is what Erik called the virtue of steadfastness in chapter 3. If I'm comfortable with my faith experience why do I need to knock down that of others? If I say I love god, shouldn't I also say I love god's creation — humankind?

People tend to avoid a person who angers easily, so this person often gets to have his or her way. At the same time, if people avoid you because of your quick temper, it's difficult to form supportive, healthy relationships. This leads to isolation and feelings of low self-esteem. If you find that you anger easily or feel angry all of the time, here are some other things you can do:

- Avoid situations that may trigger your anger.
- Focus on the things in your life that help you feel happy.
- Take care of yourself emotionally and physically.
- Exercise regularly.
- Eat a balanced diet. Don't skip meals.
- Try to get eight hours of sleep each night.

- Limit your use of alcohol, use medications only as prescribed, and don't use illegal drugs.
- Join a support group. Check with your employee assistance program or your local health department to find out what services are available in your area.

In this chapter we've addressed aggression and anger and their effects. We've shown how one can change behavior, purpose, thoughts, and emotions and work toward cooperation rather than creating distance and resistance. Assertive behavior through I-messages and negotiation when appropriate replaces aggression. Many religious scriptures speak of anger. The Bible speaks about when anger is justified — used for a positive purpose such as Jesus' anger in "cleansing the temple." Aggressive and angry behavior has effects on the body as well, such as contributing to heart disease. Learning to control one's anger reduces strain on the heart.

As you'll discover in chapter 6, anger is often associated with depression. You'll also discover how to take charge of depression.

Vitamins for Aggression and Anger

- Aggression is everywhere and takes many forms, ranging from verbal threats to physical acts to religious claims. Aggression works to elevate the aggressive person, to put him or her "on top." Fortunately, cooperation is also everywhere.

- If you're the aggressor, consider the consequences for yourself in your relationships. If you or your children are the target of aggression, protect yourself and your kids. If necessary, call your local abuse hotline or 911.

- Anger, like all emotions, is the energy behind aggressive behavior; but even if you're angry, you don't have to be aggressive.

- From a physical standpoint, angry people put their health at risk.

- You can turn around your desire to control and instead control your anger; or focus on controlling the situation by setting limits. Work for the win-win. If your anger leads you to seek revenge, counteract this by concentrating on turning your desire to get even into compassion.

- Angry thoughts are often DUMB thoughts. You can change your DUMB thoughts to REAL. In the heat of the moment, you can take charge of your anger by using the Stop, Think, and Act technique. The breathing technique tonglen also helps.

- A host of feelings lead to anger. Sometimes it's more effective to express the feelings that accompany anger rather than the anger itself. You can express your anger or the feelings accompanying the anger with I-messages. When you state your feelings, be prepared to use reflective listening. Once feelings are sorted out, you may want to negotiate.

- From a spiritual perspective, anger can be "right on" when it's used to fight for the betterment of others — it depends on whom the anger is directed against and for what purpose.

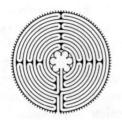

CHAPTER 6

IN THE MOOD:
DEPRESSION

Depression is nourished by a lifetime of ungrieved and unforgiven hurts.

— PENELOPE SWEET

Sara woke abruptly in her dorm room in bone-chilling terror with a knife at her throat. The evil intentions of the masked man hovering over her were clear: her choice was rape or murder.

In the mind-numbing days after, Sara fell into a deep depression. Had she forgotten to lock the door or done something else to compromise her safety? Could she ever trust men again? Would she ever feel safe again? Sara lost her appetite, energy, and motivation to do her schoolwork. Sleep was impossible; the smallest sound startled her. Her mind was tearing her body apart. Equally troubling was her fear of having been abandoned by God . . . how could He allow this to happen?

Free counseling was available from a sexual assault survivors' center, but Sara couldn't bring herself to relive that unendurable night by talking about it. Fortunately, a counselor there wouldn't give up on trying to connect, and one evening got Sara to stay on the phone. Sara poured out self-condemnation.

The counselor responded: "You are not to blame for what that man did to you."

Sara countered: "But nothing can change what happened; and because it did happen, I can't face tomorrow."

The counselor said: "Here are some words from Mother Theresa that might help, 'Yesterday is gone. Tomorrow has not yet come. We have only today. Let us begin.'" After hearing those words, Sara realized that by blaming herself she was allowing her assailant to keep brutalizing her and that her focus on the terrible past was destroying her. She admired how Mother Theresa had put her faith into action, and she had always hoped to do the same.

Sara realized she had to banish hopelessness from her mind. She taped Mother Theresa's quotation on her bathroom mirror along with this one of her own: "No one can take my hope away from me," and read them daily. Sara went on, eventually, to excel in school, become a warm and caring psychotherapist, marry a good man, and raise two healthy children.

Depression is ever present in our society. If untreated, it can lead to physical effects: fatigue, isolation, and even suicide. Many cases of depression are due to alterations in brain chemistry that alcohol and other mood-altering drugs can exacerbate. Depression can be controlled with proper help, especially with a holistic approach involving spiritual, psychological, and medical procedures. Depression and despair can also be transformed into hope by the practice of regular prayer and meditation, joining with others in worship, partnering service, and other spiritual disciplines. Physical problems often accompany depression, ranging from eating and sleep problems to physical pain. Sometimes medication is needed to alleviate symptoms. Psychological aspects involve how one can depress oneself; the purposes of depression; the thought process involved in depression; and how to think oneself out of it.

Because depression involves a loss of faith in god, yourself, life itself, or all of the above, we begin our discussion with the Big Picture — the spiritual aspects of depression. Erik discusses ways to spiritually rise out of depression.

On Dark Nights and Black Holes

Erik Mansager

One dark night . . . I went out unseen . . . with no other light or guide than the one that burned in my heart.

— John of the Cross

It's tough enough to understand depression when it invades our work-a-day worlds; in the context of our spiritual lives, depression-like moods — sometimes called "Dark Night" experiences — take on expressions that are even harder to grasp and put in context. These spiritual expressions are so marked that we wanted to discuss them first so that if you recognize them, you can explore the spiritual aspect of the feelings along with what is more commonly known about depression. After I describe depression broadly, I discuss some of the experiences that bring it about on the spiritual level, then I tease out the real, measurable differences between depression and Dark Night experiences, and finally I suggest a way of moving away from depression by means of the spiritual vitamins mentioned in chapter 3.

On Experiencing Darkness

The term "Dark Night of the Soul" has returned to common spiritual usage thanks to the attention that spiritually oriented psychotherapists have been paying to it, especially the late Gerald G. May. In his best-selling book *The Dark Night of the Soul* (2004), May harkens back to the sixteenth-century mystic John of the Cross's original treatise of the same title. May focuses on exploring connections between spiritual growth and a sense of loss.

We've all experienced loss: the passing of a loved one, the loss of a job, the ending of an important relationship, or perhaps the estrangement of dear friends over incidents that aren't altogether clear to us. With the loss comes a sense of grieving — loneliness without clear direction as to how to go on. After some time passes, however, by some ways understandable and some mysterious, we're able to function again in a manner helpful to ourselves and others.

Sometimes, but not always.

Sometimes, it doesn't work out the way we think it should.

Sometimes, we get stuck in the feeling of loss and it feels impossible to move on. We find our appetite changes and so our weight balloons (or drops surprisingly). Sometimes the loss disturbs our sleep as we try to figure things out, keeping ourselves up when we should be sleeping (or we sleep the day away because nothing much seems to matter since the loss).

Also when we can't get beyond our loss, commonly our thinking gets all messed up. Maybe it's from conjuring up all sorts of dire consequences that follow from no longer being in our familiar space. Or it might be from not being able to think of anything without the loss coming to mind. Whatever the reason, we tend to feel quite muddled in the midst of it all.

Then, as the muddle drones on and on (and on), we tend to get annoyed with the whole situation and people experience us as irritable and testy. Little do they know that inside we're quite likely feeling guilty about not doing something (*anything!*) about the loss. After the fact, all the things we thought-about-doing-but-didn't-do before the loss to improve the situation (or to improve our relationship with the lost one) come screaming back into our conscious and seem like *exactly* the magical thing that would have prevented the loss in the first place. So there we are beating ourselves up about what we didn't-do-but-should-have-done and feeling pretty worthless.

Sure, we've all felt one or more of these feelings at various times in our lives. But when they all (or most of them) show up at once, it's the picture of classic depression. Wayne and Gary tell you about some of the physical causes, purposes, and beliefs that may be at the root of nonspiritual depression. Here it's important to see this grouping of symptoms from the eyes of the person consciously seeking her or his spiritual path.

There is no doubt that there are physical and psychological benefits to developing a healthy spirituality; but it would be pretty inaccurate to think that spirituality protects you in *all* instances from feelings of loss and despair. The idea that "spirituality does *not* relieve one of suffering" seems backward to some, especially for some believers in god. Shouldn't the person who believes in an all-powerful and all-loving Being and who acts in accord with these beliefs be exempt from the ravages of depression? This is precisely the puzzle that Gerald May, and John of the Cross before him, sought to understand.

Are there differences between the depressive experiences of the spiritually oriented person and those of the person who isn't seeking deeper meaning? Yes . . . and No. At least on the symptomatic level, there is very little difference: whether depressed or in spiritual crisis, we experience changes in our appetite, our sleep patterns, our level of activity, and the organization of our thoughts. But that's not the end of it. Any spiritually oriented psychotherapist will tell you that although these symptoms are similar — even identical — there is a remarkable difference between experiencing them as a person who's working on a spiritually related issue and experiencing them as one who's not. That is, how we interact when we're depressed compared to when we're experiencing a Dark Night is as different as, well, night and day.

Before getting into the different ways you interact with others, I'd like to be more specific about the types of incidents that bring about the feelings of spiritual loss and then lead to a Dark Night rather than depression. After spelling these out, I return to the issue of distinguishing the difference between what you experience within a spiritually oriented Dark Night and what you experience within the more common appearance of depression.

Spiritually oriented people have the same kinds of emotional issues that others do — of course. When they run into the "limit setters" or "barrier experiences" such as the death of a loved one, as I discussed in chapter 3, spiritually oriented people are likely to take a Big Picture view of the matter and try to make sense of it that way. Still, you surely suffer when your sense of coherence and faith in the continuity of life is shaken (Sperry, 2001). And, if you're prone to seek outside reasons for mishaps, when you experience turmoil and upheaval in your spiritual life, you're more likely to blame the issue on something really important to you — god or higher power or the like. Any number of personal issues can result in "spiritual crises" or develop into full-blown "spiritual emergencies."

Spiritual Crises and Emergencies

Spiritual crises and spiritual emergencies are related to be sure, but we can tell the difference between them. The spiritual crisis that occurs is very likely to arise from crises that we all face — the loss of a friend or relationship, an identity issue, or the like. It's our spiritual orientation operating during a "nonspiritual" crisis that casts a spiritual light on the matter and makes it a spiritual crisis. This is different from a spiritual emergency that arises specifically out of our spiritual practices. Let me say a bit more about each.

Spiritual crises. Relationship and family crises can come up in your life unexpectedly, just as physical illnesses and psychological disturbances can. Identity issues can be root-shaking revelations. Some identity issues are more fundamental to your self-understanding than others. To some of us, our religious identity is our most basic identity. A man or woman coming to understand and accept his or her sexual orientation surely experiences this revelation at a soul-forming level. Now imagine if he or she also identifies with a religious denomination that assesses this sexual orientation negatively. A spiritual crisis would compound the identity crisis.

Losing your faith for whatever reason or being disillusioned with your religious/spiritual or church community can also lead to a deep and painful crisis. The disillusionment may arise from different sources. To be sure, the ongoing inhumane tragedy of child abuse by the clergy tops the list of atrocities bringing about spiritual crises nowadays — not solely among those abused but regularly even among those who simply hear of the issue (Sipe, 1995).

Another thing that could bring you into a spiritual crisis is a change of denominational identity. Similarly, you may experience a spiritual crisis if you should experience your beliefs shifting while still within a given religion. Many Catholics experienced this crisis in the 1960s as the Second Vatican Council brought about an understanding of Catholic identity different from what had been experienced within that generation. Similarly, crises persist among Catholics, as well as among mainline Protestant denominations, as their church leadership — after a period of relative openness — returns to a more conservative faith expression.

And here I'd like to say a word to spiritual leaders such as imams, ministers, priests, and rabbis who are reading this. There are still other spiritual crises you might experience because of "religious burnout." The relentless nature of religious life, whether speaking of direct ministry or participation in the life of your spiritual community, can leave you depleted of self-esteem. This is especially the case if you feel ineffective in accomplishing the goals you've established for yourself. For example, many church organization personnel are called on to work with victims of natural disaster when the federal government is unprepared to provide assistance. When working with the traumatized, the less effective you find yourself, the less you'll be able to recognize when you actually *are* effective; and so your sense of personal effectiveness — so important for everyone's self-esteem — can spiral down and out of control into full crisis.

Spiritual emergencies. If spiritual *crises* develop during "normal" crises in the context of your spiritual path, spiritual *emergencies* result directly from your spiritual expressions. For example, should your process of spiritual growth and change become chaotic and overwhelming (Grof & Grof, 1989), this constitutes a spiritual emergency. As you'd guess, these emergencies are as varied in personal expression as are the persons who follow spiritual paths. Generally, however, they can be characterized as the extreme highs and lows that you experience when you are newly practicing your beliefs.

Peak experiences of whatever description (such as the emotional high from having a baby, completing a graduate degree, or completing a rigorous fast or meditation regimen) are profoundly disorienting. Although usually positive, peak experiences can leave you feeling disconnected from others who haven't had such experiences. They can also leave you longing for the brief but intense intimacy that the experience provided. It's the same with near-death experiences, which, though related to measurable physiological changes (Kung, 1982/1984), are experienced as if your body is somehow disconnected from your mental processes. Numerous "life after life" experiences have been reported since R. A. Moody (1975) first began tracking them in the 1970s and are recounted as variously inspiring, upsetting, and, at times, disorienting.

On a more dramatic note, "possession" states and past-life experiences are among the experiences that lead to spiritual emergencies. It's primarily, but not solely, conservative Christian believers who relate experiencing possession by evil spirits, whereas it's mostly members of Hindu-related spiritual paths (or New Age related expressions) who address concerns about past-life experiences. All these experiences are related to the scriptural traditions of the religion in question.

Waiting/Wading through the Darkness

It's clear, then, that a wide range of experiences leads to depression. When you experience depression-like symptoms related to loss amid your search for deep meaning, the experience is what May calls the Dark Night of the Soul. And, although there may be little or no difference in the presentation of the physical symptoms, the place and psychological space that engendered those feelings are vastly different. Different, too, is the experience of those you love and interact with.

Gaping black holes. When people are depressed, interactions even with their long-standing friends or acquaintances can test the friends' patience and push them to the absolute limits. It often seems that no matter the amount of caring we expend toward our depressed acquaintances, their depression persists. Week after week, month after month with little or no gains to be shown, we experience a frustration with depressed persons — along with a good measure of annoyance. Even with great patience, our sense of "bother" with these friends rises. If not checked, this rises to irritation and eventual exasperation with them. Adlerians and the more cognitive of the helping professionals recognize this as the purpose behind the depression: because the depressed are experiencing a certain level of anger or even desire for revenge, they use depression to "get even" with anyone and everyone for perceived injustices that they suffer amid their depression.

At the same time, we might detect in our depressed friends a self-focused insistence that *we* get busy at banishing *their* suffering — "Right now!" When they're suffering from depression, this is the most recognizable aspect of how we experience them: they expect *others* to do something about it. Now and again, we all express and experience pleas for help; but when people feel severely depressed, their level of expectation for others to do *their* work is very high. This contributes to the experience of frustration one feels with depressed people.

A third aspect of peoples' experience of depression is the detection of cynicism or resentment. It's my opinion that it's this characteristic of depression's manifestation — a feeling of bitterness — that catapults many depressed individuals into the medication dependence that so often occurs. This is usually the case when a physician prescribes medicine without suggesting some accompanying therapy. In the midst of their depression, their loved ones may experience the depressed as desperately self-absorbed, as constantly pleading for help. Yet the depressed persons believe that no one can really help them — not even themselves. Because they feel unable to rely on themselves and depleted of any shred of self-respect, the cynicism they feel and we sense in them is wholly understandable.

We summarize the way people are experienced when depressed this way:

Loved ones' experience of you when you're depressed. Loved ones eventually feel annoyed and frustrated. They feel excluded due to your inner focus and persistent pleas for help. Loved ones experience you as cynical and bitter.

But don't despair. Wayne and Gary have much to say about how to treat even the most enveloping cases of depression. Here I want to contrast a typical clinical presentation of major depression with what friends and acquaintances typically experience from those experiencing a Dark Night of the Soul.

Passing dark nights. When our friends are depressed, we tend to experience a growing frustration with them. However, when friends are experiencing a Dark Night, we are surprisingly *un*troubled by their demeanor. We may even describe our encounter with them as if their experience of consolation positively impacts us (May, 2004). It's as if they are aware of a larger perspective from which they can view and accept, even if not wholly understand, their sufferings. Up close it looks to us that their experience indeed hurts, but in the Big Picture, which they're quick to point out, they derive great comfort. There is a sense of "we're in this together" that they tend to promote, grateful that they don't have to be alone, yet aware that it's no one's job to resolve the suffering but their own — and often in such settings, their god's.

With such an attitude, we sense a contrast with the persistent self-focused pleas for help of the chronically depressed person. When experiencing a Dark Night, people tend to show unexpected compassion for others and a wholesale acceptance of their situation. There's likely to be more talk of how they have learned to cope by watching the example of, or reading about, others who have coped with similar or worse situations. There is seldom a hint of self-blame although I've heard such clients speak of their "lot" in life. One quite spiritual friend of mine shared, for example, as we discussed her cancer diagnosis: "I hate this, but all I can see is the challenge all the women in my family have faced: the prospect of eventual breast cancer and to live fully in spite of it." My friend didn't take the diagnosis lightly. Although she initially balked at the regimen of chemotherapy and radiation, she ultimately reconciled herself to it and its effects. She became an exemplary patient in the hospital, doing what she could to support others in her situation.

She beat the cancer, and most striking to me was the sense of humor she hung onto through it all. Besides accepting psychologist Bernie Siegel's admonition to "laugh yourself healthy" by a daily dose of belly laughs, her upbeat attitude and ability to see humor in the often painful situations she found herself in sustained her as well as those of us who love her.

My friend exemplified the contrast between Dark Night experiences and depression.

Loved ones' experience of you when you're experiencing a dark night. Loved ones frequently feel a sense of consolation when spending time with you. They experience your sense of humor. They experience your compassion for others and your acceptance of the situation.

In chapter 3, I discussed vitamins for the spirit: AWARE. In grappling with depressive symptoms, it's possible to become AWARE of the difference between depression and a Dark Night and chose to experience something like a Dark Night as one sure path out of depression.

Daily Vitamins for Nightly Darkness

The essential vitamin in this case is A1, the apply vitamin. The way to loosen depression's self-focused noose is that of other-focusing. Here's how it works:

A   First, pop a vitamin A: ask about the purpose and benefit of the depressed feeling or of remaining in a self-focused state.

W   Then take some vitamin W: wait, patiently and calmly, both for an answer to arise as well as for clearer questions to emerge.

A1   In the meantime, supplement with vitamin A1: apply yourself to the well-being of others. Adler said his standard remedy for depression was to help people produce lists of how they could help others — an exercise to supplant the usual self-focused rumination that occurs with depression. His experience was that within two weeks of his clients actually doing the list, their depression would noticeably lift.

R   That's when you grab some vitamin R: reflect on where you were, how you felt, and how you feel now as you engage with others. Consider how you are taken care of within this other-focus.

E   Now you're ready to go out and soak up vitamin E, the real experience of life, being part of the greater solution.

Now that you know how to distinguish between depression and Dark Nights, Wayne will share some of the physiological aspects of depression.

Depression — Medical Condition or Opportunity?

Wayne F. Peate

> *When you don't take the world as given, but as full of possibilities, it becomes endlessly exciting.*
>
> — ELLEN LANGER

Treating depression is a significant part of modern medical practice. One in ten people consult a doctor for symptoms they believe are related to a physical condition that are really due to depression. A nonpsychological illness can also lead to depression, especially if it's severe or chronic. In this section, I explore two questions and their answers. First: "Is there a biological basis for depression?" Yes. Second: "Does the human species need the depressed and their coping skills to survive the great trials of our species?" Yes! Let's explore this duality called depression.

It was nineteen degrees Fahrenheit (minus seven centigrade) this morning and the gas at my house, along with 450 other homes, had been out all night and day. A well-bundled DeAnna from the local Fox affiliate was at the door with Jacob the television camera operator. "You seem to be taking this well. Aren't you angry?" she asked.

"It could be worse. Some people are living in a cardboard box," I said, taking it in stride.

"What are you going to do about it? You won't be able to take a shower. It's too cold."

"I guess we'll just be smelly."

"You people are just too nice," she said, nonplussed at my make-the-best-of-it attitude. She persisted with my eleven-year-old daughter: "How would you feel if you had to take a shower in cold water?"

"I wouldn't like to, but if I had to I would just grin and bear it."

On the nine o'clock news all you heard was the "smelly" and "I wouldn't like it" parts, not the "it could be worse" or "grin and bear it."

"If it bleeds it leads," they say in journalism. The sensational, the extreme, and the angry are sought out at the expense of the positive. Don't believe me? How often have you heard the television anchor say: "Today's leading good news story..."? Certainly DeAnna had experienced plenty of others who took a darker view of negative events than my family. Certainly her editor exhibited those traits in his or her choice of what to show the public. So it is with psychology and medicine: both fields focus on the depressed and the diseased, not the buoyant and the well.

Recent research points to some intriguing findings about the origin of positive influences in the brain. Scientists now know that certain emotions are biologically based. People are surprised to learn we are hard wired for happiness through the opoid (or opium) receptors in our bodies.

Likewise, depression is closely related to brain function chemistry. Many people with depression are unable to fully experience emotions; their life, like old soda, is flat.

Think of the brain as a computer with electrical signals that send information. Our "brainwaves" travel on neurons that act like electric wires. In between the neurons are gaps known as synapses. Neuro-transmitters are enzymes that help messages cross the synapse. Without them our brain ceases to function. To push on the computer analogy, our "head" hard drive crashes and we hope our purchase warranty includes a service contract!

There are six neurotransmitters and each is specific to a different type of brain cell. People with depression have low levels of two neurotransmitters, noradrenaline (also called norepinephrine) and serotonin (another name is 5HT or 5 hydroxytryptamine). Decreased levels of these two neurotransmitters contribute to the "blue" or low mood of depression and related symptoms of decreases in sleep, energy, appetite, and interest in activities of daily life.

So is depression simply caused by low chemical levels? Is the condition similar to anemia, caused by a lack of iron, or diabetes, caused by insufficient insulin utilization? Like most health conditions, it's more complicated. Many factors lead to low neurotransmitter levels and depression, including emotional events such as a loss, certain drugs, and communicable diseases, like AIDS, that lead to brain infections, neurologic disorders, cancer, nutritional deficits such as vitamin B6 and vitamin B12 deficiencies, stress, and anxiety. For further details about these biological grounds of depression see the table below.

Depression is more common in women, partly due to hormonal event fluctuations postpregnancy and during menstrual cycles. It's also more common in certain families. However there is no clear genetic component, rather a predisposition that may have a significant *environmental* basis. Children raised in a home where love is conditional — for example, based on academic or athletic performance — may suffer depression if their achievements don't equal expected results.

The following table (next page) outlines various roots of depression. Extended discussion of each contribution is beyond the scope of this chapter. If you believe you're experiencing depression, be certain to consult a professional.

How Do Antidepression Drugs Work?
After a neurotransmitter crosses a synapse, it's reabsorbed for reuse, which is called reuptake. Several antidepressant drugs block the reuptake of serotonin (known as selective serotonin reuptake inhibitors or SSRIs, for example, Prozac, Paxil, and Zoloft), noradrenalin (Vestra), or both serotonin and noradrenalin (Elavil). All antidepressants have a time delay before effects are felt; it takes one to four weeks before you

Things That Cause or Contribute to Depression		
Hormone Disorders	**Conditions of the Brain**	**Side Effects of Drugs**
Addison's disease	Brain tumors	Amphetamine withdrawal
Cushing's syndrome	Concussion and other	Alcohol
Parathyroid hormone	head trauma	Antipsychotic drugs
elevation	Cerebrovascular	Beta-blockers
Pituitary hormones	accidents (stroke)	Cancer drugs (Vinblastine,
deficits	Dementia	Vincristine)
Premenstrual	Epilepsy, temporal lobe	Cimetidine
syndrome	Multiple sclerosis (MS)	Cycloserine
Post-pregnancy	Parkinson's disease	Estrogen replacement
Thyroid hormone	Sleep apnea	therapy
deficit or		Methyldopa
elevation		Narcotic withdrawal
Connective tissue		Oral contraceptives
conditions		Reserpine
Rheumatoid arthritis		Steroid use, prolonged
Lupus		Thallium

experience the effects. This is why the risk of suicide in some patients will not be reduced for some time and why they will require other therapy. This finding is the torment of drug companies, which struggle to show the benefits of their products, and a demonstration of the power of the mind-body-spirit connection.

But depression is more than chemistry. Its treatment is a complex interplay of biology, neurotransmitters, psychology, and spirituality. How so?

Jackie suffered the loss of her mother after a prolonged illness. A member of the clergy told her she had been in a grieving process for the past two years. Jackie had been so involved in her mother's daily needs that she didn't realize the impact of her mother's condition on her personal and professional life. Her work performance declined as did her relationships with family and friends. After the funeral she was filled with grief, an emotion that was exacerbated by her growing recognition of how much her life had deteriorated because of her mother's illness and death.

Her depression spiraled out of control as thoughts of ending it all consumed her. (Up to one in eight with severe untreated depression commits suicide.) To make matters worse, she was placed on probation at work and her oldest daughter walked out in anger at a family gathering. Antidepressants along with cognitive behavioral therapy (an approach similar to the methods Gary talks about) and suicide precautions were initiated by her caregivers.

Not all antidepressants work in everyone, and some are better for those with associated sleep problems. Side effects such as weight gain can occur, a disturbing problem for many especially because of the prolonged period of use for these medications.

How Is Depression Diagnosed?

First seek professional help. In the Internet age, some self-diagnose by completing online standardized questionnaires that measure depression, such as the EAP Depression Survey — http://www.novanthealth.org/eap/surveys/depression_test.htm. A medical examination and laboratory tests may uncover a physical disorder, but most cases of depression are psychological in origin, and there is no test for serotonin level in the synapses. The health provider will look for underlying physical causes, as outlined in the table: Things That Cause or Contribute to Depression.

When no physical cause is found, depression is managed by medication and therapy, either alone or in combination. We believe it's best to involve therapy when antidepressants are prescribed so that the person will learn how to manage his or her depression and eventually not need the medication. Also, Erik and Gary give ways for self-management of depression.

Mind as a Healer

> A poor man was so famished that he resorted to eating leaves to ease his hunger. Some leaves were so dirty that he cast them on the ground uneaten. "No one can be as unfortunate as I," he thought as a wave of depression engulfed him. Suddenly, he heard a rustling on the ground behind him. He turned and saw a crippled man crawling on the ground hungrily chewing the leaves he had just discarded.
>
> — SPANISH PARABLE

Can you will yourself into a positive outlook? Does optimism, an "antidepressant" found by looking in the mirror, improve with practice? The power of positive thinking, self-help books, reading a good novel, religious or spiritual practice, and a circle of friends or supporters have lifted many out of depression. A friend of mine whose mood was down spent a summer reading the works of Jane Austen, and her energy and interest in life recovered. The effect was so profound that when she seemed low, her husband would tape her library card to a dozen roses. Losing herself in her delight with Austen's biting social commentary, wit, and wisdom was the mental balm she needed.

Her experience led me to a logical question. How did people cope with depression in the premedication and counseling era? It's been said that before there were psychiatrists there were clergy. But even in times of higher levels of religious participation, many were indifferent or were nonbelievers. How is it that some famous depressed personalities like Winston Churchill and Abraham Lincoln were able to overcome their melancholy without medication or cognitive behavioral therapy? Both were the greatest political leaders of their respective centuries, yet each was so depressed at times, they could hardly get out of bed. Was it because of positive psychology or what some call resiliency?

Black dog days. Churchill described his frequent depressive episodes as his "black dog" (Jenkins, 2002). I love the analogy. The family hound is familiar and ever present and its peculiarities and remedies are understood by the observant owner. Unloved and neglected by his parents as a child, Churchill developed a resiliency that overcame his black dog days. And he had plenty. He was blamed for one of the worst military disasters in World War I at Gallipoli. His escape from an Afrikaner prison during the Boer War, which made him the toast of England and a viable candidate for Parliament, was due to his depression.

He was so melancholic from his imprisonment that he made a desperate and foolhardy leap through an unguarded window. He was free but without food, shelter, or hope for rescue. Fortunately, he knocked on the door of the only townsman who was British, a man who hid him in an ore train headed out of Boer lands. That prison window was the metaphor for Churchill's life. When he was down and depressed, he pulled up his courage, nurtured a vision, fought the tide, and believed in an escape — most famously from the annihilation of his country by the Nazi war machine.

Each victory under Churchill's watch became "our finest hour." Who else but Churchill could be seen picking his way through the rubble of the Blitz, which killed 10,000 in London during the first month of German bombing (and 48,000 civilians in the UK during the entire war) with his fingers held aloft in a "V" for victory sign? How absurd! How Churchill!

His black dog, his depression, was always present, and because it was so, he had honed a lifetime of skills to overcome it. Those skills translated into lifting the spirits of a nearly defeated Britain standing alone against the terrors of fascism. Churchill learned how to believe in the impossible and how to convince others that democracies — including the neutral (in the early years of the war) United States, which lent material that kept his island nation afloat — would defeat the monstrosity of Hitler. If Britain had fallen, a vital launching pad for the liberation of Europe would have been lost while Hitler completed the annihilation of non-Aryan races and the development of nuclear weapons.

The great depressed emancipator. If Churchill had a black dog, Abraham Lincoln had a life draped in black crepe. His life was a long list of deaths — his mother, a sweetheart, three sons, and friends — accented by repeated failures. His depression descended into near suicide on more than one occasion. "I am now the most miserable man living...," the thirty-one-year-old Lincoln confessed. "Whether I shall ever be better I cannot tell; I awfully forebode I shall not. To remain as I am is impossible; I must die or be better..." (Abraham Lincoln Research Site). Depression is often associated with such physical symptoms as sleep troubles, and Lincoln noted that his nighttime rest was troubled to the point of being "light and capricious."

How is it that an untreated depressed politico from the backwoods rescued America from dissolution and its greatest crisis? Like Churchill, Lincoln coped best when he found a cause that pushed him outside of his depression and into the light of a greater need. What's more, Lincoln had become so adept at overcoming his depression and its emotional extremes that he was the most successful antiextremist in the history of American politics. Without Lincoln's centrist approach, his government would never have unified against the storms of dissent. Lincoln took the unheard of and much criticized course of creating a cabinet that included his political rivals, including three powerful antagonists. In so doing, he converted his enemies into nationally focused allies! His stirring words that appealed for peace and cooperation to "the better angels of our nature" were not idle poetry. Lincoln's nature ached with the bitterness of depression, but he believed in angels of his own making and of Americans' making under his guidance that could heal a nation that had descended into war against itself.

Is Finding Your Mission the Best Antidepressant?

Again, how is it that two men with recurrent depression each saved their respective countries a century before modern medicine and its popular adoption? And this *without* psychotherapy? Although Freud and Adler and other psychologists were contemporaries of Churchill, their methods were not widely used in Britain in his time.

Churchill and Lincoln had long years of experience with depression. Like the Biblical story of Jacob wrestling and overcoming his angel, they had their depression in a headlock and had learned how to make it behave. Both were consummate humorists who could tickle a laugh out of the darkest hours. Each was able to subsume his depression into a greater cause than his self-interest. Both were much maligned in their time and endured it because of their vision, and both are admired by the ages. They would have agreed with Albert Schweitzer, the theologian, musicologist, and mission doctor who observed: "The only ones among you who will be really happy are those who have sought and found how to serve."

My admiration of Lincoln and Churchill stems from the dissection of how depression managed may well have saved humanity. We social animals who walk upright — whether ape or human — need many biological group tricks to endure the jungle. For example, there may be a biological reason that some of us are early risers, others late. Because predators prowl 24/7, if everyone were alert in the morning, more would be eaten at nighttime; and if we were all wide awake late at night, many would be easy prey in the daylight.

In a similar way, depression can be seen as but one tool in a collection that aids our survival as a group. A medicated Lincoln or Churchill would have been more effective in the ordinary duties of their daily lives, but they might have been unavailable, unskilled at rescuing us when all seemed lost because they had never learned to overcome the dark. If medicated, they might have lacked the intuition and clearheadedness to propel us into the light against slavery and fascism when others had succumbed. Their vision might have been numbed, and we all might have suffered more because of their lack of creativity.

I began this section with an observation that the health professions have focused on the deficit, the disease, rather than on the resiliency and the positive attributes that allow us to overcome the near fatal condition we know as depression. Who knows? Perhaps the condition is essential, so that a certain few will inspire us all with the resiliency of the human spirit.

Next, Gary discusses how we talk ourselves into depression and how we can talk ourselves out of it.

Head-Tripping into Depression

Gary D. McKay

We must accept finite disappointment, but we must never lose infinite hope.

— MARTIN LUTHER KING

Whether you're experiencing a "Dark Night" or a "black dog," the material in this section will help you "lift" yourself out of depression or help a loved one or friend who's depressed.

When he encounters a client who he suspects is depressed, a friend of mine in Columbia, Missouri, psychologist Dr. James Straub, asks the client: "How do you go about depressing yourself?" After getting over the shock of James's question, the client will ask him what he means. James then explains to the client how we think ourselves into depression.

It's the Thought that Counts

"I can't stand it"; "It will never change"; "I can't go on"; "This is so awful"; "I'm worthless"; "It should be different — but it won't be" — and on and on with negative, self-deprecating, hopeless thoughts plunging us into depression. Although life is tough at times, it doesn't mean it's impossible, even though it may seem that way. You may be down, but you don't have to be out. Consider the story of Caitlin.

Twenty-eight-year-old Caitlin felt she was in a dead end job. She'd joined this firm right out of high school and never went to college. She served as an administrative assistant, but she wanted more and didn't think she would get it. Her mother suggested Caitlin go to college, assuring her that she would help her financially. But Caitlin was reluctant; she felt she was "too old" to be around those college kids. Also, she'd recently broken up with a long-term boyfriend, so she didn't see a future in relationships either.

She continually engaged in depressive thinking: "Life sucks. I'll never get anywhere. I'll end up alone and stuck in this worthless job." The more she told herself these things, the worse she felt. She found it nearly impossible to get up in the morning and called in sick frequently. Her boss spoke with her and expressed displeasure at her absence and her lack of performance when she was there. Of course, this just contributed to her depression.

Her best friend noticed how down Caitlin was and how many times she'd cancelled out on plans. She talked with Caitlin and convinced her to seek therapy.

The therapist helped her see that her self-deprecating thoughts and behaviors were not solving her problem. What did she want for her life? She was so depressed, she couldn't answer the question.

"What if you changed your thinking?" the therapist asked.

"What do you mean?" asked Caitlin.

"Well, you're constantly telling yourself how awful life is, how bleak your present and your future are and that you're powerless to do anything about it." He showed Caitlin how these thoughts created her depression. He then proposed that she move from what I have been calling DUMB thoughts to what I call REAL ones. He taught her how to talk to herself in a different, more encouraging way. She could tell herself something like: "Life is tough, but it doesn't altogether suck. I can still get someplace. Although it's difficult to change, I don't have to stick with this job. And I can still meet someone. There's still time; I'm not that old!"

"You have to really believe these new thoughts, not just say them," the therapist said. He suggested she keep a journal of her depressing thoughts and list ways to change her thinking. He asked her to concentrate on taking the "less" out of hopeless. "There is always HOPE," he told her — "Healthy Optimistic Possibilities Exist!"

The therapist encouraged Caitlin to focus on the positive aspects of her life, such as her relationship with her best friend, a caring mother, and her willingness to seek help and work on her depression. He also suggested that she work on her sense of humor — as down as she felt, humor along with his other suggestions would help her lift her spirits. He asked her to focus on whatever she found funny — movies, sitcoms, stand-ups on TV, cartoons, and, especially, laughing at herself. If she had difficulty finding humor that induced her laughter, he suggested she just laugh several minutes a day.

Then the therapist helped Caitlin explore the purpose of her depression. It turned out that her sadness and anger was a way to back out of a life she didn't like. The more depressed she felt, the more of an excuse she could give herself for not showing up at work or for poor performance. Dwelling on her failed relationship and avoiding her friend reinforced her misery and rationalized her work behavior.

In addition, the therapist suggested she incrementally change her behavior, including getting up earlier in the morning and making an extra effort at work. He taught her the "Act as if" technique (Mosak, 1995). That is, no matter how down she felt, she was to act as if she felt better. Combined with analyzing and changing her thinking, looking at the positive and humorous side and encouraging herself to behave differently would alter her mood. The therapist also suggested she not avoid going out with her friend; again, no matter how she felt, act as if and convince herself to go out.

Caitlin — along with the encouragement of her friend and her therapist — followed the therapist's suggestions. It took some time and lots of discussion, but she began to feel better, to have more hope. She knew she would have to get a degree if she wanted to advance in her job or seek another, more satisfying job. She still didn't want to attend a university with "college kids" younger than she; but she found some online courses she could do at night and on weekends. She continued to go out with her best friend and eventually met a guy who showed some promise.

If you're feeling depressed, follow Caitlin's example: examine your thoughts. How are you demanding, underestimating, maximizing, and blaming? How do you revaluate your demands, eliminate your excuses, accept disappointments in your life, and stop blaming yourself, someone else, or life itself? Refer to chapter 2 for a fuller explanation of DUMB and REAL thoughts. Also, the techniques reframing, deep breathing, and imaging discussed in chapter 2 help lessen depressive thoughts, along with the suggestions Caitlin's therapist made.

When you're analyzing and disputing your depressive thoughts, also ask yourself the following questions:

- Am I confusing a thought with a fact?
- Am I assuming every situation is the same?
- Am I overlooking my strengths?
- What do I want?
- How would I look at this if I weren't depressed?
- Am I asking myself questions that have no answers? E.g., how can I redo the past?
- What difference will this make in a week, a year, or ten years? (Emery, 1988; McKay & Dinkmeyer, 2002)

If You Expect the Worst, You May Get It

Expectations are powerful. When we expect something, we tend to move toward it. Expecting things like the following set you up for disappointment and lead to or increase depression (McKay & Dinkmeyer, 2002):

- When you want something, you should get it.
- If you work hard, you will succeed.
- It's unfair when people don't do as you think they should.
- People should think and act as you do.
- You must be perfect; if you aren't you're a failure.

These expectations are a real setup for failure — who's perfect? In addition, people who are depressed may be overly invested in approval. They believe others must approve of them and that they can't stand it if they don't. When you depend on others' approval to define your worth, you're giving them absolute power over you, your feelings, and your behavior (McKay & Dinkmeyer, 2002).

When you're examining your depressive thoughts, see if any of the above discouraging expectations apply to your thinking. Also, consider your "need" for approval from others and if this applies, ask how that contributes to your depression.

Purposes of Depression

As you learned in chapter 2, emotions serve a purpose; they give us the energy to behave in certain ways. As for Caitlin, sometimes our purpose is to excuse ourself and back out of a life we don't like. So giving yourself an excuse for your behavior is one purpose. Other purposes include reducing people's expectations and taking off the pressure on you to perform, excusing yourself for failure, defending yourself against criticism, and getting others to protect or take care of you, that is, you shift your responsibilities to them. Another purpose for depression is to express anger — not directly, but through a "silent temper tantrum" — and, as Erik pointed out, to get revenge.

So when you're analyzing your depressed thoughts, look for your purpose. As said before, it's often revealed in such self-talk as: "People expect too much of me." In this case your purpose is to reduce people's expectations of you and to get them to back off. Or, it may be like saying to yourself: "I just can't do this anymore." Here, your purpose is to get others to serve you.

When you're rethinking and changing to REAL thoughts, consider how your purpose can be changed as well. For example, instead of "People expect too much of me," decide what you're willing to do and what responsibilities actually belong to others. In this way you change your purpose to taking care of your responsibilities — but not to trying to save the entire world!

To Feel Better, Behave Better

As we learned from Caitlin, changing your thoughts and purposes is one thing; to complete the process, you need to change your behavior. As Erik and Wayne have mentioned, humor is a good antidepressant. So from a humorous perspective, to change your behavior — get off your Acquired Suffering Syndrome and move toward others!

As Erik pointed out, one of the ways to change your behavior and alleviate your depression is to help others. Writer Arnold Bennett said: "The best cure for worry, depression, melancholy, brooding, is to go deliberately forth and try to lift with one's sympathy the gloom of somebody else." When you focus on someone else's problems and offer to help, you have less time to concentrate on your own!

You don't have to seek out someone who has problems to focus on others. And you don't have to be a Lincoln or Churchill, saving countries. Contributions in daily life are important too. For example, you can volunteer for church activities or you can volunteer for local agencies; do whatever it is that gets you focused on others instead of retreating into depressive thoughts.

And don't forget fun; spend fun time with your family and friends. If necessary, compel yourself to do it. And while doing it, concentrate on the activity and the other people involved, rather than ruminating on your feelings.

In Addition to Feeling Blue, Are You also Seeing Red? — Depression and Anger

Depression is merely anger without enthusiasm.

— UNKNOWN

People who are depressed may also be angry. Sometimes they don't realize that they are angry. This type of anger often stems from the inability to improve your life. It could also arise from the misconception that you have to be perfect; but because you can't be, you're depressed and angry with yourself.

Examining the purposes and beliefs that create the anger help you alleviate it. Using the techniques discussed in chapter 5, you can take charge of your anger. You can decide whether it's best to express it or let it go. If you deal with your anger, you may also find your depression lessening.

Caitlin was angry as well as depressed. Her therapist helped her see that she was mad at life, at the job, at herself. He helped her talk through her anger. Once she got in touch with her anger, expressed it to her therapist, and worked on her beliefs that created the anger, the anger lessened along with her depression.

Recognizing the feelings associated with your anger also helps. Are you angry because you're disappointed, hurt, stressed, afraid, or frustrated? Feeling let down can go way beyond dissatisfaction and into despair to the extent that you believe nothing will ever change. Hurt can lead to anger and extreme sadness. With too much stress, you shut down — with the added advantage of getting others to take care of you. Fear and anxiety stop you dead in your tracks, and eventually you give up. Frustration is another action-stopping emotion: you can feel so frustrated that you believe there's nothing you can do to improve the situation.

Anger can also be used to cover up depression. This is especially true with men due to differing cultural expectations for men's versus women's emotions and behavior. Some men think that although it's okay for a woman to be depressed, it's not so okay for men. Men learn they are supposed to be tough, so *anger's* okay, but withdrawing into *depression* — that's another story. So, if you're male and angry, examine your anger to see if it's related to depression. If it is, accept that and work on your depression as well as your anger. If you're female, might your angry man also be depressed?

Avoiding Responsibility by Popping Pills

In the year 3535 . . . everything you think, do, and say is in the pill you took today.
— ZAGER AND EVANS, "IN THE YEAR 2525 (EXORDIUM AND TERMINUS)," 1969

As the line from the Zager and Evans song predicted, there's a pill for practically everything — and we haven't reached 3535 yet! I once heard what I thought was a commercial for a psychotropic medication on National Public Radio. I thought it was odd to have an ad on NPR. Turned out it was a joke, a spoof on drug ads. The pill was called "Noprobatall!" Because real drug ads always mention side effects, I imagined that this one had the side effects insomnia, loss of appetite, and loss of libido. So I thought: "You can't sleep, can't eat, and can't have sex, but you won't have any problems!"

When it comes to mental health conditions — especially depression — doctors sometimes overmedicate. When irresponsibly prescribed, such a medical regimen removes responsibility for the depression from the person. Wayne has pointed out that certain types of depression benefit from medication combined with cognitive behavioral therapy. So, I'm saying: don't overuse it! Get a second, and a third, opinion because in certain circumstances medication is not needed at all if a person changes his or her depressive thoughts and purposes.

Some people are on antidepressants for years and never receive any therapy. In a way, they are "addicted" to the drugs because if they stop, guess what, they're depressed again. There are also side effects to contend with and interactions with other drugs. Again, the basic idea of antidepressants is to use them *in combination with* therapy and eventually the drugs will become unnecessary.

Part of the problem with medication is the pressure physicians feel due to the amount of advertising by drug companies: "Depressed? Take this"; "Anxious? Take that." More and more today, people go into their doctor's office demanding meds. Many physicians (and some psychologists licensed to prescribe) yield to the pressure. Also, many insurance companies authorize medication but only approve limited therapy.

What I'm saying is, if you're feeling depressed, by all means get some help! See your doctor; and if there are no physical indicators, decide to work on your purposes and thoughts. Realize that the more you take responsibility for your depression, the better chance you have for mastering it. Use the methods we discuss in this chapter that help you take that responsibility. Just for the record, we advise therapy if you're not making progress or if you're considering suicide. If you decide to see a therapist, seek one with a similar approach to that described in this book.

Depression and Suicide

Some people are so depressed that they think suicide is their only way out. Some even try it and are lucky if it doesn't work out! One thing is for sure, if you kill yourself, you've ended your problems, but you've also created problems for others in your life. Suicide is sometimes associated with revenge — you want to get even with someone in your life you believe is "causing" your problems. If you're having suicidal thoughts, consider the possibility that you want to punish someone. But first, get yourself some help. Check the phone book for a suicide hotline. Call them immediately.

If someone close to you is depressed, watch for signs of intended suicide. Some of the signs are talking about death or suicide, withdrawal from social interactions, wanting to be alone, changes in routine, avoiding favorite activities, giving away favored possessions, reckless driving, excessive drinking, mood swings, telling people goodbye as if it's the final contact with the person, and, of course, actual suicide attempts (Dinkmeyer, McKay, McKay, & Dinkmeyer, 1998; Suicide: Understand Causes, Signs and Prevention). If you notice these signs in yourself or others, seek help. See the next section for what you can do to help a friend or loved one with depression.

What if You're on the Receiving End?

If a family member or close friend is depressed, do your best to encourage the person to get help. You may want to share the ideas in this book with the person. If she wants to talk, listen. Use the reflective listening technique discussed in chapter 5. Help the person explore alternatives, too (see chapter 5). Ask her to think about areas in her life that she enjoys, for example. Explore with her where to receive help. Don't be afraid to help, but don't try to get involved beyond your skill level. There are plenty of professionals out there to help!

Whatever you do, *don't* feel sorry for him or her, *don't* feel hurt by the behavior, and *don't* get angry. Sympathy, hurt, and anger just reinforce the person's negative feelings and behavior. Also, don't take over the person's responsibilities — unless it's something for the family that absolutely must be done and your loved one isn't doing it.

Depression, like the flu, can be "contagious." You could slip into depression because you can't help your depressed loved one. Depressing yourself won't help your loved one, or you. Do what you can to help the person, but realize that the depression is his or her responsibility.

In this chapter you've seen that depression is related to spiritual issues such as Dark Nights and to a host of medical conditions. All three of us believe that humor and positive involvement with others help alleviate depression. It's important to note the purpose of your depression and your DUMB thoughts — your beliefs about life and your situation that create your depression. Anger is often related to depression. Getting in touch with and working on your anger helps you master your depression.

In the next chapter we discuss addiction, which is often related to depression because depressed people may self-medicate in an attempt to control their depression. Chapter 7 helps you determine if you have a problem with a substance or behavior and what you can do about it. If you're not an addict but a loved one is, you'll also learn what you can do to assist him or her.

Vitamins for Depression

- In the context of our spiritual lives, depression-like moods are sometimes called "Dark Night" experiences. It's possible to become AWARE of the difference between depression and a Dark Night and choose to experience something like a Dark Night as one sure path out of depression.
- People with depression have low levels of two neurotransmitters. Decreased levels of these contribute to the low mood of depression and related symptoms of decreases in sleep, energy, appetite, and interest in activities of daily life.
- Depression involves a complex interplay of biology, neurotransmitters, psychology, and spirituality. Certain types of depression benefit from medication combined with cognitive behavioral therapy.
- If you're feeling depressed, examine your thoughts. How are you being DUMB? How can you get REAL?
- Look for the purpose of your depressed feelings. Purposes for depression include indirectly expressing anger and seeking revenge.
- In addition to changing your thoughts and purposes, change your behavior. Look for humor in your life, and focus on others rather than yourself.
- If a family member or close friend is depressed, do your best to encourage the person to get help.

CHAPTER 7

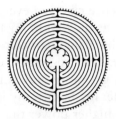

THE SUN WILL RISE TOMORROW: ADDICTION

You do anything long enough to escape the habit of living until the escape becomes the habit.

— DAVID RYAN

Instead of arriving by ambulance, the man walked through the back door of the emergency department as if he owned the place and then collapsed from a heart attack. As the staff performed the life-saving procedures, they realized their patient looked disturbingly familiar. It was Seth Sloane — a hospital staff physician. At thirty-five, he was unusually young to have a heart attack, and no one recalled him having any health problems.

His drug screen revealed all. It was positive at dangerous levels for cocaine, a frequent cause of fatal heart conditions. More startling, Seth was one of the hospital's most popular and well-respected doctors. He had won teaching awards, was always available for his patients, and was the "go-to-guy" for difficult diagnoses. How could such a skilled professional have used enough cocaine to cause a heart attack? How could a doctor who knew all the risks succumb to drugs?

Through hard work and determination, Seth had risen from a working-class family to an esteemed position as a sought-after specialist. His success, though, soon led to arrogance. After casual experimentation with cocaine, he felt confident that addiction was simply impossible for him.

His near-death experience changed everything. "All my life I have been a take-charge guy: I was the first in my family to go to college, got top grades, and earned a scholarship to medical school. Suddenly I found I wasn't in charge anymore. The drug was in charge of me. I spent every moment planning how to get more and not get caught. I nearly lost everything important to me: my family, my job, and my life."

Seth concluded that a higher power than his own self-interest was really in charge of his life. He was able to recover by drawing on his newfound and more deeply felt spirituality. A friend observed of Seth: "He found God when he found out he wasn't God."

There are many types of addictions and compulsions: gambling, sex, alcohol, illegal drugs, and misused legal drugs. You name it, we can become addicted to it. And while addictions are increasing, the average age of addicts is decreasing. The drug destroys addicts physically, and the addict's behavior destroys relationships with family, friends, and co-workers.

In this chapter we explore the purposes of addiction — what's involved in making the decision to use and how to use the power of your mind to break the habit. This includes using reframing, deep breathing, relaxation, imagery, exercise, and humor to avoid addictive and compulsive thinking and behaviors.

There are varied approaches to addiction recovery. Faith-based approaches to overcoming addiction are one way to stay clean and sober. And yet religion itself can be an addictive process that at times also needs monitoring. This chapter explores combining spiritual approaches, rational techniques (based on the work of Albert Ellis and other cognitive therapists), and addiction-avoiding behaviors to keep the addict "clean."

Body of Evidence

Wayne F. Peate

In this section I cover the physical basis of addiction and exciting discoveries that use brainpower to overcome addiction.

Addiction experts tell us there are two types of addiction: psychological and physical. For the addict, the difference is moot; they feel hooked and out of control. Many develop both forms of addiction. Narcotic addicts become psychologically addicted to the euphoria of the drug, and then they develop a physical addiction as they begin to require more and more of the substance to achieve the same effect. Sex addiction is an example of a psychological addiction. This might surprise you. As physical as sex is and as necessary as it is for physical continuation of the species, it's not a physical addiction like that experienced by alcohol, tobacco, or heroin users.

Attitude Is Fortitude

As a young medical student, I did an addiction medicine rotation at the Brattleboro Retreat in New England. While there I was impressed by Skip, one of the attending physicians who seemed to have it all: brilliance, charm, and empathy toward his patients. At last, I'd found a role model.

To my surprise, during one of the group therapy sessions Skip said: "When I was an untreated alcoholic I used to drink mouthwash in the clinic to get my alcohol fix and not get caught with the smell of whisky on my breath." (The wintergreen mouthwash smell masked the 25 percent alcohol in the product.) I almost fell out of my chair! Later in private, he revealed how medical school had been his undoing. Unable to sleep at night because of worry over his class performance, he had turned to alcohol. Soon a soothing "one drink nightcap" became an all-day addiction.

What was revealing was his conflict with the disease model of alcoholism. "I made a choice every day to drink. That's not a disease, it's a decision." Nonetheless, he did share that brain scans show alcoholics suffer permanent physical change in their brains that does not recover with sobriety. Some sustain liver damage. He continued: "Bad decisions can lead to disease. Our job is to inform the public of the dangers of alcohol addiction." Skip had considered a career in anesthesiology. He instead chose psychiatry because he feared that he would succumb to the temptation to abuse the painkillers that are so readily available to anesthesiologists.

"Propinquity breeds familiarity," he warned. "Don't risk bad decisions by placing yourself in proximity to bad options. That's why my wife doesn't keep beer in the fridge. The temptation for me to relapse is too great." Then he offered me a jelly bean. "They're gourmet. I always keep some in my office. You have to be addicted to something." We laughed.

Skip also sent me to an AA (Alcoholics Anonymous) meeting. "What did you think?" I told him that the organization might be called SSS for the "sincerity, support, and smoking" of the participants!

"They seem to have replaced alcohol with smoking [Most AA meetings now are smoke free]. Here have another jelly bean."

Skip taught me a lot about addiction and the body-mind-spirit connection. Here's what I learned from my addiction mentor.

Attitude truly is fortitude. He shared that he had family members who were alcoholics: "One of my siblings is still abusing alcohol, another never touches the stuff." Same family, different decisions. "I could say I have a disease. I say I have a decision. Do you know why God has a Chosen People? Because every day we choose His way or another way."

Temptations are tempting. Skip's attitude was that he was susceptible to substance abuse. So he chose a specialty that was less likely to lead to the temptation to misuse drugs. Did you know that half of all anesthesiologists who become addicted to narcotics die from that abuse? He shared his concerns with his wife, which led to the decision not to keep alcohol in the house. You might think: "If Skip were strong, it wouldn't matter." The way Skip looked at it was some days he wasn't so strong, so why risk the chance of a relapse by keeping temptation close at hand?

One is a lonely number. Skip got help from others when he needed help. Unfortunately, many get into difficulties and feel they have no one to turn to for support. I learned from Skip's experience that it's better to build a support group *before* I need it than after. This doesn't have to be complicated. Keeping in touch with friends, joining a congregation or club, and participating in a reading club all count. Someday when you're down and tempted with an addictive substance, you won't be left out and vulnerable, because you've already developed supporters. There's another benefit, too. The best exercise for your heart is to lift up another.

Some days we're up, and others we're down. Within a circle of support, the day we're feeling down and earthbound, there'll be those who are not and who can give us our wings again. And the day they're out of sorts, there's a good chance we aren't and can bring them out of their funk. Our physiology, our body chemistry and functions, works that way. The hormones that help us deal with stress fluctuate in our bodies every day. Plan on their swings and you won't get discouraged if you or your family and friends aren't always as strong as Hercules. Don't forget: even he got plenty of help from the gods on Olympus.

Physical Addiction Field Manual

In physical addiction, the body develops a need for the addictive substance that becomes stronger than other life requirements — even food and water. Some addicts are so hooked they'll skip meals for drugs. Methamphetamine or "meth" users often go *days* without food.

What is the physiological origin of this physical "need" of the addict? Part of the answer is that your brain is hard wired for addiction. Everyone is actually a potential addict. How so? As I mentioned in chapter 6, each of us has opoid receptors in our brains. (No, that isn't the same as the drug opium!) These receptors act like brain Velcro that latches onto any opium type pain-blocking drugs whether morphine, codeine, oxycodone, or hydrocodone.

Where do these receptors come from and why do we have them? Most are surprised to learn that the body makes its own opium-like substances. They're called endorphins, or natural pain relievers. These can be up to ten times more powerful than morphine ("Pain Management: Fighting Back." American Pain and Wellness)! Endorphins increase with exercise and other forms of physical force — such as treatments like acupuncture.

These endorphins were mighty handy for our pre-pharmacy ancestors, whose legs hurt like hell while chasing down dinner or who were trampled on by that dinner and had to crawl home with a broken leg. Interestingly, chronic pain patients have low levels of natural endorphins, an indication that their bodies may not appropriately inhibit pain. This can be a question of which came first, the chicken or the egg. Are some people in pain all the time because they don't make enough endorphins? Or has constant pain caused a depletion of their endorphins?

A related question is why does pain in one form decrease other pain? For example, an acupuncture needle pressed into the skin causes pain, so how does the procedure *diminish* pain? Even more interesting: Why does acupuncture work for addictions in some individuals? There are several intriguing answers. Acupuncturists claim the needles, if placed correctly, block a meridian, a nerve pathway, to the brain. Researchers have found, in fact, that acupuncture needles in specific body areas trigger endorphin production. Naloxone is a drug used to reverse opium drug overdoses. If it's given to a patient receiving acupuncture it also blunts the effects of the acupuncture, thus lending credence to the "increased endorphin theory" as the explanation for the benefits of acupuncture.

But the questions remain: Why is recovery from physical addiction so difficult that it often requires a multifaceted, "full court press" approach to succeed? Why do addicts relapse so frequently? The reasons are many.

First, the brain has a preprogrammed addiction tendency: all our neural receptors are hungry for opium or endorphin action. Second, genetics plays a role in addictions. In certain alcoholics, there's a "familial tendency," a genetic predisposition for alcoholism. It's not as strong genetically as eye or hair color, but it's very real nonetheless.

Third, as shown by brain scans, there is a permanent physical change in an addict's neurons that may well alter her or his ability to ever use the abuse substance again without stumbling back into addiction. Fourth, concurrent with the physical addiction are psychological triggers, such as being with friends who smoke, drink, snort, or inject.

To further understand the psychological aspects of addictions, consider the power of placebo. Studies have shown that if a doctor says a particular drug is going to have a big benefit, the patient is more likely to respond. In a fascinating study of the power of mind over matter (Koman, 2005), a researcher pumped up a blood pressure cuff on volunteers' arm until they experienced pain. The volunteers exhibited sweating, grimacing, and an increase in blood pressure. Volunteers were then told they would receive morphine and would feel no pain, though they only received saline. No pain was reported. The next time, after the cuff was pumped up, nothing was given and the volunteers again reported pain.

The "placebo effect" shows the power of the brain — through *expecting* relief, one *gets* relief. Addicts tap a similar psychological effect when they expect a drug to relieve all their ills. The body-mind-spirit connection works similarly to heal addictions. The healer helps the one seeking healing from addiction by lassoing the power of the brain to heal the body, by reinforcing innate healing abilities that have previously been untapped.

Natural Highs

Are people addicted to a substance that could be replaced with natural endorphins? If so, addicts could work to replace medicinal or recreational endorphins with their own opium-like substances. Physical activity has several advantages in this regard. It promotes endorphins, is a good stress reliever, and keeps you in good physical shape.

Endorphins are most often produced with long workouts of great intensity. You should be slightly short of breath. It's during this level of exertion that your muscles consume the glycogen stored in your liver and you start to go "aerobic" — burn oxygen at a higher rate and most effectively produce endorphins. Jogging, swimming, bicycling, aerobics, skiing, and team sports like basketball are all endorphin-production factories.

Recruit others to join in recovery. Studies have shown that if your spouse participates in tobacco cessation, you both are more likely to quit (Rennard, 2008). Group recovery approaches described later in this chapter are successful because the many support the one, with each supporting the others.

Brain Fingerprints

Functional magnetic resonance imaging shows the areas of the brain that respond to the effects of certain drugs and other stimuli. By focusing on these areas, researchers are finding new drugs that block a particular brain function or work in a specific area of the brain that is involved in addiction. Damage to the insula, for example, disrupts addiction to cigarette smoking (Naqvi et al., 2007). Someday soon, we may send people to brain labs to track the benefits of psychological or physical therapy for curbing addictions.

Effects on the Brain

In the following, I provide information about the effects of several popular drugs on the brain.

Alcohol. Just about everyone knows that excessive alcohol slurs your speech, wobbles your walking, destroys your liver, causes nerve damage, slows your reaction time, impairs your thinking, leads to traffic deaths, and promotes promiscuity (or as Shakespeare observed: it provokes the desire, but it takes away the performance). What isn't widely known is that heavy drinking over time also causes *permanent* brain damage. And there's no recovering from the loss — even if you quit abusing alcohol. The range of such mental impairments varies from short lapses in memory to complete mental debilitation. The effects can be subtle and not readily recognized; many former alcoholics become quite adept at covering up their memory shortfalls with apologies, humor, or lists (Hommer, 2003).

This research is particularly important to the body-mind-spirit connection. High tech tools such as magnetic resonance imaging and positron emission tomography are currently available to assess the extent of alcohol-caused brain damage. It's now known, with the help of these procedures, that heavy drinking leads to shrinking in the cells that transmit signals to our brain's gray matter, the structure that processes and stores memories (Rosenbloom et al., 2003; Wong et al., 2003). These studies also offer hope that future tools will be available to help former alcohol abusers recover the damaged parts of their mind function.

Tobacco. Tobacco is one of the most commonly used psychoactive drugs in the world. The nicotine in tobacco increases heart and respiratory rate, blood pressure, and metabolism. Heavy doses produce tremors. When chewed, tobacco causes gum disease, tooth erosion, and mouth and throat cancers. When smoked, tobacco causes cancers of the lung, larynx, mouth, esophagus, bladder, kidney, pancreas, and cervix.

Used long term, smoking leads to pneumonia, chronic bronchitis, and other respiratory infections, lung complications following surgery, emphysema (loss of elasticity in the lungs, which makes breathing painful), elevated blood pressure, blockage of blood vessels in the arms, legs, and brain, impaired sense of taste and smell, loss of appetite, and shortness of breath. In males, it causes reduced fertility, abnormal sperm production, and erectile dysfunction. In pregnant women, smoking harms the fetus by inducing stillbirth, premature birth, miscarriage, and low birth weight.

Opiates. Opiates (derived from the word opium) like morphine, heroin, oxycodone, and hydrocodone are narcotics that affect the central nervous system. Morphine relieves pain, creates a euphoric feeling, and impairs mental and physical abilities. Opiates' effects also include constipation, decreased hunger, diminished cough reflex, slowed breathing, reduced sex drive, and menstrual cycle abnormalities. The most insidious thing about opiates, however, is the increased tolerance for the drug that develops the need for increased amounts to get the same results — resulting in physical and psychological dependence.

Ecstasy. Ecstasy is known as a "feel good" drug, which users — mostly college- and high-school-aged students — take because it induces euphoria, extreme relaxation, and intimacy and connectedness with others. It reduces the need to eat, drink, and sleep, allowing users to remain active for all-night "raves," where the drug is commonly taken. Short-term effects include nausea, chills, sweating, tremors, high body temperature, and rapid heartbeat. Prolonged use leads to kidney failure, blurred vision, grinding teeth, jaw clenching, heart palpitations, hallucinations, disorientation, impaired coordination, confusion, severe hyperthermia, and dehydration. Long-term effects include prolonged depression, anxiety, and flashbacks. Heavy use causes liver and brain damage. Ecstasy has a high addiction potential.

Methamphetamine. Meth use has soared in the United States. Why is it a problem? Meth is highly addictive. Believe it or not, some people become hooked with one use. So think twice before using it. It's often used in combination with alcohol and other drugs. Meth is swallowed, snorted, smoked as crystals (known as glass, crystal, or ice), or injected. Users include 6.2 percent of high school seniors, who account for 18,000 emergency room visits and 550 deaths each year (National Institute on Drug Abuse, 2002).

Health effects — or the five "Bs" of meth abuse — include:

1. Body — The body can't keep up with what is happening to it. It's like going 200 miles per hour. Blood pressure increases, and rapid heart rate can cause stroke or heart failure. You can develop "meth mouth"(losing teeth from grinding, dry mouth, and excess intake of sugars). Body temperature increases, which can cause convulsions. The risk of contracting HIV/AIDS is greatly increased if you inject meth with a dirty needle. There is loss of appetite and sleep, nervousness, and itching as if there were "bugs under the skin."
2. Brain — Meth is highly addictive. You crash hard when it wears off. Mental conditions caused by meth include anxiety, mood changes, depression, paranoia, and psychosis.
3. Behavior — Meth users experience many confrontations with others and possibly the police. There is a tendency toward violence.
4. Baby — The likelihood of premature birth and congenital abnormalities is increased.
5. Bystanders — Family and neighbors are affected by exposure to chemicals used to make meth, including drain cleaner, lye, battery acid, lantern fuel, and antifreeze. Seven pounds of hazardous waste from meth production are dumped in backyards or down drains for every one pound of meth produced (National Institute on Drug Abuse, 2002).

Cocaine. When I hear a twenty- to thirty-year-old male has died of a heart attack, my first reaction is to ask: "Was it cocaine?" Cocaine is a water-soluble drug. That means it's absorbed rapidly in your system like a cold drink of water on a hot day. Its rapid absorption is the key to understanding cocaine's profound addictive qualities and its adverse effects. Cocaine causes a rapid euphoria and jolt to body systems. Blood pressure and pulse rise, blood vessels constrict, pupils dilate, and temperature increases. Larger amounts can cause paranoia, erratic and violent behavior, tremors, vertigo, restlessness, irritability, and anxiety. Sudden death can occur with the first use of cocaine (or soon thereafter) from cardiac or respiratory arrest or seizures.

So there you have the main substances and what they do to the human body. Don't despair altogether, however. Name a substance and there's a detoxification (detox) program available.

Detoxification Programs

Most detox programs incorporate the body-mind-spirit synergy. For those addicted to opiates (morphine-related drugs like heroin), rehabilitation will include physical support (methadone, a drug that takes the place of the opiate without causing its euphoria followed by its lows), mind-healing counseling, and — if you're in a faith-based center — spiritual guidance. Alcohol and other drug detoxification programs follow a similar approach.

It's essential to remember that detox is only the first step in drug or alcohol rehab. Outpatient detox alone may not be sufficient treatment for dependency on drugs and alcohol. Many addicts will require participation in long-term rehabilitation and medication. Consult your doctor to learn specifics.

The goal of detox is to restore a life that's no longer dependent on drugs or alcohol. At the same time, detox prevents the severe physical symptoms of withdrawing from the substance — symptoms that cause death or other ill effects such as a stroke, seizures, delirium, and hazardous changes in blood pressure.

If you (or a loved one) have been using alcohol or drugs for a while, it'll be difficult to quit without help. Your body, mind, and spirit will react to going off the drug or alcohol in what is known as withdrawal. That is, your body mistakenly recognizes the substance as necessary for its survival. When it doesn't have the substance in its system, it literally acts as if it will die without it! Consequently, you might find it hard to relax, go to sleep, or maintain sleep for enough hours to feel rested during withdrawal.

Worse still, your mind may become troubled, confused, anxious, or upset. Your body might experience trembling, sweating, and rapid heart rate. For alcoholics, delirium tremens (the DTs) can occur from three to four days after they have had their last drink of alcohol. DTs can include very high blood pressure, heart rate, and temperature, sweats, and delirium (seeing, hearing, or feeling what isn't there). The DTs are nothing to trifle with; in their midst the alcoholic can die from heart conditions, infections, trauma, and fluid and electrolyte problems.

There are certain medications that help with withdrawal symptoms. Take alcohol withdrawal for example. Medications such as longer-acting benzodiazepams (chlordiazepoxide (Librium)) and diazepam (Valium) are used in preventing the withdrawal seizures and delirium that can kill you.

You might ask: "Doesn't Valium cause addiction? So, why use it for treating addiction?" The answer is, so that a person doesn't die from the severity of withdrawal symptoms. Addiction is like being on a speeding train: if you jump off suddenly and hit the ground, the sudden stop can be fatal. These drugs are used to taper the body off alcohol's effects so it can adapt to a "slower" speed without alcohol's "runaway" ill effects.

A short-acting benzodiazepine (lorazepam (Ativan) or oxazepam (Serax)) can be used by those who are more sensitive to medication effects — like the elderly person — or those with liver problems who can't metabolize medications well and who would be more sensitive to the build-up of longer acting medicines. Sedatives are useful for central nervous system excitation. Antipsychotics (for example, haloperidol (Haldol)) are an option for treating delirium, but because they can decrease the threshold for seizures, this class of medicines shouldn't be used until the patient has been first treated with a benzodiazepam. The vitamin thiamine, to prevent Wernicke's encephalopathy (a condition common in alcohol abusers and characterized by loss of short-term memory and even coma in severe cases), and multivitamin supplements should be given to the malnourished abuser.

I know the above paragraph is pretty technical and may be a bit mind-boggling, so again, it's best to consult your doctor. Next, Gary discusses the psychological aspects of addiction in more detail and different types of recovery programs designed to help addicts get sober and maintain sobriety.

People Choose to Use

Gary D. McKay

Just 'cause you got the monkey off your back doesn't mean the circus has left town.
— GEORGE CARLIN

Whether people drink, smoke, snort, or shoot, they choose to take substances. Many have influences such as alcoholic parents, a demanding job, or peer pressure. But these are influences, not causes. As Wayne's mentor Skip taught him, the bottom line is if you're an addicted person, whether to substance or behavior, it's up to you — it's your decision. If being addicted to substances or behaviors doesn't involve choice, how do people manage to quit?

People addicted to alcohol tell themselves things like: "I can't stop drinking." "I need a drink." "I must have a drink." "I deserve a drink." "I shouldn't have a drink, but . . ." With this kind of DUMB thinking, guess what, it's "bottoms up!" But what if they developed REAL thoughts instead and told themselves — and really believed — "I can stop even though I don't want to."

For example, suppose you're addicted to alcohol and you've decided to quit. It's been a rough day at work and as you're driving home, you pass your former favorite bar. You tell yourself: "Boy it's been tough today, if I could just have a drink, it would help me relax. Just one, just this once, can't hurt." So you turn your car around and head for the bar's parking lot. A couple of hours later you're drunk as a skunk. Thank god you've still got enough sense about you to call a taxi and worry about getting your car later.

Okay, let's change the scenario. "Boy it's been a tough day, if I could just have a drink, it would help me relax . . . Wait a minute; although it helps me relax, I know I won't stop with just one and then what? I'll end up drunk again. So I'm NOT going to do that. Now, what else helps me relax? Exercise, a warm bath, snuggling with my spouse . . ."

Learn to recognize things that trigger your desire to engage in the addictive behavior, like a tough day. Make a list of what triggers you — if you let it. Remember, just because there's a trigger, doesn't mean you have to pull it!

Think Yourself out of It

Psychologist and author Albert Ellis developed rational emotive behavior therapy (REBT), a form of cognitive behavior therapy in 1955. For over fifty years, REBT has helped people with all kinds of psychological problems, including addiction. My concepts of DUMB and REAL thoughts are based on Ellis's REBT.

Ellis said: "The desire for altered consciousness and moods is at the bottom of addictability. . . People prefer certain pleasurable feelings and relief from discomfort" (Ellis & Velten, 1992). But people who are addicted go beyond just preferring certain feelings; they believe they "must" have those feelings, and the substance (or behavior) is the only way they can achieve them. Placing demands on life by "shoulding" on themselves or "must-erbating" — as Dr. Ellis called it — also creates the belief that they just "can't stand" not feeling this way and that they "need" the substance (or behavior). Therefore, it's just "awful" if they can't get what they "need." Or life or circumstances are so "awful" that they "must" have _____ to survive, even though they usually condemn themselves for such behavior.

People can conquer their addiction if they accept that they have a problem with a particular substance or behavior and are first willing to accept themselves as they are — condemning their behavior, but not themselves. In other words: "separate the deed from the doer." If they're willing to, they can see that although they want a certain thing, this doesn't mean they *have* to have it. They can admit that although they actually *prefer* the feelings derived from the substance or behavior, a preference is just that, it's *not* a requirement. As Ellis asked:

"What's the evidence, where is it writ

That one must have something just because they strongly prefer it?"

True, people don't like the unpleasant side effects of their addictive behavior, but they're quite willing to put up with them to get the short-term high.

Ellis suggested people identify their addictive thoughts, which he called "stinking thinking," and actively dispute them. In other words, create REAL thoughts. In his book (written with Emmett Velten) *When AA Doesn't Work for You: Rational Steps to Quitting Alcohol*, Ellis (1992) said you can use six questions to dispute your irrational or DUMB thinking.

1. Question 1: What irrational Belief or stinking thought do I want to Dispute and surrender?
2. Question 2: Can I rationally support the Belief or stinking thought?
3. Question 3: What evidence exists of the truth of this Belief or stinking thought?
4. Question 4: What evidence exists of the falseness of this Belief or stinking thought?
5. Question 5: What are the worst things that are actually, factually likely to happen to me if I give up this irrational Belief and act against it?
6. Question 6: What good things could happen or could I make happen if I give up this irrational belief?

Other Techniques: Reframing and Imagery

In chapter 2 you learned about reframing — changing perspective by finding what's positive in a situation — the opportunity in the obstacle, or what we can learn from a mistake. Ellis' question 6 is actually a way to reframe. It's what's positive about giving up your DUMB thinking about addictive thoughts.

You can also use imagery. Imagine yourself no longer drinking, for example. See you and your spouse cooperating, having fun without drinking. See yourself interacting in a positive way with your children.

Search for and Change Your Purpose

Like all thoughts, emotions, and behaviors, addictive behavior is purposive. In the 1930s, Alfred Adler had already discovered several purposes of addiction to alcohol or narcotics. These purposes, paraphrased below, apply to other addictions as well (Adler, 2005).

Purposes of Addiction

- Relief from stress
- Avoiding responsibility
- Immediate gratification
- Getting even (as when spouses join in addiction)
- Avoiding interaction with others (the lone drinker)
- Avoiding connection with others (similar to avoiding closeness — seen as control)
- Demands for satisfaction
- Getting others to take care of the addict
- Avoiding expectations
- Seeking courage in order to "function" and meet challenges

If you or a loved one has a problem with addiction, do any of these purposes apply? We can achieve some of these purposes by more healthy means; we should give up others and pursue new purposes. Take, for example, stress relief. There are many ways to relieve stress that are healthy — such as exercise and relaxation. In chapter 2 we discussed the benefits of physical exercise and gave examples of deep breathing and relaxation exercises. You can get satisfaction from many activities that don't involve addiction. Following are some other things to think about regarding the purposes of addiction:

- Courage can be obtained through belief in yourself: resolving to do your best and to not demand perfection.
- Avoiding responsibility often means that you expect perfection from yourself. Why do you have to be perfect? Who is? Nobody!
- Why is interaction with others a problem? Find people you enjoy being with — but not people with addiction problems.

- For now, avoid people who have harmed you. Don't seek revenge. Getting even always backfires. The person on whom you're seeking revenge will turn it around.
- Focus on controlling yourself and not others. Why does being close to someone have to involve control? You can be close to someone and remain in control of yourself — you are anyway!
- Learn to delay gratification. Who says gratification must be immediate? You do, if *you're* the one feeling it — you're the one demanding it.
- Why do you have to have a servant? By now you probably realize that trying to get others to take care of you creates resentment, even if they do it.
- Avoiding expectations relates to expecting yourself to be perfect.

Some people addict themselves to try to "cure" psychological problems such as depression, fear, and anxiety. Alcohol, for example, is a depressive drug. It may temporarily relax you and distract you from your depression, but in the long run it'll make you even more depressed. Facing fear and anxiety helps you conquer them; trying to mask them with booze does not. Instead use imagery to prepare meeting a situation that you fear.

Am I Addicted? How Do I Know?

If you think you have a problem, then you probably do. Or, if you don't think you have a problem but others close to you tell you that you do, then you probably do. Here are some other things to consider regarding alcohol abuse. These are posted at the Drug and Alcohol Resource Center: http://www.addict-help.com/alcoholism-signs.htm.

- Have you ever felt you should cut down on your drinking?
- Have people annoyed you by criticizing your drinking?
- Have you ever felt bad or guilty about your drinking?
- Have you ever had a drink first thing in the morning to steady your nerves or to get rid of a hangover?

If you answered "yes" to one of these questions, then you may have a problem with alcohol. Answering more than one of the questions with a "yes" indicates a strong probability. Don't be fooled, though. Answering "no" to all the questions doesn't necessarily mean you don't have a problem if you've had drinking-related problems with your job, relationships, health, or the law (Drug and Alcohol Resource Center).

What if you suspect, based on the above information, that a loved one has a problem? Later in this section, I discuss what you can do to help. But for now, let's continue as if you have a problem or wonder if you do. If you're still in doubt, there are more extensive online self-tests you can take. (See the appendix for suggested websites.) And when it comes to other kinds of substance or behavior abuse, there are online self-tests you can take for these too. We list their websites in the appendix as well. Although most of the self-test websites direct you to AA-type treatment centers or groups, if you test "positive" for addiction, you can choose other types of recovery if AA doesn't appeal to you.

Next, I discuss treatment alternatives.

Okay, I Think I Have a Problem. What Do I Do Next?

There are many ways to seek treatment. Some people prefer therapy or a treatment center. If you're addicted to a substance, it's best to talk with your physician first to see if there are detox issues such as those that Wayne discussed above. Your doctor may be able to prescribe medication to help you detox. She or he can also steer you to treatment options.

If you decide to see a therapist or check into a rehab center, be sure to check their philosophy to see if it fits with your belief system. For example, an Adlerian, rational emotive behavior therapist or other cognitive behavior therapist will have approaches similar to what you've been learning in this book. See the appendix for websites that help you locate therapists.

You may prefer to seek treatment on your own through self-help groups or by using an individual approach, such as REBT — Albert Ellis's work mentioned above — or Rational Recovery, discussed below. Following are three popular approaches for dealing with addiction: 12-step programs (such as AA), SMART Recovery, and Rational Recovery. After reading a description of each approach, you'll find an example of a person who has used the approach.

12-Stepping It

12-Step groups like AA, NA (Narcotics Anonymous), and GA (Gamblers Anonymous) are well known for the treatment of addictions. You can find a list of the 12-steps in several places, such as Wikipedia (http://en.wikipedia.org/wiki/Twelve-step_program). The steps involve admitting that you are powerless to control your addiction and that a higher power, such as god, is in charge. The 12-step philosophy views addiction as a disease.

Following is Doug's story. Doug belongs to a Christian recovery group in his community called "Celebrate Recovery" that is based on the 12 steps.

My addictions will never go away, but I'm now able to live with them and have them not control my life. God is in control of my life; when thoughts about old behaviors start appearing in my mind there are five things I'm probably not doing: 1) praying, 2) reading my Bible, 3) being accountable to my sponsor, 4) listening to God, and 5) writing in my journal.

I have been so blessed over the past thirty years to have these struggles because it has made me compassionate toward others who are hurting in life's daily struggles. I have been attending Celebrate Recovery since October 20, 2004, and have realized just how important God and his son Jesus Christ are to me and what a huge part they both play in my daily life.

I'm a grateful believer in Jesus Christ. I'm in recovery for depression and addiction to food, alcohol, and pornography. Pornography has been the worst addiction to battle, because it is a hidden addiction based on secrets and lies. I always knew what I was doing was wrong in my mind and heart, but I just needed my fix after a stressful day at work or at home.

I always thought I could handle the addiction by myself and that I didn't need anyone's help; but when I tried to control things it usually made a mess of my life. It wasn't until I allowed God to fill the hole in my heart that my life started changing. I was at peace when God started loving me, which I was never able to do before because of the guilt, shame, and anger in me.

Doug's strong Christian faith is very helpful to him. But what if you're not a believer in Jesus as God or are of another faith? What if you don't believe you're powerless to control your addiction? What if you don't see the addiction as a disease? What then?

There are other approaches, some group based, and some individual. Next, we'll look at another popular group approach called SMART Recovery.

Get SMART

You can use the self-management and recovery training (SMART) program whether or not you're a religious or spiritual person. In

SMART, addiction is not viewed as a disease and it is believed that you have the power to help yourself. SMART, based largely on Dr. Ellis's REBT, is a four point program involving:

1. Motivation to abstain — enhancing and maintaining motivation to abstain from addictive behavior
2. Coping with urges — learning how to cope with urges and cravings
3. Problem solving — using rational ways to manage thoughts, feelings, and behaviors
4. Lifestyle balance — balancing short-term and long-term pleasures and satisfactions in life (SMART Recovery)

SMART Recovery has meetings in many communities. Check their website (http://www.smartrecovery.org) to see if there are meetings in your area. If not, you can "attend" online meetings through SMART Recovery chat rooms.

Here are some excerpts from Melissa's story, which is posted on the SMART website along with several others. You may want to check out the posted stories to find out more about how SMART has helped people.

> When I heard the knock on the door, I had no idea my life was about to change. "You're the worst of all of them. You're the mother. You should know better." That's what the detective who came to my house that day said to me. I can still see him standing in front of me, judging me.
>
> As I sat on my couch, the other detectives searched through my house and found pipes, dope, and forged documents. I was in utter shock and denial. My little girl was clueless as to what was going on, but she felt something was up. My oldest was at school and to this day I am grateful for that.
>
> I lost my home, my kids, my job, my friends, and basically my life to that drug. It had reached inside and taken over, and I had allowed that to happen. I mean, I've used some substance or another since I was about fifteen. I suppose you could say that the only way I knew how to cope with anything was by taking one mind-altering substance or another.
>
> I found the SOL [SMART On Line] community by doing an Internet search, and I decided to try it out because it made sense to me. There was this huge emphasis on self-empowerment,

and for myself, the thought of not having control over my behaviors seemed hopeless. I figured that if I had gotten myself into this mess, then I had best learn how to get myself out.

I began to attend meetings and post on the message board, and the replies that I received were encouraging and heartfelt. I made myself a home on the boards those first few months, and let out every thought that crossed my mind. I have no doubt that had it not been for the amount of time I spent posting and in the chat room, I would have slipped far more times than I did those first few months.

With each slip came a new recognition, and with each of my recognitions came a newfound strength. For each step back I took two steps forward. I learned the tools and how to apply them, and with some trial and error, I began to really get it.

There have been many times when I wanted to give up, or just let go of the fight, and those are the times when SMART was the most useful to me. I would show up in the chat room late at night, and there would be a listening ear available. No judgments were ever made regarding what I was saying, and there was not a single moment in which I did not feel as though I were a member of this community.

If you would prefer to do it on your own rather than joining a group, you could use the techniques in this book to change your DUMB thoughts to REAL ones. You could get Ellis's book mentioned above (*When AA Doesn't Work for You: Rational Steps to Quitting Alcohol*), and follow his advice. You can also use these techniques while attending a 12-step or SMART group.

Another approach that's similar to Ellis's work and SMART is Rational Recovery. It's designed to be an individual recovery process.

Managing It on Your Own — Rational Recovery

In 1985, social worker Jack Trimpey and his wife, Lois, created Rational Recovery. Jack had attended AA meetings and didn't find them helpful, so he developed his own approach. In the beginning of the development of RR, Trimpey believed in groups — trained in his approach. But now he doesn't believe in groups and thinks that addiction is strictly the individual's problem and up to him or her to solve it.

RR is based on the Addictive Voice Recognition Techniques (AVRT). He says that thoughts of drinking or using are the addictive voice in our heads. He calls the addictive voice "the Beast." It's "the Beast" that wants us to drink or use so we get pleasure from the substance or behavior. Trimpey suggests you call your addictive voice or Beast "it." So, when you recognize those thoughts, you know that "it," the Beast, is out to get you to do what "it" wants. (No, you aren't becoming schizophrenic; it's just a helpful technique!) Through combating and defeating the Beast, you resist addictive thoughts and behavior.

Trimpey's book *Rational Recovery: The New Cure for Substance Addiction* (1996) and website http://www.rational.org give detailed information on AVRT. Here is how Tony used RR to handle his alcohol addiction:

> *My adventure through recovery began in the late 1980s as best I can remember it. I was receiving promotion after promotion, raise after raise and began celebrating my victories, drowning my failures, and using alcohol as a tool for creativity (or so I thought).*
>
> *I didn't have a drinking problem; there were a lot of good times that came out of that bottle, never mind the bad ones, as they were just part of living life in the fast lane. As the years ticked by, the drinking became what I worked for — but I didn't have a drinking problem. I came to realize much later that was exactly the case — I didn't have a drinking problem. On the other hand, anyone who came into contact with me had a drinking problem — me. My former employers finally made the decision to solve their drinking problem; so, the day after Christmas in 1991 they returned all my stock monies (which they didn't have to do) and proceeded to terminate me after fourteen years of service.*
>
> *I would spend my time finding a job then figuring out ways to get to the bars, get more money to get my precious drink. Everything else took a backseat to my drinking. I would only hold a job for a short time as those employers had much less tolerance for drunks (go figure). My next-door neighbor was my kind of guy as he too had a wife (just like mine) who would not tolerate the drunken stupidity. Our drinking endeavors took a great deal of time and effort to stay below our spouses' radar screens. I had everyone fooled: wife, children, family, neighbors, employers, police, etc.*
>
> *The reality of it was I wasn't fooling anyone. The people who were in direct contact with me just hadn't taken the*

initiative to solve "Their Drinking Problem" yet! My wife being the closest to the epicenter of this little nightmare I had created started attending Al-Anon meetings, which pushed me to attend the AA counterpart, but I was nothing like those people. I didn't have a drinking problem. In fact, after hearing all the horror and war stories of the speakers, I'd need a drink and it was off to the nearest watering hole.

It didn't take long for my wife to figure out that the only thing she had in common in the Al-Anon circles was a drunken spouse and that she could either accept it or not. She realized that she did not have a "disease" called codependency. She was not enabling her drunken husband. She had a drinking problem and she was ready to solve it.

After catching up with me on a sober moment, she made her case and took her stand. Her ultimatum was quite simple; I could keep on drinking and staying out late doing whatever it was that I did, of which she would no longer be tolerant. As she put it, she married me because she loved me but the following would come to pass if I made the choice to continue drinking. We would end up in court, the judge would side with her, she would get the house, the cars, the kids, and half of whatever paycheck from whatever jobs I might be able to hold. If that's what I wanted, that's where we were going.

She had just solved her drinking problem. Me. On the other hand, I now had a drinking problem that needed to be solved. I had already been to AA and it just wasn't my cup of Kool-Aid. I happened to see a list of Recovery programs (most of which were 12-step based) but one really caught my eye: Rational Recovery.

I began attending and in a few short weeks the addiction was over. The premise was self-reliance; recognizing my irrational thoughts and inclinations to drink were my addiction (not me). I am responsible for my choices and actions, period. With that I make much better decisions and choices overall. Sure I still make mistakes (it's human) and for the most part enjoy learning from every one of them.

If Your Loved One Is Addicted

Suppose it's not you who has a problem with a substance or behavior, but a loved one. What can you do? First, let's talk about what *not* to do. First, *don't* put yourself or your children, if you have kids, in danger. Safety first. If your loved one tends to get violent, plan escape routes and safe places to stay — such as with relatives or friends. Or find "safe houses" in your community. See the appendix for websites on domestic violence and child abuse.

Do you nag, plead, lecture, threaten, or otherwise act negatively toward your loved one when she or he is using? If you do, I'm sure you've noticed this doesn't work. So stop. Look below for some other ideas and do some research.

Alternatives to nagging, pleading, lecturing, and threatening. You can talk to your loved one about his or her addiction in constructive ways using I-messages (see chapter 5) when he or she is not using, for example: "When you drink, I feel sad because you draw into yourself and we have no positive contact. I love it when you're not drinking and we can be together."

Take action for yourself. Tell your loved one what you'll do when he or she is using, such as leaving the house to visit a friend. Take your kids. Respectfully refuse involvement with the loved one when she or he is using.

In their book *Get Your Loved One Sober: Alternatives to Nagging, Pleading, and Threatening* (2004), Drs. Robert J. Meyers and Brenda L. Wolfe discuss the CRAFT — Community Reinforcement and Family Training — approach. CRAFT basically involves using positive ways such as I-messages to encourage your loved one.

Another thing Meyers and Wolfe suggest is that you be careful to *not* take over your loved one's responsibility when she or he is using. For example, arranging to be the chauffer so the addicted one can engage in drinking, making excuses (like calling his place of work to say he's sick when he has a hangover), or cleaning up her messes. Let the drinker experience the consequences of the behavior.

CSO support meetings. CSOs — Concerned Significant Others — can join groups like Al-Anon to get support in dealing with the addicted loved one. SMART also conducts online meetings for CSOs. There may also be SMART CSO meetings in your area. Check the SMART website and contact them for information.

Interventions. Some addiction therapists offer "interventions." An intervention involves the therapist and loved ones confronting the addicted one in a meeting. The meeting takes place at a time when the addicts don't expect it, so that they have no opportunity to back out. They may be thinking they're going somewhere else or to meet someone else rather than to an intervention meeting. The meeting can also be held in the family home. The addicted one doesn't know others will be talking to her or him about the addiction. You know your loved one, so choose a time when he or she won't be drinking, drugging, etc.

The intervention involves the therapist and significant others. The meeting is confrontational, but in a respectful way, and usually involves participants writing out their comments in advance and reading them in turn to the addict. The content is neither accusatory nor lecturing; instead, it simply states how one feels when the person is engaging in the substance or behavior, while perhaps citing examples. The intent of the intervention is to get the loved one to seek direct help.

Contact addiction therapists in your area to find out if they do interventions. The therapist will meet with significant others to go over the process and help them plan the intervention. See the appendix for websites on finding interventionists.

Failing all else, you may want to give your loved one a choice, similar to what Tony's wife did in his story above. In effect she told him that if he kept drinking, she'd leave him and what the consequences of the divorce would be. This is a pretty drastic measure, but if the drinking continues and the addicted one is determined not to do anything about it, it may be your best choice.

Next, Erik discusses the spiritual aspects of addiction, including the problem of being addicted to religion.

Overpowered by Your Higher Power?

Erik Mansager

> ... *the reign of God is within you.*
> — LUKE 17:21

Wayne and Gary have helped you understand the physical and psychological aspects of addiction. Wayne acquainted us with the effect of drugs on the body, and we learned of our ability to produce something like it ourselves (endorphins) rather than rely on addictive outside sources. Gary has explained about choices and the DUMB thinking that tends to underlie our addictions, no matter the substance or behavior of choice.

Here I want to share with you the emotional, craving aspect of addiction. There's that aspect of addiction that seems to grab us by the knees when we're without our substance or behavior — it's like we long for something very precious to us. I talk a bit about how you can address that deep longing with spirituality — and how spirituality is included in many recovery plans. But I also do something a bit out of the ordinary here.

I come at the addiction issue a little differently. That's because I aim to tackle one of the "solutions" to addiction and show how that can become the problem itself. I discuss how what is suggested as a *remedy* to addiction ("Go to your 'higher power' for help") can also *be the addiction itself*. It's ironic, but true that god, too, can be treated as a drug (Booth, 1992).

So I address what it is about addiction that is so attractive in the first place and how that relates to "religious addiction." Then I share how the predictable stages of addiction look when we're dealing with religion as the problem, rather than the solution it's intended to be. Next I offer an overview of how the symptoms of religious addiction look as the stages progress. After that, I explore ways out of religious addiction and then finish up by suggesting ways for developing a healthy, nonaddictive spirituality.

Root Bound or Flying Free?

Without a doubt, the traditional path of spirituality (for example, Alcoholic Anonymous' emphasis on a higher power) is helpful to millions of recovering addicts. Gary and Wayne have made this point very well. When we're in a mental space and physical condition in which we feel ourselves dependent on a substance or behavior beyond our control, there's great relief in "letting go, and letting god" take the burden for us. Having proven ourselves ineffective, it's wise to do something actually different rather than expecting a difference from our habitual behavior. And yet, as addictive problems have grown, concern is expressed about the remedy confounding the cure (Kasl, 1992).

How can it be that . . .

. . . people seek *wings* to escape their feelings of inadequacy, yet become *root bound* in a quagmire of polluted soils?

. . . the one thing that many people believe is the only way to fix their brokenness — their reliance on god — can itself be experienced as an inescapable trap of hopelessness?

. . . those who believe they are tithing faithfully sometimes experience financial ruin due to excessive tithing?

. . . those who seek to be accepted and forgiven as "sinners" still find themselves in a chronic state of discontent similar to the very sinners they are trying so hard to separate themselves from?

... people can become so fixated on being fixed that they are trapped in feelings of guilt, shame, and fear?

... people experience such dysfunctional feelings in the very name of god that they find themselves at times abusing others — emotionally, physically, and even sexually?!

These questions are not as puzzling as they seem at first — if we see that the underlying belief "I'm inherently broken and need to be fixed" is actually the issue. We all experience our limitations and littleness in the world; I spoke about that at length in chapter 3.

This feeling of littleness, of insignificance, of inferiority is really our friend because from it springs our desire to overcome that feeling. Such overcoming has led to all the great contributions of the world and to the great religions and spiritual pathways; overcoming has ennobled the human species. But it's how we characterize our littleness, how we perceive our small selves in the wide, wild world that really determines the way we'll act to overcome the feeling.

Depending on the influences of our early lives, and how we perceive them, we learn how to cope effectively or ineffectively. How we cope depends on equal parts of our biology (nature), our environment (nurture), and our perceptions (nuance). The more we learn about these, the more we're able to influence our lives. As we learn that we're *part of* the same group that's here to be helped and here to help others, the more effective and *interdependent* we tend to be.

The more we're taught to rely on things *outside* ourselves — people, feelings, substances, or whatever — the more *codependent* we tend to be. And then to a large degree, the variations of a codependent outlook on life (whether I feel I have to depend on others or on a special feeling) will identify which substances or behaviors I lean on in life: alcohol, drugs, sex, or — as we'll soon see — even god.

So, herein lies the root of all forms of addiction: the belief that we're "broken" and need to be "fixed." I'm pretty sure this is why the term "fix" has been so widely accepted within the addiction world. "Give me 'a fix'; make me better. After that I can run until I get broken again, then I'll get my 'next fix' or I'll 'get fixed' and no longer be 'in a fix.'"

The language of being broken runs throughout religious scriptures of all sorts — but especially among the Abrahamic religions — Judaism, Christianity, and Islam. These are often called "religions of the Book" because each has its, sometimes overlapping, scriptural testimony (its Book) that records the efforts of its prophets to turn people away from one way of life (a broken way of life, one of sin, falling short of the mark, and the like) to another life (one fixed and better, one of holiness or completeness).

Each of these religions has a long history of good and effective interventions in the lives of its followers and a long history of doing things that have helped better humanity. Each also has a historical tendency to abuse their prophets' "call to holiness." These and other religions, when perceived and experienced through the eyes of those who have been hurt and abused — and who *at the same time* mistake themselves as *deserving* such hurt and abuse — can use the prophets' call as proof of everyone's brokenness and absolute depravity, not just inadequacy.

Already you can see the either/or thinking I've referred to before: *either* we are saints *or* sinners; *either* healed *or* broken; *either* angels *or* devils; *either* bound for heaven *or* hell — and so on. People of these religions see themselves in this light / dark schema and tend to deal with themselves and others in one of two ways as the following illustrates:

- *Either* they believe they can't help themselves and must get someone or something more powerful than themselves to help pull them up and out of their predicament and continue to affirm them. (And who could be more dependable and powerful than god?!)
- *Or* they believe they can show how *good they are* by showing how *bad others are*. Rather than dealing with their feelings of inferiority by admitting they're really a lot like others and then working bit by bit on improvement, they point out how the others are even worse than they are. Their thinking goes something like this: "At least by comparison I'm better off than the unholy doubter." And presto! They feel a small measure better without having lifted a finger to change themselves.

Maybe you see how conveniently these damaging religious messages fit into an addictive scheme: God is angry and vengeful, sex is dirty and degenerate, doubters are unclean and responsible for God's wrath. This wrath they are quick to locate in all the social woes that they listen for in the news. From such a position, there really is no need to do anything differently. Rather, like all dependencies, the religious addict believes that by doing more of the same activities, things will change: "If only others would believe as I do, everything could really get fixed."

Such thinking allows addicts to believe that their compulsive behavior has some heavenly merit: long fasts, mindless repetition of prayers, distancing themselves from "unclean" others, obsessive, financially damaging tithing, equally obsessive TV evangelist watching (or its equivalent: priest/nun/rabbi/imam consultation) — all perceived as the right and righteous thing to do. These outward activities are confirmed as the right thing to do by all those they associate with. From such a position there's no need to go inward to do personal work.

You see the insidiousness such a pattern takes on: The more religious addicts try to be better and do better, the more imperfect their efforts are exposed to be — because "according to scripture" everything is arrogance and egoism: "Vanity of vanities; all is vanity!" (Ecclesiastes 1:2). The more they condemn others for unholy behavior, the more these addicts are distanced from others. Religious addicts' feelings of isolation and oppression increase. So it's a vicious cycle. The attempted solution to rely on the Power higher than they comes to *over*power their sense of connectedness with other "mere humans," and they find the only way to feel good about themselves is by a rigid perfectionism that's intolerant of any difference.

This is the horror of addiction of any sort. Although thinking that participation and indulgence will help them soar to greater heights, addicts end up digging themselves into a deeper and deeper hole.

So, those are the roots of the problem. Now I explore the predictability of the stages of addiction as religious addicts experience them.

Stages of Religious Addiction

Addictions don't arrive full blown. They start gradually, and at first the use of a substance or involvement in an activity seems innocent enough. But at some point it occurs to us that we can't turn back. No longer can we *not* do what we *wanted* to do as if it were just good, clean fun. And that's just how it is with religious addiction.

The church or meeting attendance, or the scripture reading, the imam/priest/nun/rabbi visits, the TV evangelist watching, all start out bringing order and solace to our lives. And, indeed, when adhered to from a perspective of connecting us with others, such activities serve in a marvelous way to help us place our littleness in perspective: we find we aren't alone; we are among others as our helpmates.

If, on the other hand, religiously involved people begin to doubt their connections with others and the worthwhileness of others and themselves, their religious activities are pursued to shore up their faltering self-esteem. This is stage one, where the trouble begins. Soon, in the next stage, the activities — whether rituals or readings — emphasize that because others don't perform the approved rituals or embrace the right readings, those people are evil. The final stage is when the addict is caught up in an endless attempt (by doing the activities "religiously") to avoid the damnable fate awaiting the uninitiated. Here's a closer look at the stages of religious addiction:

Early stage — Seeking control. You can see at the beginning of the downhill slide that it's not the initial level of involvement in a belief system that's addictive. Rather, religious involvement becomes a disintegrating disease process instead of an integrating healing process when the involvement is used to be in command of one's flagging self-esteem or one's impact on one's friends, at work, or in one's intimate relations.

People who have been abused in the past, and who believe they deserved this abuse, tend to feel life is generally out of control. Such people can become desperate about gaining some sense of control. Ironically, by conjuring up all sorts of fears about how "out of control" everything is, people heighten the need for their religious activities and then feel, in an odd way, *more in control* because they're among the few who know "the right thing" to do. They get the idea that the "fix" is within their reach; so they won't need to feel broken for long.

Middle stage — Careening out of control. Becoming more and more certain about how to get fixed, addicts make the classic mistake: "If a little works well, a lot will work better." So they plow forward, engaging in more of the religious activities, for example, tithing to excess, attending services that interfere with other obligations, and finding fault in those close to them. And what follows is pain. Financial hardships don't go away, the jobs avoided by attending more services remain undone, those loved ones who are told that they must be holier (that is, more like the addict) retreat further and further from the growing condemnation — until the addict finds his or her pain of low self-esteem increasing.

What to do?

They tell themselves: "I've got to do more of the same!"

Late stage — Tightening the circle and losing control. Following the middle stage comes the circular thinking so familiar in addiction. Rather than seeing their involvement in the offensive religious behavior as even a slight bit of the problem, the addict sees others and others' behavior as the problem. What attitude could facilitate addicts' troublesome behavior more than the belief that their troubles are caused by others? They are then exempt from rethinking the available options!

George Vaillant (1983), a leading addictions researcher, sees in this tightening circle the "dis-ease" of the addiction. Instead of seeking to be "at ease" in the world, addicts become hypervigilant and see the need for, and righteousness of, continuing their dysfunctional behavior. Their repetitive ways feel like control to them. Illusory though it is, it's all they have: compulsive, addictive behavior. Escape from the vicious cycle isn't easy. Recognizing you or a loved one is stuck, or approaching "stuckness," is the most important thing to be aware of. Only then can intervention occur.

Next, let's take a look at what the symptoms of religious addiction look like within the stages I've just discussed.

Symptoms of Religious Addiction

I've written much about healthy spirituality in the previous chapters, and we'll return to it in just a bit, but it's important to take a clear-eyed look at the symptoms of unhealthy religiosity as they relate to the progressive disease of religious addiction. In his innovative book on religious addiction, Father Leo Booth (1992) provides a comprehensive list and thorough discussion of each symptom.

Given what I've shared above, take a look and ask yourself if you recognize any of the following symptoms in yourself or your friends or a family member. Although any given one may not be an indication of a religious addiction, don't kid yourself: a combination of two or more isn't healthy. It's a safe bet that if you're experiencing two or more, the middle stage, Careening out of Control, has kicked in and addiction is waiting around the corner. Here's the list:

- inability to doubt or question information or authority
- black-and-white, simplistic thinking
- shame-based belief that you aren't good enough or you aren't doing it right
- magical thinking that god will fix you
- scrupulosity: rigid, obsessive adherence to rules, codes of ethics, or guidelines
- uncompromising, judgmental attitudes
- compulsive praying, going to church or crusades, quoting scripture
- unrealistic financial contributions
- believing that sex is dirty — that our bodies and physical pleasures are evil
- compulsive overeating or excessive fasting
- conflict with science, medicine, and education
- progressive detachment from the real world, isolation, breakdown of relationships

- psychosomatic illness: sleeplessness, back pain, headaches, hypertension
- manipulating scripture or texts, feeling chosen, claiming to receive special messages from god
- trancelike states or religious highs, wearing a glazed happy face
- cries for help; mental, emotional, physical breakdown; hospitalization

Quest: Leaving the "Right Answers" Behind

Now we know the stages of religious addiction and the symptoms that indicate an addiction is in progress, it's time to look for ways out of the dependence.

If you've understood the dilemma so far, you'll understand why in this section I must commit self-help heresy. That is, I suggest that the means by which many individuals overcome their addictions, the traditional 12-step program, won't exactly fit for dealing with a religious addiction.

You've just reviewed and perhaps found some of the symptoms of religious addiction active in your life or that of a loved one; so it should be clear that simply finding another "religious answer" to the "religious problem" may not do the trick. What is needed is an approach that, without discounting religion or a concept of god or higher power, allows the possibility of finding one's way to health *without* such tangible beliefs. The needed approach would allow one to sense the power for healing as wholly within and to experience oneself as being as whole as one can be at any moment — knowing there are many moments ahead into which one must grow. The approach needed to counter religious addiction is one in which one imagines oneself as not so much perfect as "good enough" and quite able to make the type of personal decisions that Gary has taught us is a REAL way of thinking.

So, I suggest that in dealing specifically with religious addiction, the 12 steps as constructed (or only slightly modified) need *not* be adhered to. Gary has mentioned some other approaches that better fit the bill for religious addictions (such as Dr. Ellis's ideas, SMART, and Rational Recovery), and I want to put forward a couple more here.

One of the most creative and effective non-12-stepping approaches to addictions is presented in *The Miracle Method* by Scott Miller and Insoo Kim Berg (1995). I won't go into detail, but if you enjoy and understand the approach we're presenting, you'll find the "miracle" approach both refreshing and empowering. The book emphasizes a look at *solutions* rather than at *problems* and provides "keys for success," "clues for finding your way along the path to solutions," and even "rules for dealing with setbacks." The remarkable power of the book is that it helps individuals find the strength to admit their difficulties *before* they hit a brick wall. It also offers a path of encouragement all along the way to the effective solutions.

Another approach that's an alternative to 12-stepping comes from Charlotte Davis Kasl's *Many Roads, One Journey: Moving Beyond the 12 Steps* (1992). This groundbreaking critique of why the 12 steps don't work for everyone thoroughly explores the controversy over whether the 12 steps of Bill W. and Dr. Bob (the founders of AA) are the only or best way for recovery for all men and all women of all cultures. The book also discusses common aspects of addictions and "the way out." Here, Kasl approaches the twelve steps from a feminist perspective and shows how they may be applied by a broader range of addicts than they typically are. Here's where the religious addict can begin to understand *alternatives* to turning one's life over to a Power greater than oneself.

In the last section of the book, Kasl presents a series of "new roads," including her own "Sixteen Steps for Discovery and Empowerment." It's these that I believe are wholly compatible with a self-empowering movement away from addictive religious behavior and outlook. They can be embraced without displacing the healthier aspects of one's religious or spiritual beliefs, but they inherently challenge the unhealthy symptoms listed above. I'll list them, slightly modified for religious addicts. See what you think:

1. We affirm we have the power to take charge of our lives and stop being dependent on religious behavior or religious people for our self-esteem and security.
2. We come to believe that the healing wisdom within us awakens when we open ourselves to that power.
3. We make a decision to become our authentic selves and trust in the healing power of the truth.
4. We examine our beliefs, addictions, and dependent behavior in the context of living in a hierarchal, patriarchal culture.
5. We share with another person and thereby the whole universe all those things inside of us for which we feel shame and guilt.
6. We affirm and enjoy our strengths, talents, and creativity, striving not to hide these qualities to protect others' self-interests.
7. We become willing to let go of shame, guilt, and any behavior that keeps us from loving ourselves and others.

8. We make a list of people we have harmed and people who have harmed us and take steps to clear out negative energy by making amends and sharing our grievances in a respectful way.
9. We express love and gratitude to others and increasingly appreciate the wonder of life and the blessings we *do* have.
10. We continue to trust our reality and daily affirm that we see what we see, we know what we know, and we feel what we feel.
11. We promptly acknowledge our mistakes and make amends when appropriate, but we don't say we're sorry for things we haven't done and we don't cover up, analyze, or take responsibility for the shortcomings of others.
12. We seek out situations, jobs, and people who affirm our intelligence, perceptions, and self-worth and avoid situations or people who are hurtful, harmful, or demeaning to us.
13. We take steps to heal our physical bodies, organize our lives, reduce stress, and have fun.
14. We seek to find our inward calling and develop the will and wisdom to follow it.
15. We accept the ups and downs of life as natural events that can be used as lessons for our growth.
16. We grow in awareness that we are interrelated with all living things, and we contribute to restoring peace and balance on the planet.

Spiritual Freedom: Looking for Questions

There's plenty of research evidence and practical wisdom that I've referred to in earlier chapters that speaks of the healthy interconnection of spirituality among people who help people. I strongly recommend exploring the "Sixteen Steps for Discovery and Empowerment" and finding those that are meaningful to you. Share them with your trusted friends and colleagues who know you're struggling to overcome an addiction or who themselves may be suffering from one — religious or otherwise.

By exploring the steps' contents, you can arrive at a new set of functional values. Rather than *either* judging others as less than ourselves *or* judging ourselves as less than others, we can find a way to achieve unconditional acceptance of ourselves and others in our imperfections. We are, after all, "on the way." We haven't arrived yet, and the arrival time isn't yet certain. (This is the "team orientation" I addressed in chapter 3.) Rather than embracing the rigid *truth* of one's own religion, one can start to see that a truth can be right and binding for oneself and yet not for another — because each individual perceives his or her biology and environment uniquely. (This is the "steadfastness" I addressed in chapter 3.) Rather than *isolation* (whether by being *apart from* others or by being *within* a dominant religious group), one can start to value *connection* with others outside one's religious identity. (This is the "community focus" I addressed in chapter 3.) We don't know the full measure of the time before we die! *Only then* are we really done, finished, and complete. *Until then*, we must continue to learn from our mistakes, not avoid them rigidly at all costs.

In all this, we're learning to ask better questions about life, rather than strictly adhering to prescribed, preformed answers. The list of good questions is endless. Here are some to consider:

- What will life be like after addiction?
- Who will care if I live through this?
- How can I do my part so that others won't suffer as I have?

In all this, we learn to be comfortable with not knowing rather than to grasp at "sure answers" that can't possibly address all the complexities of the life we lead in the twenty-first century. It's in the activity of "better questioning" that we learn to grow the roots that bind us to our planet earth. Better questions help us make that world better at its very roots. And these roots can be set in deep, rich soil that is life giving even if it's a bit messy. And just as important, we learn that the wings we fly with, the ones we use for seeing the Big Picture, are our own wings; and they are capable of taking us and others higher than we have ever dreamed. This movement, after all, is healthy spirituality.

In this chapter we addressed addiction as a physical and psychological process. Wayne discussed physical problems that substance abuse causes or contributes to. He also pointed out how the abuse of some substances creates physical addiction. Detox from physical addiction must be done very carefully or more physical problems can result. Gary helped us understand that much of our addictive experience is in our minds. Not all of them, of course, but we can go a long way in thinking differently about what we "need" and so change our experiences of dependency. He introduced several ways of seeking recovery, ranging from traditional AA groups to more independent ways of finding our way to a healthy dose of life.

Then Erik showed us, contrary to our typical training, that even the escape route of many addictions — our higher power — can become an addiction if we're not attentive. He suggested several ways of avoiding this while seeking recovery from other addictions. All in all, this chapter encourages us to be aware of ourselves in such a way that we don't give ourselves wholly over to a self-focus but rather think in terms of how we fit into a broader picture where we truly belong and need to be sober and alert to do our part.

Next we'll take a look at chronic illness. You'll see there are ways of dealing with it that do, in fact, lighten the burden.

Vitamins for Addiction

- There are many types of addictions and compulsions. You name it; we can become addicted to it.
- Physical effects destroy the addict's body and mind. The addict's behavior destroys his or her relationships.
- In physical addiction, the body develops a need for the addictive substance.
- Natural endorphins may be able to replace medicinal or recreational endorphins with their own opium-like substances. Physical activity promotes endorphins.
- Detox is only the first step in drug or alcohol rehab. Many addicts will require participation in long-term rehabilitation and medication.
- Addictive behavior serves a purpose, such as relief from stress and avoiding responsibility.
- There are many ways to seek treatment. See a therapist, check into a rehab center, participate in twelve-step groups like AA, NA, and GA, or use SMART. If you prefer to do it on your own, use the techniques in this book to change your DUMB thoughts to REAL ones and/or use RR.
- If your loved one is addicted and tends to get violent, plan escape routes and safe places to stay. Discuss your loved one's addiction in constructive ways using I-messages and detailing what you'll do when he or she is using, such as leaving the house to visit a friend. Join a group such as Al-Anon or SMART's CSO for support. Consider an intervention led by an addiction therapist.
- It's ironic, but true that certain types of belief in god can act on us like a drug.
- As in all dependencies, the religious addict believes that by doing more of the same, things will change. Religious addicts often find the only way to feel good about themselves is through their intolerance of others. Symptoms of religious addiction often revolve around an inability to think clearly about the benefits of religion.

(Cont'd.)

Vitamins for Addiction (Continued)

- The way out of religious dependence involves allowing oneself to experience being as whole as can be. When we neither judge others as less than ourselves nor judge ourselves as less than others, we find a way toward unconditional acceptance of ourselves and others despite imperfections. Rather than embracing the rigid truth of one's religion, one must see that a truth can be right and binding for oneself and yet not for another. Rather than isolation, one must value connection with those outside one's religious identity.

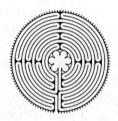

CHAPTER 8

WHEN LIFE SEEMS TOO MUCH: CHRONIC ILLNESS

I did as much research as I could and I took ownership of this illness, because if you don't take care of your body, where are you going to live?

— KAREN DUFFY

Dan Newburn was a young firefighter with a promising future. Life couldn't have been better. He was married to an intelligent, sensitive woman, and their first child was due soon. One day on the job, through no fault of his own, he suffered a devastating foot injury.

The doctors advised amputation — a career-ending procedure for a firefighter. The alternative would leave Dan crippled by a chronically deformed foot that he could never use.

Dan compared all he would no longer be able to do with all he had previously been able to do. There were about 200 physical activities he lost with his injury, but he still had 800 others he could do. He told the doctors he wanted to keep the foot and began a long, painful rehabilitation process. Vocational specialists looked for other work for him. But Dan couldn't give up on his dream: he wanted to remain a firefighter. Through his perseverance, alternative duties at the fire department were found. He also took advantage of every department educational opportunity.

Dan had always had a deep spirituality and strong core values, but his disability acted as a crucible that strengthened his "internal metal." It wasn't long before his fine character and leadership qualities became widely known. Today, Dan is the highly respected fire chief for the twenty-seventh largest department in the United States. What characterizes Dan is his belief that every crisis and every negative, whether a burning building or a crippled foot, are opportunities to make the world better. For him there are no chronic disabilities, only chronically available opportunities.

This chapter doesn't apply to you directly if you don't have a chronic illness and aren't a caretaker of a chronically ill person, but you may know someone to whom this chapter does apply. Share this chapter with that person if she or he is interested.

In this chapter we discuss medical management of chronic illnesses. We give advice for caregivers. We address where to put your focus: dwelling on the positive rather than dwelling on the problem, living the fullest life you can, and getting involved with others. You'll read some amazing stories of people managing their illness. Such stories are a tribute to the human spirit to be sure. And although spirituality may not cure, it strengthens our inner resolve, which makes the suffering manageable. Let's begin our discussion here, with the role of spirituality and chronic illness.

Optimism

Erik Mansager

You have to be an optimist, because the pessimists are right.

— HEINZ ANSBACHER

I know a sense of humor is a real help in coping with chronic illness, but still, it's no laughing matter. When faced with a chronic illness, in fact, we often find ourselves facing a brick wall. Having a chronic illness is one of the "barrier experiences" I mentioned in chapter 3. How can one ever explain to someone else the total unfairness of a cancer diagnosis, the seeming injustice of being struck with multiple sclerosis, the unfathomable hardships involved in living with HIV/AIDS, the unrelenting pain of any chronic illness?

Many of our religious ideas and perhaps whole religious traditions sprang from this very puzzle: why do bad things happen to good people? Surely many religious views developed from trying to make suffering understandable to the one suffering and to that person's loved ones. When we run into things, like chronic illnesses, that we just don't understand, we find ways to *make* them make sense. We tell our stories. The Hebrew Scriptures tells the story of Job, the Christian Scriptures make ultimate meaning out of Jesus' suffering, and the Buddhist Scriptures contain the Four Medicine Tantras, which teach adherents how to endure suffering.

Yet, although religious views satisfy many, for many others the questions persist. To fully appreciate this issue we'll need to search, and search hard, for its positive parts. And that isn't easy. No, life is tough. It can get us down, way down; that's for sure. I thought twice before changing my section heading to this chapter from my first idea: "Life's Hell: Then You Die." That, however, seemed altogether too pessimistic.

Then, I thought it might be appropriate to name this section after Rabbi Harold Kushner's 1981 bestselling book *When Bad Things Happen to Good People*. Kushner's very personal account of coming to terms with the fatal illness of his son Aaron is heartrending. The faith-filled rabbi showed great courage in grappling with an unanswerable question. In the end, he admits the issue of bad things happening is beyond him. I won't presume otherwise.

The quote above, "You have to be an optimist, because the pessimists are right," is vintage Heinz Ansbacher, a wise and kindly recently deceased psychologist who had cared for his beloved wife as she suffered the long death of Alzheimer's. Heinz shared the phrase while talking about the responses people make when coping with the complexity of life. Given these difficulties — the "hell," the "bad things" that keep happening — optimism is essential, he insisted, lest we give up on doing our part to make the world better. Call it hope if you want, but cultivating a "Here's what I can do about it" attitude is, from the spiritual perspective, both the starting point *and* a goal, at least when dealing with chronic illness.

In the following, I first tackle some of the negative aspects of chronic illness and what, from the spiritual perspective, we should avoid; then I share what good research tells us about spiritual coping with chronic illness.

Rewards or Punishments?

There are several very negative ways to understand chronic illness that share a reward-punishment theme. Some see personal health — along with abundant harvests, pleasant weather, and financial security — not so much as blessings but as personal rewards for staying within the guidelines of religious behavior. From this point of view illness is righteous punishment for *not* walking the narrow path, *not* following the right way. Not only do conservative mainline religions hold this outlook, but it also is found in any number of religious and spiritual books and websites.

The various religions differ on just why the illnesses occur and just what "not following the way" involves. Some of the more popular reasons include the following:

- Sufferers are not following commandments, edicts, rites, and the rituals faithfully enough.
- Suffering is evidence of "the sins of the parents being visited on their children."
- Suffering results from individuals daring to question god or be angry with god.

You also find similar themes in New Age spiritual guidance, where there is much said of the "oneness" of body and spirit. But this dualism — talking as if there are two parts to the individual — doesn't really mean "oneness." People who talk of "body and spirit" typically favor one (usually the spiritual) approach over the other (as if the body isn't quite as good). And if you've chosen the wrong horse (that would be your body), you are held fully responsible for any suffering you experience.

Those who suffer illnesses are too often held responsible for... you name it: being out of harmony with the universe, overemphasizing a *yin* aspect, or underemphasizing the *yang*. If ill persons would only "think right," if these people are to be believed, they would not experience the evils of bodily suffering. Whether from the Eastern point of view or the Western, too often the blame is the same: the ill person is of lesser value than the healthy person due in large part, they insist, to the ill person's own devices.

These "unholy" approaches to chronic illness are what spiritually oriented psychotherapist Daniel Helminiak (2001) says we must counter if mental health is to be part of established religion. There are many health-giving spiritual beliefs that we should *affirm*. Among these are belief in a loving god, trusting one's neighbors, and committing to honesty and compassion. Similarly, there are those beliefs we do better to *reinterpret* when they warp our interactions with others. These include neglecting work in hopes of a miracle, slavish obedience to the demands of a faith community, and the like.

More hotly debated but nonetheless important, Helminiak insists, is our *rejection* of wholly negative beliefs. Beliefs he thinks we ought to reject include blaming evil spirits for our misbehavior and forbidding ourselves to question god.

I hope I've said enough about the many downright mean attitudes and approaches you can find toward chronic illness. To say the least, they point out an "unwell" approach to spirituality that, in one form or another, keeps us from awareness. As I pointed out in chapter 3, they represent an arrogant attitude toward others and usually involve competitive striving and an inflexible insistence on narrow "truths." Luckily, this is far from the truth, the whole truth. There is another way to approach chronic pain in our lives.

Acceptance

Yes, there is another way to approach chronic illness, a beneficial way, one that doesn't blame the suffering individual. It's a positive way. It's the way of acceptance. Acceptance may not change the outcome of the illness, but it very well changes the quality of life that the chronically ill person experiences. "Quality of life" is a phrase I'll unpack in a bit for practical use. It appears in the medical literature for many issues that, when seen from a spiritual perspective, help deal with the toughest illnesses. For now let's explore the bad news and good news about research related to the spirituality of acceptance.

There has been much uproar about the prayer studies that have been conducted over the past five to ten years. Researchers have tried to prove that people who are prayed for, to get better, actually do — in some way or another. These studies haven't fared well under scrutiny, and many of them have been proven to be out and out hoaxes (see, for example, *Free Inquiry* magazine or its website, http://www.freeinquiry.com). In 2006, Benedict Carey of the *New York Times* reported that a "long-awaited medical study" seriously questioned the power of prayer. This comprehensive longitudinal study involved a group of 1,802 coronary bypass patients from six hospitals who were broken into three groups: two groups were prayed for; the third group was not. "Half the patients who received the prayers were told that they were being prayed for; half were told that they might or might not receive prayers," Carey reported.

The study, which originally appeared in *The American Heart Journal*, indicated that "a significantly higher number of patients who knew they were being prayed for — 59 percent — actually suffered *more* complications, compared with 51 percent of those who were uncertain." Carey also reported that the study "found that more patients in the uninformed prayer group — 18 percent — suffered major complications . . . compared with 13 percent in the group that did not receive prayers."

That's the *bad* news.

But I want to add that the study doesn't conclude that intercessory prayer is altogether ineffective. Rather, the problem with studying religion scientifically (according to Dr. Richard Sloan, a professor of behavioral medicine at Columbia, whom Carey quotes) is that by trying to reduce prayer to measurable elements you come up with something that doesn't look like prayer to anyone who actually prays.

The *good* news is that there has also been some really good science focused on religious and spiritual practices. By good science, I mean research that when done over and over reports very similar findings. Research on religious and spiritual practices almost always reveals positive results. For example, the *Handbook of Religion and Health* (Koenig, McCullogh, & Larson, 2001) reviewed practically all published research in the twentieth century related to religion and found statistically significant relations between religious and spiritual involvement and the following factors:

- better mental health
- improved well-being
- greater social support
- less substance abuse

Larimore, Parker, and Crowther (2002) also reported the findings of several studies that accurately predicted fewer heart attacks, reduced hypertension, higher rates of survival, and longer survival among religious patients.

So although the specific effect of intercessory *prayer* isn't measurable in scientific terms, the benefits of religious and spiritual *beliefs* on one's overall health are quite verifiable. And this applies directly to the chronically ill population as well. In one such group, Dr. Gail Ironson and her colleagues (2002) found four religious and spiritual factors to be significantly higher among long-term survivors of chronic illness than among their comparison group:

- sense of peace
- faith in god
- religious behavior
- compassionate view of others

These studies go on and on but I don't need to catalog them here. More important for those enduring chronic illness is the issue of quality of life and how spiritual awareness enhances it.

Quality of Life

Long ago, research on the effects of chronic illness identified four primary domains of well-being: physical, functional, social/family, and emotional. In more recent research, a fifth domain was added: spirituality. Attention to this domain has become necessary because of the baby boomer generation. When researchers ask people in this group about their religious standing, they tend to claim they are spiritual rather than religious. Where once religion was thought to have a uniform effect on those who adhered to it, the different expressions of peoples' spiritual journey have made it necessary to measure spirituality separately from religion.

As I've noted before, although many people's religion influences their spirituality, more and more people today practice spiritual exercises and travel a spiritual path quite apart from religion. This path is so different that researcher Dr. Amy Peterman and her colleagues (2002) developed a special scale to measure it as it relates to chronic illness patients.

In the remainder of my section I discuss the five domains that make up quality of life and comment on how spiritual awareness, by enhancing coping ability, enhances quality of life for the chronically ill person.

Spiritual

First let me visit the domain of spiritual well-being from Dr. Peterman's perspective. She and her colleagues found two dimensions of spirituality to be most important to their chronically ill patients. One dimension emphasizes "a sense of meaning in life, harmony, and peacefulness." This is quite in line with my earlier description of spirituality in chapter 3 as a meaning-making venture. But it also captures the *inward movement* of authenticity that I spoke of. It's in this movement that we root ourselves in a remembered past, one in which we functioned more or less effectively and learned much about who we are. This is called "agency" or "effectiveness." This understanding of ourselves is constantly challenged when we're faced with a chronic illness. Getting in touch with our "sense of meaning and harmony" enhances our well-being in many ways, as you'll see in the other domains.

The other aspect of spiritual well-being is "a sense of strength and comfort from the person's faith." This sense captures the *outward movement* of being connected to something greater than ourselves — a faith or set of spiritual beliefs, in Dr. Peterman's language. This is a future-oriented movement — a movement outward toward the "even now but not yet" sense of connectedness (Küng, 1976) with the world. In it we sense that life just isn't over until it's over, not until our last breath, our spirit, is gone.

Now let's see how this dual movement, *inward* and *outward*, past and future, remembering and anticipating, affects the other domains of our quality of life.

Physical

The domain of physical well-being deals with the number of physical symptoms you currently endure. The symptoms vary from illness to illness, but physical well-being depends on whether or not the symptoms interfere with your daily activities: are you "ambulatory" (can you get around on your own) or is bed rest (much or little) needed to get through the day?

Spiritually speaking you can *look inward* to what the symptoms mean to you.

- Are they helping identify who you are?
- Do they say something more about you than you've known about yourself in the past?
- Do you believe they make you less than what you are?

Pause here to reject any negative beliefs about physical symptoms being punishment for something you did. You've done nothing "deserving of" a chronic illness. Fate is mysterious; you can't explain it in terms of past events.

And from this perspective, you can *look outward* as well. Look boldly into the future with the strength of your convictions. Your symptoms, whether increasing your need for rest or not, are opportunities to see yourself differently. Might there be comfort in knowing you aren't alone in your illness? That, in spite of the possible incurability of your illness, "lack of cure" does *not* result from a lack of interest?

The medical and scientific communities, in fact, are united in seeking to cure you. This army of women and men, spanning the last several hundreds of years, is arrayed against your illness. You're not alone!

Functional

The domain of functional well-being deals with the quality of your normal daily activities and how well you participate in and enjoy them.

The spiritual *inward glance* looks at what you once were able to do.

- What does it mean to you that you're no longer as capable as you once were?
- Remember your earlier physical capabilities and sensibilities, or await a developing harmony with your newfound inner capabilities.
- Although not physical, these new capabilities may be more meaningful to you now.

Pause here to reject any negative beliefs about being only what you can *do*. We are *not* "human doings" but "human beings." Herein lies the opportunity to remember that you're more than the sum of your functioning — or malfunctioning — parts.

Then allow the *outward glance*, a glance into the future.

- Who knows what that will bring?!
- Might there eventually be a new, more effective treatment?
- Or is realism more useful at this stage and optimism out of place?
- Check again, perhaps optimism is still beckoning? Optimism that the future can and will be different from today.
- What skills will you need for that dawning future, what qualities and characteristics?

Patience is surely worth cultivating, along with "accepting what is unavoidable." But along with this might also come a fresh, plucky attitude that says: "In my future I can still be fully a part of, and can still experience, a rich life."

Social/Family

The domain of social/family well-being deals with support and communication with your social group and your loved ones.

Looking inward:

- Can you make sense out of the changes you notice in your support network?
- Can you understand the falling away of fair-weather friends?
- Can you feel the depth of concern from those true friends you never knew you had?
- Are you overly identified with your job, as you might have been with your capabilities? Your "do-abilities?"

Pause here to reject any negative beliefs about your worth if you base them on the number of people in your support system. It takes *quality*, not quantity, to enrich us.

Looking outward:

- Have you found any new support groups to be part of?
- Who is there to help you manage the difficulties?

The new community you find yourself in the midst of may be just the right substitute for the missing family members and friends who have fallen away from you over the long months (or years) of your illness.

Emotional

Finally, the domain of emotional well-being focuses on your moods and day-to-day emotional responses to your illness. In this domain, feel free to go wholly *inward*. Tune in to your all-encompassing moods at this point, but don't try to change them. Not yet.

- Get in touch with these structures and ask what they mean. What are they telling you? These moods are the structure of how you evaluate your overall quality of life.
- Have your moods changed from your healthy days of long ago?
- Are they darker than before, or are they, in fact, richly colored by an acceptance that lets you go with the flow?

Pause here to reject any negative beliefs about god punishing you with depression or feelings of despair. Such moods go with the territory, the illness, and are *not* measures of who you are in your totality. From here you may also find it possible to turn wholly *outward* with your emotions. Be aware that certain emotions are meant to join you with the larger meaning of things:

- joy that wants to be shared
- empathy that feels and appreciates that it is shared
- humility that makes room for others to share

Your *joy* of life, and the love you're still able to experience, shows that you're still capable of being part of the greater whole. Your empathy knows no bounds now. You understand the chronically ill who are experiencing what you're experiencing. At the same time, you know what the physically healthy are going through. They, like you so many years ago before you were ill, don't have a clue about what chronically ill people are going through. What delight it is to *empathize* with people as ignorant as you once were about chronic illness!

And surely the experience of *humility* isn't new to you! In due time, others may face what you're facing now. In that moment, allow them their space, wisely, gently, and willingly. Step aside and be ready to assist them as best you can, full of empathy, full of joy.

These are the domains that make up your quality of life. Spirituality, at its healthiest, informs them each and offers depth and expansion to each of them. In deepening and expanding your life — lived even in the face of chronic pain — you have the opportunity to make meaning, profound meaning, out of the otherwise unfathomable things of life.

Now let's take a look at what Wayne has to say about living with chronic illness.

Living with Chronic Illness

Wayne F. Peate

Everyone has an MS, a miserable something.

— JAMES HINE

The body-mind-spirit connection is particularly evident in those who suffer from chronic illnesses. The toll of dealing with pain and other symptoms, loss of control over body functions, hassles with getting and paying for medical care, dependency on other family members for assistance, and loss of self-esteem as one becomes "a person with _____" (fill in the blank with the disease).

Amid all the negatives are bright lights of hope. The most remarkable thing I've discovered as a physician is how different people handle the same illness. Although one becomes demolished in mind and spirit because of physical problems, another is invigorated by the challenge. Consider William Tang, M.D. As a boy in Singapore, he contracted polio. He became crippled from the waist down and wheelchair bound. I first met William on the Antarctic Marathon of 2007. His goal was to be the first person in a wheelchair to complete a marathon on the forbidding White Continent, a place where top athletes struggle to finish a twenty-six-mile race amid freezing temperatures, forty mile an hour winds that blow stinging ice crystals, dangerously slick glaciers on the course, steep hills, and treacherous mud that could pull off a shoe or mire a wheelchair wheel.

What sets William apart from others with a chronic illness who succumb to discouragement? Well, quite a long list, it turns out:

1. He never defines himself as a polio (or chronic disease) victim. He is William: "I'm here to finish the marathon."

2. Life is not for him a loss of "what might have been" if, for example, his legs worked. Rather life is a permanent adventure — he's going to be the first to complete a marathon in a wheelchair where no other human with similar restraints has dared try.
3. He doesn't quit; February 26, 2007, was his second attempt!
4. William has a community of support. This race, he brought his brother Albert along, who ran *his* first marathon in Antarctica!
5. He maintains a positive attitude in spite of setbacks. He was able to finish only half the marathon (blowing snow that decreased wheel traction made a full marathon impossible for him) but is already planning a return.
6. William always gives the credit for his accomplishments to others. After the race, when the marathoners reconvened back on the icebreaker that had brought them to the race site from Tierra del Fuego, William received a standing ovation. His response? His first words were how impressed he was with the accomplishments of the other runners and the support team.
7. In spite of what you might think, he's a happy person. He doesn't dwell on his chronic illness. His conversation, concerns, and joys are the same as others. As a fellow physician, he shared that it's tough to see enough patients these days to pay the bills, a universal concern among health care professionals.
8. He has a vigorous sense of humor that helps him not only to cope but also to build relationships with those around him — an important skill for the chronically ill, who must rely on others. On the icebreaker in Antarctica, space was at a premium. During the buffet dinners, it was a custom to let William go first in the line for ice cream. When he wheeled up to the large platter of ice cream scoops piled three feet high, he didn't take a single or double scoop. Instead he lifted the entire platter, placed it on his lap, and wheeled off with a "Thanks for letting me go first!" Any resentment for his "special" treatment vanished with the laughter of the other passengers.

For me, William's sense of humor captures what 1800s comedian Josh Billings said about medicine: "There ain't much fun in medicine, but there is a heck of a lot of medicine in fun."

There's no question about it: William is extraordinary. But so are patients I've had with chronic illness who have dealt with the most serious of conditions with ample doses of the body-mind-spirit connection. Think about William's ability to succeed as a happy, productive, balanced human being where others have failed. The key element is all mental. He's not a wheelchair-bound man blessed with biceps the size of tree trunks that enable him to race. His build is slight, though he has developed maximum strength with what muscles he does possess. He follows the great truth that your mind will give out before your body will IF you quit trying too soon because of attitude and never reach your potential. He knows that if he trains his mind to keep trying, his body will go the distance for him.

I've seen the mind use chronic illness as an escape. Many men (women seem less susceptible) use a serious illness as a long-awaited excuse to retire. Unhappy in their jobs, they practice bad health habits until they have a heart attack that buys them a ticket out of the work force. Hopefully, it isn't fatal. Their chronic condition is their badge of honor that allows them to quit with machismo. "Real" men don't just stop working; they need a life-threatening reason.

Once again the mind is in charge — even if you're unaware of your purpose or irrational beliefs, or DUMB thinking, as Gary would call it. Instead of saying: "How can I best live out my remaining years and make the best of them as long as possible by maintaining a healthy lifestyle my entire life?" they do everything they can to sabotage their doctor's and their family's hopes for them. Women seem to be more aware of the benefits of long-term health maintenance than men. They are also less in need of an excuse ("I had to quit because of my heart attack or diabetes") than men.

My strategy with men with chronic illness and health habits that will lead to a chronic condition is to find a trigger in their work life that relates to their longevity. An easy one is the manager approach. I'll tell someone in management that if their body were their business it would be bankrupt (high cholesterol, excess weight, and inadequate physical activity will lead to body failure). If they're into cars, I'll say to them that if their body were a car, it's about to blow an engine. The latter turns a health maintenance schedule into an auto maintenance program.

But what about those whose illnesses aren't only chronic but are also worsening? How does one use the body-mind-spirit connection in those cases? It's remarkable how many people with a terminal illness will hang on until a significant family event, say a grandkid's graduation or a milestone birthday. Clearly, it's mostly mental factors that help them hang in there.

The Chronic Illness Roller Coaster

What really discourages those with chronic illness is the disease roller coaster. Even though their condition is chronic, they have their good and bad periods. What gets many down is that during the better days, a faint hope that they'll recover builds. Then the bad days return, and a feeling of failure and hopelessness compounds the negative impact of those symptoms. Not all of us are a William, a remarkable chronic illnesses "thriver." And by thrive I mean he more than survives. Most of us need a toolbox of mind-spirit-body strategies to help us thorough the bumps on the illness roller coaster. Here are some things you can do:

Help others worse off than you or in need of something you have. Alton has a debilitating spine condition. He can barely get out of bed some days, the pain is so bad. Worse, he walks funny and he's embarrassed to be seen in public or to socialize for fear others will stare. Fortunately, he was encouraged to become a reading mentor. One hour a week he reads to a girl named Antonia from an impoverished neighborhood and school. Doing so has made all the difference for him and for her. He says, in spite of his illness, after meeting Antonia he feels incredibly lucky. He grew up in a stable home with supportive parents who encouraged him to learn and succeed in school. Her father is in jail and her mom has a host of social problems that limit her involvement in Antonia's education. Before Alton started working with her, she was a third grader reading at first grade level. Now she's reading above grade level and teaching Alton Spanish!

Value short-term successes. "Today I was able to go to the store myself and shop when most days I can't," said one patient. Honor success. Give yourself a reward. One woman buys herself a rose when she is able to meet a goal, no matter how small. "Sure the day was mostly a big pain in the patootie, but I made the best of it." She calls this "retail therapy."

Be you. "I'm not the heart attack in room 410." One of the toughest tasks for those with a chronic illness is not to be so identified with the illness that you become the guy with heart disease or cancer, instead of _____ (your name). Find an outside interest that has nothing to do with your illness: garden, write limericks, sing, write emails or letters, help others — just about anything will do.

Dealing with Chronic Pain

Normal pain sensors are like fire alarms that alert us to danger to our body. Chronic pain is the smoldering fire that never goes away and that flares red-hot unexpectedly. Unlike acute pain that resolves when the injury heals, chronic pain persists for months, for years, or for life. The cause of chronic pain is usually an injury, arthritis, infection, immune disorder, or cancer. Sometimes there is no identifiable cause; this is called "psychogenic pain." If there is damage to the nerve fibers, neurogenic pain occurs. Pain itself can cause permanent changes in nerve fibers in what is known as "wind-up" — a pathologic process that lowers the threshold for feeling pain. Those nerves then even begin to generate pain themselves. Once this occurs, it's difficult to eliminate chronic pain.

To make matters worse, chronic pain leads to stress, depression, and anxiety, which complicate pain treatment. If you're depressed, you're less likely to be engaged in pain management methods. If you're anxious, you'll feel pain more strongly. As a physician, I've ordered relaxation, acupuncture, biofeedback, medications, electrical stimulation, and surgery as well as cognitive behavioral and other therapies for my many chronic pain patients. Those who respond best have one thing in common, a powerful body-mind-spirit connection. If they feel supported psychologically by friends and family, they suffer less. This has to do with the issues of quality of life that Erik addressed above.

Scientific advances hold great promise for better treatment of chronic pain, including improved medications that are more selective at blocking pain with fewer drug-related side effects. Much prejudice exists about medication for chronic pain. An individual with diabetes or high blood pressure or asthma is rarely condemned for taking medication for life. Those on long-term pain medication are too often branded "addicts" or "weak." This lack of understanding leads to further discouragement — or worse. When I was a child, a neighbor suffered from chronic crippling back pain. The doctor's opinion was that medications were overused. Unable to cope, my neighbor committed suicide and left two young sons without a father.

Sometimes OTC (over the counter) medications help. Commonly used OTC pain medicines should be used with caution. Acetaminophen (Tylenol), if taken over the recommended amount, can cause liver failure. Nonsteroidal anti-inflammatory drugs (ibuprofen, naproxen, etc.) can lead to stomach ulcers and bleeding, and taken long term in large doses can damage the kidneys. Consult your health care provider on the use of OTC pain medications.

Guidelines for Caregivers, Friends, and Family

Chronically ill people wish to be accepted as people, not as sick people. William wants to be athletic like anyone else. And when he's treated as any other person crazy enough to do a marathon, the joy in his face is evident to all. One of my students has to miss class because of a cardiac condition. We've arranged a virtual classroom so she can experience lectures just like other students.

Sometimes you'll have to deal with anger — the chronically ill person's anger and yours. It's not easy being chronically ill. If the symptoms don't get you down, the treatment might. Medication side effects can be worse than the disease. Many chemotherapy patients after losing their hair, their energy, and sometimes their lunch from nausea wonder why they submit to taking drugs for their illness. Anger can well up at the loss of a bodily function, irritation at the health system, or the thinking that god gave them a sickness that won't go away. Anger can cause the release of body stress hormones and cause blood pressure and pulse to skyrocket.

The caregiver who is the recipient of an angry blast may retreat, attack back, or grow resentful. As Gary said in chapter 5, you can't control the other person's anger, but you can control your response. Reflect back on an anger episode. What was it that triggered the response? Was the ill person feeling helpless? Many chronically ill patients say they feel upset because they lack control. Consider chronic pain for example. Fortunately, we now have battery operated pain control units for pain patients that allow them to manually increase a pain-blocking electric impulse to an electrode on the hurting part of their anatomy. They are in control, and as a result most report greater satisfaction with their treatment experience. If you identify the reasons for the anger, you can respond more effectively next time and perhaps even prevent the occurrence. You learned some response techniques in chapter 5.

It's essential to not force your opinions on the ill. An angry explosion or seething resentment will often follow. You may be more likely at such times to express your growing opinion: "Dad you need to be in a nursing home. I can't keep coming over here to bail you out!" Instead of trying to force him into a nursing home, a visiting caregiver may suffice for now. Think it through in advance: How much can you help? How much help does the other actually need? How will you explain all this to the ill person?

Connect in a positive way with chronically ill people. If you're resentful, condescending, and uninterested in your interactions with the ill, they're likely to respond in kind. Recent research by Dr. Daniel Goleman, the author of *Emotional Intelligence* (1995), has detected what neurologists call "mirror neurons." These act like wireless receivers between two people. They allow us to hold a conversation. When two people really connect, these neurons are working at their best. If patients surmise that the provider really is interested, is paying attention, truly cares, then they are more likely to comply with treatment recommendations, to believe the plan for them will work.

I usually make a comment about the T-shirt or other garment the patient is wearing as a way of connecting with the person, not the illness. Another strategy I use is to ask: "What are you doing for fun?" This often brings them out of their illness and helps me reconnect with them as a fellow human and not as a diagnosis. My interest is also selfish; I've learned lots about the world and its happenings because of my patients' hobbies, travels, volunteerism, vocations, and child rearing. It's too easy to assume that physical illness means mental decay. Maintain a respect for the person within or, as Erik reminded us, the soul, the "you," who persists through any sickness.

Another way to encourage chronically ill people is to let them do what they are capable of doing. If they make a request to do something, decide if their request is a preference or a safety issue. If it's a preference, then your answer is to let them decide. For example, the person can choose what to wear, how to arrange the room, and where to spend waking hours. Your help allows the person to have more energy for what she or he enjoys or can do for herself or himself. The attitude then is "I'm here to help you as much or as little as you decide." Professor emeritus Walter St. John of the University of Arizona says: "Never do for others what they can and should do for themselves."

On the other hand, expect role reversal. It's hard to deal with parents and friends whose physical and mental functions become more childlike and dependent every day — unlike your own children who become more adultlike and responsible. Chronic illness can also consume the entire family, young and old alike. It's likely you'll feel underappreciated.

It's also irritating if your loved one's illness is self-inflicted. This seems to be why breast cancer research, for example, gets more financial support than lung cancer research. Those with lung cancer may have smoked, and therefore some think: "They deserve lung cancer, and now I'm stuck with caring for them!" In reality, 15,000 to 22,000 cases of lung cancer each year in the United States (nearly 10 percent) aren't related to tobacco — radon is the most common cause in these cases (National Cancer Institute, Radon and Cancer: Questions and Answers, 2004).

Those with a chronic illness will have plenty of questions. How do you answer effectively? Many times you need more time to respond or to get help. For example, they may ask you health questions. If you don't know the answer, you could say: "I'm sorry I don't know that. But I'll help you find someone who does know." Sometimes they ask you something that requires an answer that, at the moment, you don't have time to deal with. You could say: "You've said something that's important. Let's take care of what you need now and we can talk about that _____ (state a time that works for you)." Sometimes the person actually has the answer or is able to take care of the situation. Ask: "What do you think you can do?"

The chronically ill will complain. Expect it. You'll need to respond even if you don't think their issue is legitimate. They may say things like: "It's all wrong!" "What are you going to do about it?" Don't interrupt. Sometimes just having the complaint heard is enough. If need be, ask for clarification: "Help me understand the part about the doctor keeping you waiting because he had an emergency." Listen to the feeling as well as the facts: "Sounds like you feel devalued because you had to wait."

If the complaint is real, answer how you'll respond and when. Don't leave them hanging. People often can accept bad news; they don't like to be ignored, however. Be honest: "I can't promise the nursing home will fix that, but I promise to ask that they do."

Now the tough question: those with terminal illnesses will want to know how long they have to live. As a physician I can tell you that our profession has made some whopper mistakes. Doctors told a friend of mine he would die of tuberculosis by the time he was fifteen. He made it another fifty years! You can respond: "I don't have a crystal ball, but let's get your affairs in order and get answers for you from those who might know."

In spite of the hassles, many have said that caring for the chronically ill has been an uplifting experience. One friend said: "I never really understood Mom until I cared for her. Now it all makes sense and I love her more for it." Another, after being the caregiver at home for his mother, chose to become a nurse.

The Latest and Greatest Research

Erik's reference to the army of women and men being arrayed against your illness couldn't be truer. Exciting developments are occurring in chronic illness therapies, including stem cell use for spinal cord injuries, diabetes, Parkinson's, and Alzheimer's; pancreas islet cell transplants for diabetes; and numerous chronic pain control modalities that block pain receptors tormenting patients.

Stanford scientists have used functional magnetic resonance imaging (fMRI) scans to let people with chronic pain see their individual brain function. As mentioned in chapter 7 on addiction, certain parts of the brain light up during fMRI when you experience certain feelings. Once patients see their brain activity, they can improve their level of pain by 40 percent. Dr. Sean Mackey at Stanford believes that someday we'll be able to go to a multidisciplinary pain center and use such imaging techniques to treat other conditions such as phobias, addiction, and depression (Conger, 2005).

Next, Gary will discuss more ways to use your mind to deal with chronic illness. He gives some examples of amazing people who have taken charge of their illness.

Taking Charge of Your Illness

Gary D. McKay

Attitude

Whatever may be next,
"We'll see about that!" she says to herself.
It all started with a simple question
About a just diagnosed obscure, rare disease.
"How do you spell that?" she asked the Gastroenterologist.
"Oh, you'll never find it."
Surprised, she asked what he meant.
He said, "You know, on the Internet."
"I just want to know how to spell it." was her outside response.
But, inside she thought,
"We'll see about that!"
Numb and exhausted with yet another not good news appointment,
She listened with her husband as the
Oncologist said, "The usual survival rate is 6 months to 24."
Later, she thought,
"We'll see about that!"
Tired from the surgery and PT, she heard the
Orthopedic surgeon say,
"You'll never drive a stick shift car."
And, somewhere within, the familiar refrain

Once more surfaced so loud and clear:
"We'll see about that!"
So now it is 20 months out from the
6-24 months range and the PET scan is clear.
As I drove to the appointment in my old stick shift car
And, as I incorporate the Best of the West
With the Best of the East on a daily basis,
I say to myself,
Whatever may be next,
"We'll See About That!"

(VICKI STRAUB, AUGUST 2006)

"We'll see about that!" Vicki, what a woman — she really has attitude! But it's a great attitude; she has a chronic illness, but she won't let it defeat her. You met my good friend Vicki Straub in chapter 2 when she talked about using imagery to deal with illness. Later in this chapter, Vicki shows you how she uses imagery to combat her latest challenge. For now, let's continue on how attitude helps you out.

Although you are able to do only so much medically for your chronic illness, what you do psychologically and spiritually is your choice. You can choose to dwell on the problem or see it as a challenge and focus on other aspects of your life. You can see your situation as terrible, or you can see it as frustrating and inconvenient, but not awful. You can tell yourself that you can't stand it, or you can believe that although it's certainly not pleasant, you can tolerate it. You can concentrate on how this should not have happened to you, or you can tell yourself that although you would wish this on no one, it did happen and you'll manage it. Blaming gets you nowhere either — whether you blame god, life, yourself, or someone else.

If you find yourself slipping into anger or depression or anxiety, use the techniques to challenge your DUMB thoughts. Concentrate on developing REAL thoughts: Re-evaluate your demands, Eliminate excuses, Accept disappointments, and Let go of blame.

You can say: "I have a disability." Or you can say: "I have the ability to . . ." You can choose to concentrate on your abilities and how to use them to enrich your life.

If you have a chronic illness or have a loved one or friend with one, how will you make the most of your life or help the other make the most of his or her life? Will you sit or lie around feeling sorry for yourself and become depressed? This is certainly easy to do when one's facing physical challenges. Or will you decide to dwell on other, positive aspects of your life?

Remember the example of Mattie from the introductory chapter — the boy with muscular dystrophy? Mattie chose to look on the plus side of his life. He was an International Ambassador for the Muscular Dystrophy Association. He wrote poetry, worked for peace, and had quite a sense of humor. The short time that he was with the world, he contributed greatly to it.

There are examples of many other well-known people who have chosen to concentrate on their abilities. The late actor Christopher Reeve fought from his wheelchair for stem cell research. Actor Michael J. Fox, who has Parkinson's disease, continues the stem cell research crusade.

Paralyzed from the waist down, Franklin Roosevelt depended on a wheelchair, yet he served as president of the United States from 1933 until he died in office in 1945. If Roosevelt had concentrated on his paralysis rather than his task as president, would he even have been president?

Of course you don't have to be famous to dwell on the plus side of your life. In addition to Vicki, I have other friends with chronic illnesses. One friend was in a severe car accident when he was a young man that left him physically challenged. He has to walk with a cane and drag his legs. Yet he teaches school and has acted in amateur theater.

Another friend is near eighty as I write this book. He's been on oxygen for several years. Yet he does whatever he can as long as he can conserve his energy. He is still driving as well as giving presentations for a local counseling group.

THE AMAZING STORY OF ROSE SIGGINS:
A WOMAN WITH HALF A BODY

Rose (Rosemarie) Siggins was born with sacral agenesis, a rare disease that affected her legs. Rose's legs were amputated when she was two years old. She "walks" on her arms, or sits on a skateboard to get around. For longer distances, she drives a car. In fact, she's very interested in cars and restored a 1968 Mustang that she uses as a race car. Using her arms to walk has caused some cartilage, joint, and bone problems. So eventually, she'll probably need to use a wheelchair. She doesn't like this, but she'll handle it.

Yes, Rose is an amazing woman who sees her ability rather than her disability. "A lot of people with disabilities feel that life owes them something, and I was raised in a way that, no one owes you a dime.

The world doesn't owe you anything. This is what you have, and you use your resources, and you get through life. My personal opinion is, get up and go for it; just do it," says Rose. And she does "just do it"— whatever she can do, she does.

Rose is married and has a son. When she got pregnant, she was endangering her life to keep the baby. Yet she decided to risk it and told her mother that if it came down to a choice of saving her life or the baby's, she wanted the baby saved. But it didn't come to that. She had an unusual risky type of caesarean delivery. The baby survived and so did she. In fact, Rose is the only one with her disease known to give birth.

A few years later, Rose's mother got terminal cancer and died. Her mother had been the caregiver to Rose's father, who had schizophrenia, the beginnings of Alzheimer's, and dementia. Her brother lives in the house and is mentally handicapped and sometimes has violent outbursts. Now Rose has had to take over as caregiver. She and her husband, Dave, and their son, Luke, moved into the family home. Her father also developed emphysema soon after Rose took over.

She had all these challenges, and along with the support of her husband, she met them! Whatever challenges Rose has in the future, with her health or with her family, with her positive attitude, we're sure she'll handle them (Channel Five Broadcasting, UK, 2005).

Techniques for Managing Your Illness

First, learn all you can about your disease. With greater knowledge comes more control. Ask your doctor, read books, go on the Internet. Support groups teach you about your condition as well as provide encouragement and ideas. Do what you can for yourself; this will help your caretaker. Caretakers can get overwhelmed trying to take care.

Psychologist Dr. Vijai P. Sharma suggests six tips for managing your illness:

1. Accept your illness. That word, "acceptance," gets under the skin of people who are still mourning the loss of better, happier days when [they] were far more capable [of] doing things. Those who make an effort to adapt to their circumstance understand the value of acceptance. They know it helps them to get over loss and meet the new challenges they face.

2. Like yourself as you are today, with all your problems, illnesses, limitations, and of course, your physical appearance.

3. Get over the "Why me?" attitude so you can solve the problems of today. It might be, for example, the problem of how you could be more comfortable while lying in bed or how you could still get some exercise in spite of a knee hurting so much. In order to look at the problem of today, you have to stop staring at the past and the future.
4. Take total responsibility for your health and never overlook all the help you can get.
5. Become an expert on your illness.
6. Take pride in what you can accomplish today, and don't shame yourself over what you can't.

Dr. Sharma has a helpful website: Mind Publications (http://www.mindpub.com). The section on chronic illness has several articles on various aspects of chronic illness: http://www.mindpub.com/topic16.htm.

Use ideas you've learned from earlier chapters; for example, in chapter 2 I mentioned several ways to handle your DUMB thoughts and purposes. In addition to disputing those thoughts and purposes and turning them into REAL thoughts and positive purposes, I talked about techniques like reframing.

Reframing involves finding the positive in the negative or the opportunity in the obstacle. Although your disease is certainly not positive, you can look at it in a more positive way. As Wayne said, don't identify yourself as the disease. Instead of telling yourself: "I am diabetic," reframe and say: "I have diabetes." "I am diabetic" seems to indicate a description of who you are. You're more than diabetic; you are a person with strengths and weaknesses. You have diabetes; diabetes doesn't have you. Thinking this way lets you get on with your life despite the annoying inconvenience of diabetes. When you reframe, concentrate on what you can do rather than what you can't do. So, how can you use reframing to handle your disease? Think about what you could do that would be useful to yourself and to others. For example, if you're in a wheelchair with limited ability to get out and about or housebound for another reason, volunteer to make phone calls or send emails for your church or a charity.

We've discussed how important a sense of humor is to a productive life. President Roosevelt was known for his sense of humor and his positive attitude, which this quote demonstrates: "When you get to the end of your rope, tie a knot and hang on." In the chapter on humor, we discussed ways to develop your sense of humor. What funnies can you find in your life?

You can relieve the stress you experience with your disease by using deep breathing and relaxation. Use the breathing exercise in chapter 2. Do whatever you find relaxing, such as relaxation exercises, taking a warm bath, watching your favorite TV program, or reading.

Imagery helps too. As stated in chapter 2, Vicki Straub, Ph.D., used imagery to deal with a hysterectomy as well as a chronic liver disease — autoimmune cholangitis. Other conditions have developed since that time. In addition to medication and imagery, Vicki uses a guided imagery tape — *Positive Imagery for People with Cancer* by Emmett E. Miller, M.D. — relaxation exercises, meditation, and activities like writing poetry and exercising to manage her current challenges, including stage 4 breast cancer. She's also in touch with her spirituality through the help of a friend who's a retired Methodist minister.

Vicki says she uses "... the best of the East and the best of the West. Every day I am involved in imagery at some level." She envisions animals that will attack her cancer cells, such as raptors, owls, eagles, hawks, blue jays, and other birds of prey with excellent eyesight and vigilance as well as bears, cougars, wolves, and elephants. Here's her story:

> *I begin my imagery session by putting on a CD of relaxing music. I use deep breathing and relaxation exercises and then I imagine a quiet place, take myself there mentally, step into the scene, and feel healthy and strong. Taking that healthy feeling, I go to a control center in my body, imagine what cancer cells look like and instruct my raptors and other creatures to see what the disorganized cancer cells look like. This is what the white cell cancer fighting imagery animals monitor for, dispose of, and keep in check. The final part of the imagery is seeing the future with myself looking, feeling, and being healthy. I remind myself to send this message to my immune system throughout the day. I also send a message of following through with the day-to-day decisions that are consistent with the future I am moving towards.*
>
> *I go to the gym about three times a week, eat a low fat diet, keep my weight reasonable, am socially involved, take rest breaks during the day, and consciously do creative things to help express experiences in as rich a way as possible. I*

refuse to whine and I refuse to only focus on what is wrong with me — that's not what life is about.

Imagery has not become something I do. It has become who I am: constantly being aware of the present with all of my senses, writing and painting on a regular basis and often with a fervor and passion that has to be expressed. Sharing with significant others, reading my poetry, giving my art to others and connecting with others vs. isolating myself is also a part of the coping mix of strategies and tools.

We've discussed how to apply reframing, humor, deep breathing and relaxation, and imagery in dealing with chronic illness. There are additional things you can do, such as exercising, sharing your feelings, and developing your spirituality.

Exercise increases your energy and lessens the stress you experience with the limitations on your life because of your disease. Do whatever you can do to increase your strength. Remember Wayne's story of wheelchair-bound William and the Antarctic marathon? It's a very inspiring story. Although he couldn't finish the race due to wind-blown snow, he did his best.

If you're having a bad day, share your feelings with someone who's willing to listen and sees alternatives. This helps you gain a different perspective on the problem you're facing.

Get in touch with your spiritual dimension — prayer and meditation help. The labyrinth experience discussed in chapter 3 can help you get in touch with your spiritual side, and reflect on your quality of life as Erik suggested earlier in this chapter.

Courage — The Bottom Line

The word "courage" is derived from the French word *coeur*, which means "heart." So when one has courage, one has heart — heart in the sense that you're willing to make the most of your situation. If you're facing a chronic illness or have a loved one with such a condition, how can you bolster your heart, your courage, to meet the challenges? Each of the people we've talked about possesses courage — they couldn't survive without it. For example, Rose Siggins decided she would lead as normal a life as possible given the fact that she has no legs. Vicki Straub combines medication with imagery and other activities to battle her breast cancer.

Courage means you don't give up or give in to your challenges. Senator John McCain, in his book *Why Courage Matters* (2004), tells stories of soldiers and other people who have met challenges that most of us would consider overwhelming. If you have a chronic illness, you can choose to see it as your enemy and keep it at bay. Although you may not be able to defeat your enemy, you can keep it from entering your positive territory or you can keep it in jail, so to speak, and you control the keys!

On the back of McCain's book there is a statement about courage:

> We're all afraid of something. Some have more fears than others. The one we must all guard against is the fear of ourselves. Don't let the sensation of fear convince you that you're too weak to have courage. Fear is the opportunity for courage, not proof of cowardice . . .

As McCain says: "We're all afraid of something." Perhaps we're afraid of what our illness is doing or will do to us. But if we give in to the fear, what happens to the quality of our life? Battle the illness: focus on what you can do, not what you can't. Have attitude — as Vicki said: "We'll see about that!"

In this chapter we've tackled the challenging condition of chronic illness. Erik told us of studies on the limited effects of prayer but reminded us of the undeniable strength of personal faith. He reminded us also of the power of spiritual beliefs, positive thoughts, and positive actions — all of which you can call on for dealing with such a challenge. Wayne and Gary emphasized the power of a positive mental attitude in managing a chronic illness. The amazing stories of people like William, Rose, and Vicki are most encouraging because they show that one can have quality of life even when there are limitations.

In the final chapter, we'll take a look at the future and what awaits us all there: aging. With aging may come the very chronic illnesses we've been dealing with here. But other, more positive things can come as well — grandchildren for some and other great joys as well. We can fear the future, or we can look forward to it (pardon the pun)!

Vitamins for Chronic Illness

There are many health-giving spiritual beliefs that we should affirm. There are beliefs we do better to reinterpret when they warp our interactions with others. There are also wholly negative beliefs we do well to reject.

- Research on religious and spiritual practices reveals positive results, such as better mental health. Four religious and spiritual factors are stronger in survivors of chronic illness: a sense of peace, faith in god, religious behavior, and a compassionate view of others. Two dimensions of spirituality are most important to chronically ill patients: a sense of meaning in life and a sense of strength and comfort from the person's faith.
- Chronic pain can be managed in a number of ways. Those who respond best have one thing in common: a powerful body-mind-spirit connection.
- If you are the caregiver of a chronically ill person, sometimes you'll have to deal with the person's anger and yours. Connect in a positive way with chronically ill people. Let them do what they are capable of doing. They will have plenty of questions; assure the person you will do your best to find an answer. When the chronically ill complain, respond even if you don't think the issue is legitimate. Don't leave them hanging.
- Although you are able to do only so much medically for your chronic illness, what you do psychologically and spiritually is your choice.
- Learn all you can about your disease. With greater knowledge comes more control. Instead of identifying yourself with the disease, reframe. Concentrate on what you can do rather than what you can't do.
- Humor can defuse frustrating health situations. Deep breathing, relaxation, imagery, and exercise also help. Share your feelings with someone who's willing to listen and sees alternatives. Consider how you can bolster your courage to meet the challenges.

THE AGING CURE: MAKING IT WORTH THE WRINKLES

Minister and couples and family therapist, James R. Hine, Ph.D., one of our guest authors, at the time of writing the following story, was ninety-four and still taught, preached, and wrote. We lost him in 2006 at the age of ninety-six — what a long and fruitful life! Jim maintained a positive outlook evidenced by a lively sense of humor, staying mentally active with his work, physically active with golf as long as he could, and socially connected with his faith community.

Every evening when there weren't clouds in the way (which was often, as he lived in Tucson, Arizona), Jim gazed at the heavens and let his mind explore and feel the joy of being part of the grand design of the universe. His creativity flowed and his gratitude grew for the years he had enjoyed. He started each day renewed for another adventure in living. Jim had and overcame two bouts of prostate cancer, so he wasn't blessed with perfect health. What Jim had was the ability to kick out the negative and focus on the positive. He also whistled. "It's hard to feel down when you whistle," he told me. Try it. Any tune will do.

Jim's personal story below is a compelling example of the interaction between the three dimensions.

Jim's Story: "Miles to Go Before I Sleep"
Rev. James R. Hine

During the spring of 1988, I came to a turn in my life that took me down a road that I had not anticipated. I might add that I was not sure I was prepared to take it. The story of the life of my family consisted of good health and long lives. I was seventy-nine at the time and had passed the normal life span for most men. I wanted more — many more years. My father died when he was almost ninety-six, my mother's life ended at ninety-one, and my brother lived to be ninety-five. I wanted to surpass them.

It all began at the time of an annual checkup. My very good friend, Dr. George King, upon examining me, detected what he thought was a problem with my prostate gland. He knew a specialist he hoped would see me — a Dr. George Drach, head of neurology at the University Medical Center in Tucson. It was arranged. Dr. Drach examined me and set up a time for testing. It was on that spring morning with my wife, Janet, at my side that the results came in. I had cancer.

On my way from the hospital to our car, my legs were numb and my brain was whirling. Janet supported me and we drove home. No one in our family had ever had cancer. I was the first. Questions came flooding into my mind. I knew the statistics. This kind of cancer was fatal in many cases. What would it mean for me? How much time did I have? Was there any hope for a cure?

As a minister and a therapist I had helped many persons in their times of illness. I had held the hands of those who were departing this earthly life, giving them comfort. Now what could I do — or anyone do — for me? I was not afraid of death for I had faith in a god whose nature is love, and I was safe in his love. However, I wanted to live longer, much longer. I had posted a line from Robert Frost on my desk where I could see it every day: "I have promises to keep and miles to go before I sleep."

I have a strong Christian faith. The Bible is very meaningful to me. I pray every day. Now what does this have to do with my physical condition? It seemed right that I should pray about it. Maybe this was not the kind of prayer I should have prayed, but it came out of my desperate desire to get well: "God, I have tried to serve you all my life, now what are you going to do for me?"

I am constantly mulling over my concepts of God. They have changed since my childhood when I thought of God as sitting on a throne up in the sky, from which on occasion God would intervene in some way in the affairs of the world. Now God was not some object "up there" but a living Presence — a Spirit living around me and within me. In the coming of Jesus into the world of humanity, I see God, as did the writer in John 1:1,14, "In the beginning was the Word, and the Word with God, and the Word was God . . . And the Word became flesh and lived among us, and we've seen his glory, the glory as of a father's only son, full of grace and truth." In his early life, and in his resurrected life, Jesus helps me know what God is like.

Now, I ask, would my Christian faith have something to do with my possible healing? Would it be through prayer? If so, how should I pray? I turned to the Bible and read the stories of Jesus as a healer. I read books and articles — Norman Cousins's *Anatomy of an Illness*, and Dr. Bernie Siegel's *Love Medicine and Miracles*. Dr. Siegel's book contains the story of his years of experience with cancer patients. His conclusion is that attitudes, habits, and the spiritual condition of people have much to do with the healing process and possible cure of their illnesses. He maintains that love is a powerful stimulant to the immune system. Miracles can happen to patients who have the will to love and the courage to work with their doctors to participate in and influence their own recovery.

I decided to use all the resources at my disposal to participate in and influence the healing of my body. I was fortunate to have Dr. Drach, a devout member of a Lutheran church in Tucson. To be with this kind, gentle, encouraging physician was a blessing in itself. He decided to start by having me use a drug that had shown some promise in reducing tumors in the prostate. Weeks passed and I began to improve physically. There was a spiritual change, also. I came closer to God.

My religious faith would help me, and I was determined to cooperate with my doctors in every way possible. I was fortunate to have an internist who, along with Dr. Drach, helped me in many ways. I would take my medications faithfully. I would exercise as prescribed by my physical therapist. I would eat a diet of healthy foods.

When I am in my car alone, I do something that I can't do elsewhere. I sing, mostly hymns, but other songs occasionally. I know all verses to "Our God, our help in ages past . . . " I like to read and write poetry. Once when I was ill with a head and chest cold, I composed a poem about a relationship I had with a girl named "Flu." There is therapy in poetry that can be found nowhere else. In this case, I tried to see the humor in my misery. While visiting in Santa Fe in 1993, I enrolled in a watercolor class. This brought about another profound change in my life. I became passionate about painting, and it has been great therapy for me ever since. I paint cards and send them to cheer up my friends. I organized a class of beginners who wanted to learn how to paint. I find great satisfaction in teaching, and I still teach a correspondence course for the University of Arizona. All of these activities help me anticipate the serendipities that I hope will occur in the future.

Soon after I discovered I had cancer, I started a practice of going out under the open sky to pray before going to bed. Viewing the moon, the stars, and the expanse of the sky gave a new dimension to my soul.

First, I would sing the doxology, and then utter a great prayer of thanksgiving for another day of life. Then I would remember the people who I knew needed help, then say a prayer for Janet and me and our family. Now I could lie down in peace.

Five years ago, Janet had a heart attack. This was a new challenge. I have become her caretaker, and I believe this has been good for me. She took care of me for so many years; now I could take care of her. I have also tried to help others, some who are having problems with cancer, others with family problems. For me the Bible has it right: in loving others, one comes to know God.

After about eight years of my being under his care, Dr. Drach left for a position in a hospital in Texas. I was losing a friend and a wonderful physician. At that time, I heard that Dr. Frederic Ahmann was receiving patients with prostate cancer in a program he was conducting at the university cancer center. I applied and was accepted. What a marvelous serendipity this turned out to be. In Dr. Ahmann, I found a man who had some of the same qualities as Dr. Drach: compassion, a good sense of humor, and proficiency in his field. At the very start, he showed a profound interest in helping me. At first he said: "We will just watch your condition with periodic checkups." In the year 2000, he noticed that my PSA [prostate-specific antigen] count was rising. It continued to rise until he said: "You have two choices, radiation or do nothing." He told me if I chose radiation, I would have to go five days a week for seven weeks for treatment. The treatments would weaken me. At my age, could I do that? After much thought and prayer, I chose radiation.

My experience during those seven weeks was dramatic. I approached my first day with a feeling of fear and dread. It turned out to be a period of spiritual growth. It was partly the discipline of the daily routine. It was sitting with others each morning waiting our turn to go under the big machine. Here we would share our experiences in attempting to get well. One wheelchair-bound woman made a fifty-mile round trip every day. We all cheered when someone completed treatments. The radiologists and nurses, whom we came to know fairly well, were cheerful and encouraging. Days passed and graduation time arrived. I received my diploma and gave gifts to my therapists. It was like saying goodbye to old friends. I realized more than ever that one's healing was the result of many people working together — a community effort.

It was a month later I went in to hear the results. My heart was beating rapidly. Dr. Ahmann gave the announcement: "It is working!"

It was a time for thanksgiving — to God and to all of God's servants along the way for answering my prayers. My cancer can't be eliminated, but it can be kept in remission for a longer period of time. Dr. Ahmann and I have joined in a covenant. He says he will watch over me, and if I follow his advice from now on, I might surpass the span of life of my family and possibly live to be a hundred. I will do my part, and I am confident he will do his.

Fifteen years have passed since the day I received the news that life was going to be different for me from then on. And that difference has deepened and enriched my life. And now again, I have "promises to keep and miles to go before I sleep."

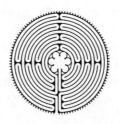

CHAPTER 9

SEE WHAT TOMORROW BRINGS: AGING AND PLANNING ·FOR THE FUTURE

If I had known I was going to live this long, I'd have taken better care of myself.

— GEORGE BURNS

Unless you die young, one thing is for sure — you're going to get older. "Okay," you may think, "I'll read this chapter when I'm old; no need to read it now." Not true. Preparing for "old age" is like preparing for anything in life. Although you're probably in your thirties or forties as you read this book — that's the age of many people who read self-help books — how you handle the fact that you will age and how you plan for it is what counts.

A healthy diet helps you age better. Physical activity is medicine: exercise delays the onset of osteoporosis, certain cancers, and heart disease — even eighty-year-olds with modest strength training can reverse loss of flexibility, strength, and balance. The more you stay in motion, the more chances you have for healthy aging. With the future will come advances in medicine, and there will be more treatments and cures for what ails ya.

Exercising your mind is also important. As Wayne said in chapter 1, keep learning: the sharper your mind, the happier your life. Your attitude will also help you create happier advanced years. Staying connected through group activities, volunteering, and support groups if needed also improves attitude.

Spirituality and the future are synonymous. Whether you believe in god or have another form of spirituality, your spiritual beliefs will continue to comfort and give meaning to life as you advance in years.

In this chapter, we not only deal with the future and aging, we discuss preparing for the future by living in the here and now, noting the power of expectations, pursuing the positive and negating the negative.

Expectation Management

Wayne F. Peate

I don't feel old in my head, but darn that mirror!
— Molly Peate

Ask elderly persons how old they feel they are and many will say: "I feel like I'm still twenty-five." Others can't even remember their name or the item they just went to the kitchen to get. A patient once told me that you're never so aware of who you are and how much your brain defines you as when you age and you're fearful of losing your identity through memory loss. In my section of this chapter, I discuss this fear by addressing both the bad news — including the brain difficulties related to aging — and the good news about preventing the difficulties. All along the way, I talk about what we can do to prevent brain decline.

"Old-Timers' Disease"?

Did you know that nearly half of those over the age of eighty-five suffer from Alzheimer's disease — a condition of brain destruction that causes loss of memory and ability to solve problems? Alzheimer's affects 4 million in the United States and that number will increase fivefold in the next four decades (Alzheimer's Facts and Figures, 2007). If the brain were a bunch of highways all sending cars with passengers with information to share with other parts of the brain, Alzheimer's would be the traffic jam. Amyloid plaques — or brain speed bumps that slow traffic — block brain messages. In Alzheimer's, signals between the brain and body get delayed. Risk factors for Alzheimer's include aging, smoking, a sedentary lifestyle, genetics, and risks to the cardiovascular system including obesity, poor diet, and high blood pressure.

Brain Calisthenics

Want to avoid Alzheimer's effects? Give your brain a regular workout. The Nun Study (Snowdon, 2001) has shed some fascinating light on the aging brain. A group of 678 nuns from the School Sisters of Notre Dame in the United States was chosen because they lack unhealthy habits such as drug abuse that harm the brain, they keep a diary (a useful tool to measure complexity of thought, such as vocabulary and logic), and they live in the same community. Also, the nuns agreed to an autopsy upon their deaths, the only sure way to diagnose Alzheimer's.

One nun had the most surprising story. She taught all her life and after retirement kept her mind active with mentally challenging activities. None of her colleagues in the nunnery reported that she had any mental lapses. After she died, her autopsy showed that her brain was riddled with Alzheimer's. The conclusion was that her history of working out the brain had built up mental reserves that counterbalanced her Alzheimer's. So as I said in chapter 1, the mind is like a muscle: keep it built up and it's always ready for action. If one muscle is injured, sometimes other muscles pick up the slack. So it goes with the brain, if one part is damaged another might have the potential to compensate.

Completing higher education also conveys a preventive effect against Alzheimer's. The more you learn, the more brain capacity you have to ward off brain function decay. Some researchers have suggested exercising your brain by doing crossword puzzles, learning a new language, starting a new hobby, and doing "mind exercises" as another way to prevent the effects of Alzheimer's. Here are some examples of mind exercises for you to work on in your "mind gym":

Proverbs: "A stitch in time saves nine." "Birds of a feather flock together." Think about what these mean to you.

Word memory: Memorize a list of thirty words in two minutes, and then write them down.

Math: Convert pesos to dollars. If you have thirty pesos and there are ten pesos to the dollar, how many dollars do you have?

Riddles: "Don't have it, don't want it, but if I have it I won't part with it." Answer: "A bald head." (To find riddles, visit sites like http://www.riddles.com or http://www.justriddlesandmore.com.)

The Aging Prevention Pill?

Imagine you could take a pill to fend off the ill effects of aging. Scientists at Harvard and the National Institute of Aging have found such a substance. It's called resveratrol — a component of red wine. Mice were given a high fat diet (increased weight leads to diabetes in humans and mice), and those that also received resveratrol were protected from diabetes and lived longer (Bauer et al., 2006). Now don't go filling your cellar with premium vintages. You can't actually drink enough red wine to obtain an effective amount of resveratrol. Your kidneys will give out long before the benefits kick in. It is, however, sold as a nutritional supplement. Resveratrol is also reported to be beneficial as an anticancer, antiviral, and anti-inflammatory substance (Faith et al., 2006; Jang et al., 1997). The studies on resveratrol are encouraging. You might want to ask: "Are you a man or a mouse?"

The research that created the gene map of the brain has shown that our head controls up to 80 percent of our body's functions (Allen). Scientists used software and robotics to learn what parts of mice's brains activate what bodily functions. The structure of the brain in mice is remarkably close to that of humans. In the future the hope is that we'll be able to unravel the foundations of various psychoses and learning disorders. That is, we're hoping to better understand the interaction of mind and body on such mental anomalies. In fact, the brain map has already borne fruit in this arena. For example, the gene known as Kibra discovered by TGen (Translational Genomics Research Institute) was found to have an effect on short-term memory loss. As you might have guessed, TGen intends to release a drug to counter memory decline.

Numerous other drugs are in the later stages of development and are expected to be released soon to help combat Alzheimer's effects on the mind. One is Alzhemed, which has been found to reduce those "brain speed bumps" (amyloid plaques) I mentioned earlier that tangle up brain cells in Alzheimer's patients.

Body Maintenance

Old age ain't no place for sissies.

— BETTE DAVIS

Body systems decline as we age. It's as if they take a rain check now and again and leave us without notice, wondering why we can't do today what we were able to do only days ago. This type of decline when it hits the immune system of elders presents a particular challenge.

As you might guess, there's plenty that can be done about compromised immune systems in our senior population! New research suggests that our brain also assists our immune system with what is known as the inflammatory reflex. Based on the work of Dr. Kevin Tracey of Boston University's School of Medicine, it appears that a stimulated vagus nerve (that's the nerve that travels from our brain to our heart and abdomen) totally suppresses sepsis — an overall body shock that can kill (Bauhofer and Torossian, 2007; Huston et al., 2007). Okay, so some day drugs may work on the vagus nerve in such a manner; but we already know that meditation can too. Those who meditate regularly can change their heart rate — a vagus nerve function — and actually control their brain to counteract inflammatory conditions in the bowel and heart. Pretty amazing, eh?!

Can Stress Cause Cancer?
With the exceptions of testicular cancer and childhood leukemia, our risks for getting most cancers increase as we age. A colleague I've run with for years once said: "I run to make sure I'm not getting stressed out by something and having that create cancer cells in my body." A recent study says he is right. Norepinephrine is a hormone that increases during stress. It has been shown to activate cancer cells to metastasize (Kiecolt-Glaser et al., 2003). But the good news is because meditation diminishes stress hormones, it very well might be a cancer fighter too.

Better with Each Year
So far we have focused on the decline in the aging brain. But an exciting body of research supports the notion that some brain functions actually improve with age. Verbal skills improve, vocabulary increases, and the related ability to understand synonyms and antonyms is heightened. Older brains carry more "expert knowledge" related to their vocation (job) and avocation (hobbies). Furthermore, our Elders carry around more mental problem-solving tools.

They have a wealth of experience to draw from that enables them to formulate solutions. That's why Elders are often considered walking encyclopedias of knowledge and our oral historians. In Africa it's said that when an Elder dies, the community loses a library. Solar astronomer at the University of Arizona Bill Livingston, age seventy-nine, is an example of a library full of "cognitive templates" or mental problem-solving road maps (outlines of how to handle certain kinds of situations). Although he retired years ago, he still shows up at "work" every day to coach younger scientists.

Thus, older people have a better mind road map even if they can't memorize the off-ramps and detours as well as they used to. No, we haven't lost all our abilities: As the 72 million baby boomers age, there has been increasing pressure to increase the age of mandatory retirement for air traffic controllers and pilots. The reason for this push is more than demographics. Good research has shown that older air traffic controllers handle complex tasks such as keeping airplanes from running into each other as well as or better than those half their age, even though they had slower reaction times, decreased attention, and decreased short-term memory (Broach & Schroeder, 2005). This seems to be because the older controllers put to use those mental templates they have developed over many years of experience.

In my own profession I can attest that the young residents and nurse practitioners I mentor have minds like steel traps. They have outstanding recall of the latest drugs and their benefits and harms. On the other hand, I'm able to recognize key patterns in a patient's history more quickly and develop a diagnosis more efficiently than they are. I've also noticed I'm more controlled in my emotions than I used to be. Dr. Leanne Williams, along with some of her colleagues at the Brain Dynamics Centre at the University of Sydney, Australia, studied 260 people from teens to elders. Subjects were shown pictures of faces with different emotions while their brains were scanned with magnetic resonance imaging to see which parts were activated. Younger people were less likely to control their mental reaction to negative pictures of anger and fear than were older subjects. In this sense, elders were found to be more emotionally stable and at peace with the world they encounter (Williams et al., 2006).

Ah, the Wisdom of Age!

My mother, Marlea "Molly" Peate has many sayings about aging. She'll tell you: "I'm not that old really; you should ask someone who's ninety." Mom was a surgery nurse, so she's seen it all and has several rules for graceful aging. Here're a few of them:

1. Don't hang around boring people; especially ones who complain about some body part not working like it used to.
2. Stay around fun people.
3. Hang around young people; they keep your mind occupied.
4. Send funny emails to your friends even if they are a little off color.

5. Volunteer at something. You'll meet people who are worse off than you.
6. Don't go to too many funerals, just the ones you want to. Instead have a drink for the departed.
7. Start a diary. Ask yourself: "Who can I strangle today?" Just writing it down will make you feel better and keep you out of jail for murder.

Her advice can be summed up as: "Keep life a permanent adventure."

Another family member, Lucia Struthers, is in her seventies. Her husband was crippled in his thirties by a fall down an elevator shaft and spent the rest of his life in a wheelchair. Lucia's attitude was she could bemoan her fate or move on and cope, which she did with a beaming smile. She says: "Life's deepest sorrows are spent in self-pity."

Don't Retire Too Early

Comedian George Burns worked well into his nineties. When asked when he was going to retire, he answered: "Retire to what?" Another questioner asked him what his doctor thought of his smoking cigars. "I don't know, all my doctors are dead," replied Burns. George Burns captured the essence of successful aging. He kept his mind active, felt useful because he was contributing to society, and maintained his sense of humor.

I'm the designated physician for 1,200 firefighters. Like those in the military, many of these brave souls retire at a relatively early age. When I ask them what they will do after they retire, many respond with a blank stare. Those are the ones I worry about. Few outside interests, sparse hobbies, and no volunteering or other activities to keep us vital, alive, and valued leads to a loss of internal vigor and self-value. I've seen the light go out in too many who retire their brains, their bodies, and their self-esteem when they retire from their job. Their mental and physical health rapidly declines. "I'm no longer of use, so what's the use of living," one said to me. I wrote him a prescription to volunteer. His next visit he said he never felt better. He loved computers and was serving as a computer coach for a senior center.

Stay Fit

Ludmila Sunova, age seventy-five, from Slovakia has run 125 marathons but didn't start competing until she was fifty-five! Why? "The Communists wouldn't let women run in races. I had to wait until the Berlin Wall fell." You don't have to be a marathoner to experience the benefits of physical activity and a mindful attitude. Your daily activities help keep you fit. Harvard psychologist Ellen Langer studied eighty-four women who worked as housekeepers in four hotels. She told those from one of the hotels that their daily work counted as a workout. There is truth to this conclusion, because activities of daily living are part of the physical activity advised by the surgeon general. After four weeks in the study, those from the hotel who received information about their work counting as physical activity reported they felt healthier, even though their level of physical exertion didn't change (Lambert, 2007).

So whatever you do, now or when you get older, find ways to stay fit, whether it's planned exercise or just moving in your daily life. The more fit you are, the better you'll feel.

Fall in Love, Again

All of us have had that intense emotional attachment to another called love. Rutgers's Helen Fisher, an anthropologist, performed a study that suggests that being in love is good for us. She showed pictures of their beloved to fifteen subjects whose brains were being scanned. The activated area of their brains was the part that releases dopamine (the pleasure- and addiction-related chemical in our brain). For those subjects shown a picture of someone who had dumped them, the areas in the brain that were activated coincided with those activated in the midst of obsessive-compulsive, angry, and risky behavior (Fisher et al., 2006). This study might also explain why relationship problems can lead to elevated blood pressure, anxiety, and even affective disorders (these include depression, mania, and anxiety).

After the romance fades, how do you reignite it? Additional research has shown the answer is to do something novel, a new activity, dinner with another couple, take up a hobby together. Psychologist Dr. Arthur Aron proposes that novel experiences activate dopamine and strengthen a flagging romance (Fisher et al., 2006).

These are just some of the things that we can do to slow down, avoid, and reverse the physical effects of aging. Before moving on to Gary's and Erik's sections, I'd like to add just a note about how the physical aspects of aging tie into the mental and spiritual aspects.

The Physical Ills of Aging and the Body-Mind-Spirit Connection

How is the body-mind-spirit connection related to the physical ills of aging? As you learned in chapter 8, physical illness affects the mind and spirit as well as the body. And, the reverse is also true. Take for example arthritis, which so frequently afflicts the aging population. If you develop arthritis, you're likely to have strong feelings about this condition. If you're fearful or depressed or feel alone or ignored, the arthritic symptoms will most likely feel worse. But if your mental and spiritual wellness is being nurtured, the physical symptoms are easier to bear. Wise healers prescribe not only pills, but also support groups, religious or spiritual connections, and communication with family and friends.

Just as there are many types of age-related maladies, so there are many different types of arthritis — and, like the other maladies, each requires a different approach if it's to be managed properly. Management isn't the same as cure, so we do well to realize that even if a cure is *not* possible, being more comfortable usually *is*. Comfort is more than physical sensations of course; it also involves mental and spiritual components.

Both your mental attitude and sense of spirituality can help you deal with any challenge that comes your way as you age. Consider osteoporosis for example. This disease occurs when bones thin and then break. Proper diet (with adequate Vitamin D and calcium) and weight-bearing exercise (like walking rather than swimming) help prevent the condition. If you develop it, you may have to take medications that slow the progression, but they aren't cheap and have side effects. So, how about increasing your comfort by dealing with it emotionally and spiritually as well?

Mentally, learn all you can about it: the effects, treatment, and what you can do personally to handle it. Learn about the right kind of exercise, food, and medicine. Spiritually, if you're religiously inclined, prayer is a comfort. Also, some faith-based communities offer walking and nutrition programs that supplement these efforts with encouraging biblical messages such as: "With God all things are possible" (Matthew 19:26).

Similar support offerings are available for other age-related conditions. For those who don't want to be involved in formal religion programs, there are other types of support groups. Ask your physician about such support groups, look in the phone book, and do an online search. There are also online chat support groups. The main point, though, is to remember that your body, mind, and spirit all work best in conjunction with one another. Now let's hear from Gary about dealing with aging from the mental perspective.

"I May Be over the Hill but I'm Still above the Ground!" — Attitude and Aging

Gary D. McKay

There are three stages of life: youth, middle age, and "gee you look good!"

— RED SKELTON

Although none of us three authors are spring chickens, I'm the oldest fowl in the flock! Compared to me, Wayne and Erik are a couple of kids! So, I know about aging and it can be a pain in the whatever: whatever hurts today (or doesn't hurt today as the case may be). But it has its positive sides too. You can join AARP (at age fifty or older) and get discounts! You can also get discounts on movie theater tickets, entrance to museums and national parks, public transportation, and even some restaurants. You can join the new government program: "No Old Fart Left Behind!" If you're retired, you now have the time to enjoy doing what you want to do. If you're still working, you can continue to enjoy your job and prepare for the future.

As you age, you may be faced with chronic illness such as diabetes, arthritis, and heart problems or chronic pain. In chapter 8, we discussed handling such issues. We included some stories of people handling their chronic illness in the most positive way possible.

Dr. Andrew Weil, a noted integrative medicine expert, says this about aging and health: "A lot of people ask me how much is genetics and how much is environment and lifestyle. I think it's always both. My way of thinking of this is that we're all dealt a certain hand of genetic cards, some good, some bad. But, it's up to us how we play them" (Weil, 2006).

Another health expert, Dr. Deepak Chopra, comments,

People have to change their concepts of aging and I am not asking them to do so based on some fanciful notion but on scientific fact. When they change that, then their perception of aging will change and it will become clear to them to grow old and to become wiser, to become more creative, to become the springboard for creativity and affluence. Once your perception of the whole phenomenon changes, your reality will change, because reality is nothing other than your perception of it. (From "An Interview with Deepak Chopra, M.D." www.intouchmag.com.)

So, like everything else, healthy aging has a lot to do with attitude — or "age-itude."

"Age-itude"

Years may wrinkle the skin, but to give up enthusiasm wrinkles the soul.

— SAMUEL ULLMAN

At this point in time, you're probably involved with your career and, if you have one, your family. Life changes; and it's best to be prepared for it. For example, remember graduating from high school? Graduating from college? Getting married? Having children? Getting divorced? The more prepared you are for future changes, the smoother they'll be.

When it comes to aging, some celebrate and are proud that they're living longer. Others dread getting older — "Oh no, next year I'm gonna be ____!" It's your decision. So, instead of "Oh no" change it to "Oh yeah." Watch your DUMB thoughts. They can be a setup for depression. Even though I don't like getting older, I don't have to dread it. I don't have to see it as awful. It's a fact of life. I don't have to like it, but I can and do accept it and decide how I'll spend my advancing years. I can volunteer, exercise, continue writing, search for humor in life, travel, and socialize with my friends.

When you look in the mirror and see that aging face, you have at least two choices: examine every wrinkle, or celebrate the fact that you see your face — that you're still here. When that new — or familiar — ache comes, realize that although it's uncomfortable, it's a sign that you're still breathing. When you catch yourself dwelling on your age, refocus — decide how you'll make the most of your life. Keep doing, moving, and planning.

Let's review DUMB and REAL thinking. If you catch yourself feeling sad, depressed, or bored as you age, examine your thoughts. Look for your Demanding statements: how life, you or others *should* be. Search for your Underestimating beliefs: those "I can't stand it" statements that emphasize your weakness rather than your strengths. How are you Maximizing this situation: why is it awful? Who are you Blaming for your feelings or situation: is it life, your spouse, your partner, yourself?

Challenge and dispute these beliefs. Reevaluate: why should it be a certain way? Where's the law that says just because you want it a certain way that it must be that way? It is what it is. Eliminate excuses:

why do you think you can't stand this? True, you don't like it, but that's very different from believing you can't stand it. Accept disappointments: although the situation isn't the way you want it, what makes it a catastrophe? Let go of blame: the fact that the situation is the way it is, is nobody's fault. Blaming is useless, unless you just want to create bitterness.

Look for ways to reframe the situation. Is there an opportunity here? For example if you're bored, that means you have time to do something. So, choose something you really want to do and do it. What humor can you find in the situation? If you're bored, at least no one is forcing you to do what you don't want to do! Another way to get perspective is to talk it over with someone. Maybe the person will have some suggestions — things you haven't thought of.

You can also lift yourself out of depression or boredom by doing something for someone else. As you're reframing, think of what you can do for others. You may want to volunteer to work with kids or other adults. Is there a neighbor or friend who needs some help? If you're a churchgoer, maybe you'll want to spend more time in church activities. It doesn't matter *what* you do, it matters *that* you do! What opportunities in your community are there for volunteering? If you're unaware of such opportunities, do an Internet search of your town or city such as "Tucson + volunteering."

Plan, Plan, Plan

Although it's true that we live one day at a time, planning for the future will help you enjoy those future years. Planning goes beyond financial planning. It involves thinking about and preparing for what you'll do with your time. How long do you want to (or are allowed to) work, for example? What will you do with your time when you have more of it? Some people can't wait to retire; they look forward to doing nothing. But for most, doing nothing gets old fast. Planning ahead gives you something to look forward to.

Some people like to start a new career, which could mean something like being a greeter at Wal-Mart or going back to college to get a certificate or degree for working at a job you've always wanted to do. A friend of mine spent his working life in factory management. When he retired, he couldn't wait to work at his passions: building, plumbing, electrical work, painting, etc. He loved to work with his hands — things he'd done on the side while he was in factory work. Now he could do as much of this as he wanted and make some money as well.

Maybe you'll do some traveling to places you've long wanted to visit. Or, there may be a hobby you've always wanted to take up but just couldn't find the time for before. Variety is important too. Having different things to look forward to and do helps fend off boredom. And there's more time for relationships too. For example, if you have grandchildren maybe you can spend more time with them.

Planning at your particular stage of life may not be just for retirement. You may have other plans for your working life. You may not like the job you're in, or you may want to go for a promotion. What will it take to make changes? Make a list and plan ways to accomplish your goals.

Another preretirement event that some don't seriously consider is how life will be when the kids grow up and leave home: the "empty nest syndrome." Maybe you feel that you just can't wait for this! An old joke illustrates this point:

A Catholic priest, a Protestant minister, and a Jewish rabbi were discussing when life begins. The priest said: "For us, life begins at conception." The minister (a liberal one) said: "For us, life begins at birth." The rabbi said: "For us, life begins when the dog dies and the kids leave home!" (Mosak, 1987)

However, for many, the empty nest is a sad event. Author Jennifer Pitzi Hellwig, M.S., R.D., points out that when the kids leave home, parents may experience:

- Sadness
- Loneliness
- Emptiness
- Uselessness, or no longer having a purpose in life
- Guilt (for example, if the relationship with the child was strained before he or she left)
- In some cases, parents may experience symptoms associated with clinical depression or adjustment disorder, including:
  - Difficulty concentrating
  - Fatigue or lack of drive
  - Inability to seek or derive pleasure
  - Changes in eating patterns
  - Excessive worry or anxiety
  - Indecision

Of course if you're experiencing depression, review chapter 6 and seek help from your doctor or a therapist if need be.

Realize that the empty nest, although it may be lonely and strange at first, has its positive side. You now have more time to do things you've always wanted to do but couldn't manage with kids in the house. In fact, you'll be better off if you prepare yourself for their exit. If you've begun to engage in activities apart from the kids rather than investing your entire free time in the kids' lives, the transition will be easier. Also, realize that your kids' moving out rarely means you'll never see them again. And, in our modern world, there's so many ways to keep in touch, via phone and email for example.

Aging with Grace (or Joe or Mary . . .)

If you're married or in a committed relationship, when you and your spouse or partner retire, just think of all the time you can spend together. But watch out, this could be a problem. You're used to spending nights, weekends, and vacations together. Full-time togetherness isn't something you're used to (unless you both work at home or own your own business, of course — but even then, you probably have time apart). For some couples, spending more time together is a blessing; for others it's a curse, possibly leading to divorce.

One way to prepare for full-time life together is to begin now. Establish a couple of meetings — where you really listen to each other, make plans, and solve problems between you. This will not only enrich your life now, it will also help you build bridges for the future.

Couple meetings work best if you first begin with a "heart-to-heart" communication model (McKay & Maybell, 2004). The purpose of the heart-to-heart is simply to get connected — to really hear each other. It's not a time to solve problems — that will come later — it's just a time to connect in a respectful positive way. During the meeting — usually scheduled once a week — the couple takes turns sharing their feelings. The topics could involve couple issues or things unrelated to the couple that one wants to share. Again, this is just a time to listen, not to try to solve issues.

Once the couple is comfortable with sharing in heart-to-heart meetings, they can establish couple meetings for planning and problem solving. The couple meeting begins with a heart-to-heart sharing and then proceeds to seeking solutions though brainstorming using the exploring alternatives model.

For couples with children who still live in the home, family meetings can be established. These meetings are for making plans and solving problems that involve the entire family — they aren't appropriate for couple issues. You can learn more about heart-to-heart, couple meetings and family meetings by consulting my book *Calming the Family Storm* (McKay & Maybell, 2004).

In chapter 5 we talked about ways to communicate and solve problems together. We suggested using I-messages to communicate your feelings in a respectful way, for example: "When I'm interrupted, I feel disrespected because it seems what I want to say doesn't count." We talked about how to really listen to another through reflective listening: "You feel angry because I'm not interested in that activity." We also discussed a process called "exploring alternatives," a technique for resolving problems between significant others that involves the following steps: connect and clarify, brainstorm solutions, evaluate solutions, and choose and use a solution.

If you and your significant other get in each other's way when you retire, arrange to do different activities. First of all, you may not always be interested in the same things. Second, having some time away from each other enriches the time you do spend together.

Stay Positive

If you keep on saying things are going to be bad, you have a good chance of becoming a prophet.

— Isaac Bashevis Singer

Many experts report that a positive attitude delays or aids the aging process. For example, a study of 500 people from age sixty to ninety-eight conducted by the University of California at San Diego discovered the following: "Optimism and effective coping styles (or attitude) were found to be the keys to aging successfully rather than traditional measures of health and wellness"(New Attitude on Successful Aging).

In other research, Dr. Becca Levy of Yale University conducted a study of 660 people fifty years of age and older " . . . those with more positive self-perceptions of aging lived 7.5 years longer than those with negative self-perceptions of aging" (Health Education Newsletter: Ageism in America).

How do you develop a positive attitude? First be optimistic — see the plus side, expect the best. Here's an old joke that illustrates the difference between pessimism and optimism (Mosak, 1987):

A pessimist is like the little child who gets up on Christmas morning, sees a new bicycle under the tree and thinks of everything that can go wrong with it. "The tires will go flat, I'll fall off and hurt myself, someone will steal it . . . " On the other hand, the optimist is like the little child who sees a little pile of horse manure under the tree and says: "Gee, there must be a pony somewhere!"

How do you remain positive? Keep searching for the pony! Positive affirmations or self-talk are another way. Consider these affirmations (Developing a Positive Attitude):

- I will think of myself as successful!
- I will have positive expectations for everything I do!
- I will remind myself of past successes!
- I will not dwell on failures; I just will not repeat them!
- I will surround myself with positive people and ideas!
- I will keep trying until I achieve the results I want!

Some of the suggestions earlier in this section will help you develop and maintain a positive attitude, such as planning things you want to do. Give yourself a reason to get up in the morning rather than dreading meeting the new day. Look for the plusses in your life each day. Begin this now around the family dinner table by asking your kids: "What good things happened in your life today?" Share your own as well. This gets everyone in the habit of looking for plusses.

Too often in life, our focus is on problems rather than on the positive. So, start your focus on the positive today. Focus on your strengths, not your weaknesses. Accept yourself as you are, not as you could be. Apply strength focusing and acceptance to others as well — particularly your family members. And remember: living in the here and now, as Wayne and I have addressed it, helps you prepare for the "there and then," which Erik addresses next.

A Time for Every Purpose — Turning with the Seasons

Erik Mansager

> We come from the earth, we return to the earth, and in between we garden.
>
> — Author Unknown

With all due respect, Gary *is* the elder among us. Still, my crossing the half-century mark has given me reason to pause, and pause again. Sitting to write my section of the final chapter, it seems there's so much I want to share and so little room to share it in, a feeling that's kin to advancing age itself. I want very much to address the aging process with those who believe in god but also to share something with those who don't.

What occurs to me as I ponder the spiritual side of things is that aging, although a kind of end, in many sacred traditions is thought of as a new beginning. Although for some it is a new beginning, in some traditions, the new beginning *isn't* an afterlife nor is it necessarily a reincarnation. Aging has also been thought of as the cycling of seasons — in all their beauty and wonder. And it's from a "seasons perspective" that I'd like to share.

That is, in so many ways we come full circle in the paths of spirituality that I shared earlier in the book. We have accomplished many of our initial strivings for mastery, and we strive instead for less material things. Our search for integration seems more or less complete, and we're aware that there's limited time to meet all our goals. Our movement of self-transcendence reaches now to thoughts of the next generation; and our images of ultimate concern (whether god or another spiritual concept) are familiar even if we still don't quite grasp them wholly.

In my sharing about seasons, I first present an outline of seasonal "stages" to see what some theorists say about entering our later phase of life, then I address specifics about gathering our lives together and readying ourselves for that stage of life. Finally, I review the process of spirituality and awareness that I shared in chapter 3. This time, though, I talk about their impact on older age — whether we're believers or not.

Stages of the Seasons

There is still no cure for the common birthday.

— JOHN GLENN, U.S. SENATOR, AT AGE SEVENTY-FIVE

There is a lot of literature out there on the idea that life can be understood as segmented into age ranges from birth to death. This area of research is called "life span development." Often these writers follow a specific development theorist, such as Erik Erikson. In the really old days, psychologists tended to think of children as more or less "little adults" who just needed to grow up. Life span development now shows us that our growth takes place as steps that follow one after the other and that each one influences the next. This "stage" approach isn't perfect, but it provides a useful way of understanding maturation.

The stages we're most familiar with come from Erikson (1950, 1982), who believed there were eight stages of life:

1. Infancy
2. Early childhood
3. Play age
4. School age
5. Adolescence
6. Young adulthood
7. Adulthood
8. Old age

In fact, it was Erikson (1959) who coined the term, "identity crisis" for what adolescents face at the onset of puberty. As Erikson saw it, crises weren't limited to adolescents. He believed we face crises in each of the eight stages. If we weather them successfully, it's proof of having acquired an essential virtue that aids us in facing the next stage. The integration of such virtues is what brings about a positive, forward-moving maturity and eventual wisdom. Failure to do so brings its own peculiar pains. Here, I only address the last two of Erikson's stages and discuss the crises found within them and the virtues that emerge if the crisis is successfully faced.

Adulthood. Leaving "young adulthood" and entering "adulthood" includes having resolved the dilemma of isolating oneself or developing a style of intimacy that typically results in the rearing of children. But raising the kids is a temporary challenge. Seeing them off into the world is the greater quandary, the one that we face in later adulthood. Transmitting our culture to our children — whether our own children or those of "the next generation" — becomes the crisis we face in adulthood. Erikson put this in terms of an inner battle in which we fight against "stagnation" and reach to become "generative."

Being generative or successfully passing on what's most precious to us, Erikson (1964) believed developed the virtue of "caring" in our adult years. Without care, we become "self-bounded" adults and experience stagnation of our hopes and dreams. On the other hand, care-filled adults want to pass on to others "what has been generated by love, necessity, or accident." Being able to do this, we feel more a part of the evolving world and tend to feel as if we're ensuring a secure future for those who follow.

Old age. As care-filled adults grow older — having by and large incorporated generativity into their lives and having benefited the next generation in that way — they face yet another crisis. In our old age, we have the opportunity to integrate the virtues of the seven earlier stages into a formidably integrated character, distinguished by its completeness and consistency. Completeness is about knowing who you are in spite of your weaknesses and strengths. Consistency is applying your virtues in a predictable and helpful manner.

Less successful older adults refuse to, or feel they can't, accept that life is drawing to a close whether they like it or not. Such older adults are more susceptible to feelings of hopelessness and despair. Rather than integrating the hard-won virtues, they are weighed down by all that's left incomplete in their lives.

The older adult who's successful in fighting off despair finds herself or himself with a "detached concern with life itself, in the face of death itself" (Erikson, 1964). This is Erikson's definition of the virtue of "wisdom." Integrated, wise elders among us exhibit not only great knowledge, but also an ability to discern in any given situation what is useful from what isn't. It's not that they feel complete unto themselves; in fact very often the wisdom exhibited by those of advanced age comes from actively participating in what Erikson (1968) called a "living religious or philosophical tradition." Indeed, no one is an island — and when we encounter the rock-steady good judgment of age, we recognize it as the virtue of shared wisdom.

This is where the seasonal aspect again becomes apparent. Historian and psychologist of religion David M. Wulff (1997), reflecting on Erikson's ideas, comments that "successful completion of the life cycle takes us full circle, bringing not despair but the fulfillment of hope." As you can imagine, this "stage thinking" also influenced those who think about spiritual or faith development.

Faith development. Psychologist James Fowler (1981) understands faith to be larger than religious experiences alone. To him it's "an orientation of the total person, giving purpose and goal to one's hopes and strivings, thoughts and actions." And he believes this faith develops over a lifetime. It starts with the story times of our childhood that speak to us of powers that both threaten and protect. A European psychologist of religion, Fritz Oser (1991) adds that the relationship children have with their god-concept is one of seeing god as all-powerful and seeing people as reacting to god rather than interacting with god.

Later, during our school-age years, Fowler says our stories develop into broader narratives — such as myths in which good is rewarded and evil punished. Oser agrees: the child can now have an influence on god, but god is still the one who decides. In adolescence, what most often follows from this is the development of a kind of grand story-of-my-stories. But adolescents don't yet have the self-criticizing ability to determine that their "my-story" is necessarily different from others' "my-story."

Our growth into an attitude of critical thinking and evaluation marks the beginning of adulthood. Understanding that my beliefs and your beliefs are different, yet each helpful to us individually, is an important aspect of "individuation." It's at this point of differentiation that a broad critique of what you've been taught and what you've accepted finally takes place. Oser, too, says those at this stage may view humans as autonomous in the world and reject religious authority. Unfortunately, many people stop actively searching at this critical stage without having resolved the critique. Instead they set aside religion and spirituality altogether.

This period serves some people as a transition, a transition from the somewhat self-bounded nature of personal "my-stories" to a broad understanding of faith in the context of many other faiths, cultures, and individual differences. This stage is highly important to the process of aging. Fowler calls it a joining experience or "conjunctive faith." In spite of similarities and differences with others, the individual at this point sees his or her faith as having deep personal meaning.

At the same time, these tenets don't embody unshakable, universal truths. Like Erikson's virtue of wisdom, conjunctive faith for Fowler is embodied in a living faith tradition or religion. But such faith is "worn loosely" and accommodates the realities of life lived among contradictions and paradoxes. It involves a "second naïveté" (Ricoeur, 1978) that I addressed in chapter 3 — realizing that our childhood explanations, if no longer accurate, still aren't any more harmful than other explanations we use today.

Readying for the End

> *Eternity is not something that begins after you are dead. It is going on all the time. We are in it now.*
>
> — Charlotte Perkins Gilman

The point of sharing these seasons or stages was that, as Wulff (1997) pointed out, when we're attentive and strive for awareness during our aging process, our life cycle comes full circle. Healthy spirituality allows you to hope deeply in the successful outcome of your life — however you measure that success. Earlier researchers of religious responses to aging (for example, Pratt, 1920) thought that as we get older we naturally cling to traditions because our later developed faculties, such as logical thinking, fail us. From this perspective, because we're unable to retain later developed processes, our lack of security pushes us back to cling to the things we've "known" longest and found most reliable. We now know that isn't necessarily so!

Closer research into the stages, such as that of Levin and Chatters (1998), researchers on spirituality and aging, gives a profoundly different picture of spirituality in old age. They found that despite diminishment of physical capabilities and the decrease of more "otherworldly" experiences (like déjà vu, ESP, and clairvoyance), that's not the whole story. Rather, at the same time that our bodies are slowing down, deeply personal, nondelusional kinds of mystical experiences actually increase. This is another practical way of measuring hope. In your older age, as some faculties fail, maintaining a realistic optimism is still called for.

Of course, not everyone experiences advanced age as a blessing: our energy will wane, strength will elude us, coordination fail us, and friends will leave us. Still, most of us have been touched by remembering loved ones who didn't make it this far in life. We may have had childhood friends who succumbed to disease, high school chums killed in auto accidents, family members or workmates lost in a war. Life seems uncaring and cruel if a child departs before the parent. From such a perspective, aging is a privilege — even if it's a difficult one to bear. It's time to ponder what lies ahead, as more and more of your life's percentage lies behind you.

Transitioning from adulthood to old age can threaten our sense of power and permanence. The list of potential threats is a long one: estrangement from family members, bankruptcy, possible separation from one's native culture, forced retirement, and changes in our environment. You needn't kid yourself — worst case scenarios can hurt. But you needn't face them unprepared.

Now is the time to face the possible scenario and plan a course of action. Perhaps the worst won't happen; perhaps your best-laid plans won't either. But you do well for your peace of mind to accustom yourself to the difficulties ahead so that you're not thrown into disarray when the inevitable unfolds. Let's explore just three potential threats: finding the empty nest grown cold, the loss of our life partner, and moving out of our comfortable atmosphere (which usually means into nursing homes built as more of a convenience for the *caregivers* than a comfort for the *cared for*).

Empty Nests Grown Cold

Children grow. That's what they do. They're doing just what you're doing: aging. Already in adulthood we suffered through their leaving the nest. We comforted ourselves remembering we'd done well by preparing them to live strongly and to contribute to the world as they left our safety bounds. That was the aim of so many good democratic-style parenting programs — from Gary's *STEP* programs to the *Positive Discipline* collection and *Active Parenting*. Keeping such principles in mind now will help you remember that as the already empty nest grows cold, you too can still contribute in the world.

Thinking how you want to contribute is a two-pronged approach: use the couples' meetings Gary talked about earlier in this chapter and talk with a trusted counselor (professional or otherwise) about a living will. The couples' meetings will help with the practical "what to do with ourselves" questions. If you plan ahead as Gary suggested, you'll have some ideas on what to do when the kids exit. The living will helps with the spiritual concerns. After all, who will *care for* the things you *cared about* when you're gone?

Something that I know has brought great peace of mind to many is to distribute precious material items to loved ones — children, grandchildren, trusted friends, and relatives — long before they're too old to do so. Here's an example:

My friend, eighty-one-year old Naomi, has been busily gathering up her Native American jewelry over the last year or so and finds great joy in sharing it with those she knows will appreciate it. Her quiet meditation before each "gifting" allows her to give it graciously — sometimes with a simple note, always with a big hug — and to let it be a sign of her abiding love for those she presents it to. She has been a gift to many. They will remember her more vividly when they remember the gift.

To be sure, only you can determine what "precious" means. It need not be of monetary value at all. For example, the item most cherished by my brothers, sisters, and me after our dad's death was his copy of *One Hundred and One Best Loved Poems*, from which he used to read to us as kids. Mom's retained the original, but we all have copies to read from when we gather together.

Loss of life partner. Whether by death, late-life divorce, or the ravages of senility, losing a lifelong companion is like losing half of your soul. There are no easy answers to this and I won't be glib about it. Still, we can plan well for this possibility by speaking with our dearest relatives and our friends, by pledging to be available for them, and by accepting their pledge that they will be available for us should one of us experience such loss.

The pact is to be present to the other, to "sit Shiva" with them in honoring the passing of their loved one. While this is more or less a formal process for those who embrace Judaism, there is great wisdom in it for others as well. During the year that follows our loss — as the seasons and celebrations come and go without the beloved — it's a welcomed gift to have a trusted friend checking in on us, processing the feelings we're having, and assuring us that we're not alone.

I hasten to add that working through feelings of grief also includes subtle and not-so-subtle feelings of relief. This is especially the case when the death of a loved one has followed prolonged physical or mental suffering. At such times, we do well to remember that the circumstances at the end of one's life are not a summary of that person's life. The vibrancy and contributions, the laughs and the sorrows that made up our loved one can't be contained in the sometimes painfully slow demise of a parent or partner.

Moving from "Our House" to "the Home"

Although there are undoubtedly some very fine care facilities, there are also some assisted-living facilities and nursing homes in North America and Europe that have brought negative attention to themselves. The groundbreaking sociologist Max Weber (1958) wrote long ago that the roots of capitalism could be found within the Christian traditions. Much good has come from this, as well as the sometimes-devastating belief that we're worth only what we produce.

What follows from this production orientation is a disregard for who we are, especially when we no longer produce at our former level. And if we're not able to do for ourselves, we're placed among those we can pay to do it for us. Employing others to look after our elderly in a physical way, without teaching them to care for the whole person in a spiritually consistent manner, is a setup for abuse. If we don't teach others to truly "care" for our elders in the virtuous way Erikson speaks of, we will more and more frequently find the elder abuse cases hidden on the back pages of our newspapers.

Other cultures, and specifically faiths other than Christian, are radically different in their approach to aging. In Muslim and Hindu countries, for example, homes for the elderly are all but unheard of. For Muslims to go outside their extended family to care for elderly parents is shameful. In one study, almost three quarters of Muslims asked had mixed feelings or outright rejected the possibility of eldercare outside the extended family (Haddad & Lummis, 1987).

Anu Sharma, a research psychologist formerly at the Minnesota Institute on Public Health, maintains that among the varied Hindu populations aging is a venerable and highly respected process. In fact, the persons most beloved in India are children and the elderly. Those in the middle generation are least valued; their function is to support these two age groups. She says that there are no nursing homes or childcare centers in India. The extended family provides these services.

Christians, too, have at times provided something similar. In addition to denominationally oriented nursing homes, there is the growing phenomenon among Christians of interconnected communities in which folks care for one another across the life span. This is the theme of Thomas P. Rausch's *Radical Christian Communities* and Jean Vanier's *Community and Growth: Our Pilgrimage Together*. Rausch (2000) presents the broad overview of many such communities and Vanier (2001) presents the specifics of what can be healthfully expected from such Christian communal life. Spiritually considered, exploring such communities is very appealing to some.

Eternity is now! This is the time to act on behalf of ourselves and of those we love; now is the time to map out our current portion of eternity in mindful awareness.

Spiritual Processing

Sing your death song, and die like a hero going home.
— MOHICAN CHIEF AUPUMUT, 1725

Given what I've just shared here about preparing for the end portion of life — realistically and optimistically — and given what we've learned about the life cycle and its completion and ripening in our older age, I want to come full circle as well. In my final section, I'd like to review the stepwise process for understanding spirituality that I first introduced in chapter 3. I think you'll see that this is a summary of how, through the seasons of life, we come to greater understanding of our life and how we make ultimate meaning of it.

The way into spirituality included the step of distinguishing between spirituality and religion. This step focused on the meaning-making function of spirituality, which can now be seen as a primary component of the later stages of faith development.

Another step covered the idea of "Big Questions" and "Big Answers." The point was to begin opening ourselves to new conceptualizations of God or whatever our ultimate value is. We're served well when we remember that what we have worked so hard to nail down will also pass. Things are different from what our limited minds can grasp.

At the center, we were able to see how our perceptions of the world we live in were formed. We were also able to view how our perceptions of the world many believe we're going to originated. We formed our perceptions by making sense of our unique families, geographies, and physical imperfections. In this way, we found that "the divine world" was rooted firmly in "the human world." Such a view was intended to draw together two important aspects of "knowing" those worlds: the individual and the community. From the perspective of old age, our community is seen to have consisted of many, many individuals, most of whom have gone before us and whose contributions we have benefited from.

Within the center we also explored knowing the world on what was called a holistically spiritual level. It introduced a nondualistic understanding of "soul" and "spirit" — they were seen as movements of the individual, rather than as parts. That is, the terms soul or spirit weren't add-ons to the human person. In the sense of "second naïveté," we did not need to deny the view of the soul's surviving death. But the broader center-look helped us become aware of our distorted view of the world — a distortion that arises as we grow from childhood to adulthood. This distorted view, however, can be "corrected" with the wisdom of old age.

Leaving the center, we came to understand acceptance and "awareness" as the healthy result of walking a spiritual pathway. In light of the current chapter's subject, these are the fruits of generativity and wisdom: accepting "what is" and passing that way of acceptance onto the next generation as well as awareness of it all being bigger than ourselves and that our lives play a part but don't altogether determine the future.

Finally, reentering the world distinguished healthy spirituality from various unhealthy varieties. We defined spirituality in this way:

- Striving to integrate our lives in a self-transcending way in the direction of whatever value we hold as ultimate in our lives relates deeply to the aging process. This is what Erikson termed "a coming to wisdom" through an integration of all the virtues learned in a life lived imperfectly, but lovingly.
- Striving emphasizes mastery of the Big Questions, whose answers are not dependent on ourselves alone but occur *among* others: those who view the world from a perspective newly awakened in light of old age.
- Integration, understood now in light of the stages of life and faith, is an appreciation for variety while adhering to specific beliefs without needing to impose them on others.
- Transcendence of the self is understood as seeking the wisdom "deep within myself" and passing it on to the generation "far beyond myself."

Ancient AWAREness

Wake up!

— ANTHONY DeMELLO

So we did it! We came full circle around the subject of spirituality by addressing the aging process. And now it's time to wake up — pay attention — be aware! Reviewing the prescription for spiritual "vitamins" for the wise and caring individual would be helpful:

A   stood for *asking*, and in the wisdom of our years it also means *awakening* —awakening to the wonders we work so hard to understand yet now know there is no ultimate grasp of.

W   stood for *waiting*, and now it takes on the deeper meaning of *wondering* — wondering about the growing need and desire to let things go, to let them unfold at their pace, without hurrying the answers.

A¹   stood for *acting*, and now it means preparing for endings and the new beginnings that follow. Here what is most important is *absolving*, absolving our family and friends of their transgressions, no matter how big, so that we might absolve ourselves in turn and face our last stage with a pure and strong heart.

R   stood for *reflecting*, and not only in the sense of reviewing how our actions have impacted our world; it now takes on the urgency of *resolving*. Resolving, finishing whatever is possible in our remaining years helps us keep our eye on fulfillment.

E   stood for *experiencing*, and now surely represents experiencing integrated strivings toward self-transcendence; and it beckons us to fully engage that experience by *en-JOY-ing* it! We're not just talking fun and games here, but infusing the experience with joy, no matter the cost.

As the eighteenth-century Algonquin chieftain Aupumut was purported to have said: "When it comes time to die, be not like those whose hearts are filled with the fear of death, so when their time comes they weep and pray for a little more time to live their lives over again in a different way. *Sing your death song, and die like a hero going home.*"

This chapter gave you ideas on how to age healthily and plan for the future. Exercising the body, mind, and spirit keeps you healthier longer. The Nun's Story that Wayne discussed showed how keeping one's mind active could actually help one deal with Alzheimer's! Wayne's mom, Molly, gave some great advice on handling aging. Gary showed how your attitude toward your future or "ageatude" would help you get the most out of it. If you think of getting older as a negative, it will be. But if you concentrate on how to enjoy your advancing years — you'll feel better and do better. And as Erik pointed out: "Eternity is now," not something that occurs after you leave this life. Your sense of spirituality, whether you believe in an afterlife or not, will help you gain meaning.

Okay, You've Finished the Book — What Now?

In this book you've learned how the body, mind, and spirit are connected in a holistic way; they aren't "parts" of us. Our mind affects our body. Having positive perceptions affects not only your psychological health but your physical and spiritual health as well. For example, when you look for opportunities rather than focusing on obstacles, you feel better. When you decide to eat a healthy diet and exercise, you improve your mood. Whether you believe in god or not, your sense of spirituality — "What's it all about?" — will affect your attitude and your physical health.

We suggest you continue to journal on what you found essential for you in this book. Review the book from time to time to see how to apply the ideas to your life. If you'd like to read more about some of the topics we've addressed, see the appendix for recommended readings and websites.

Live well; take care of your body, mind, and spirit; replace any negatives with positives; and enjoy your life!

Vitamins for Tomorrow

- Nearly half of those over the age of eighty-five suffer from Alzheimer's disease. To avoid Alzheimer's effects, give your brain a regular workout.
- Body systems decline as we age. Those who meditate regularly change their heart rate and actually control certain brain functions.
- Some brain functions actually improve with age. Elders have more mental problem-solving tools because of a wealth of experience to draw from.
- Elder advice: "Keep life a permanent adventure"; "Life's deepest sorrows are spent in self-pity." Don't retire too early and don't have few outside interests. This leads to a loss of internal vigor and self-value. And whatever you do, find ways to stay fit, whether it's planned exercise or just moving in your daily life.
- After the romance in your marriage fades, reignite it by doing something novel together.
- If your mental and spiritual wellness is being nurtured, physical symptoms are easier to bear.
- Healthy aging has a lot to do with "ageatude." If you catch yourself feeling sad, depressed, or bored as you age, examine your thoughts. Look for ways to reframe the situation. Look for humor in the situation. Get perspective by talking it over with someone.
- Planning for the future will help you enjoy those future years. Think about and prepare for what you'll do with your time.
- Realize that the empty nest, although it may be lonely and strange at first, has its positive side. You now have more time to do things you've always wanted to do but couldn't manage with kids in the house. If you're married or in a committed relationship, think of all the time you can spend together. One way to prepare for full-time life together is to begin now.

(Cont'd.)

Vitamins for Tomorrow (Continued)

- Many experts report that a positive attitude delays or aids the aging process.
- Transmitting our culture to our children — whether our own children or those of "the next generation" — becomes the crisis we face in adulthood.
- Older age serves some people as a transition from the somewhat self-bounded nature of personal "my-stories" to a broad understanding of faith in the context of many other faiths, cultures, and individual differences.
- Healthy spirituality allows you to hope deeply in the successful outcome of your life.
- You do well for your peace of mind to accustom yourself to the difficulties ahead so that you're not thrown into disarray when the inevitable unfolds.
- Apply the new AWARE model to aging: vitamin A = awakening; vitamin W = wondering; vitamin A^1 = absolving; vitamin R = resolving; vitamin E = enjoying.

RECOMMENDED BOOKS, ARTICLES, AND WEBSITES

Recommended Books and Articles

AA Services. (2001). *Alcoholics Anonymous — Big Book* (fourth edition). New York: Alcoholics Anonymous World Services.

Ainsworth, M. D. S., & Eichberg, C. (1991). Effects on infant-mother attachment of mothers unresolved loss of an attachment figure, or other traumatic experience. In Parkes, C. M., Stevenson-Hinde, J. , & Marris, P. (Eds.). *Attachment Across the Life Cycle*. New York: Routledge.

Al-Anon Family Group Head. (1992–2006). *Courage to Change: One Day at a Time in Al-Anon II*. New York: Al-Anon Family Group Headquarters.

Albom, Mitch. (1997). *Tuesdays with Morrie*. New York: Doubleday.

Armstrong, Karen. (1993). *A History of God*. New York: Ballantine Books.

Armstrong, Karen. (2000). *The Battle for God*. New York: Ballantine Books.

Bergin, P. L. (2002). *Holy War, Inc. Inside the Secret World of Osama bin Laden*. New York: Simon and Schuster.

Blakely, T. D., van Beek, W. E. A., & Thomson, D. L. (1994). *Religion in Africa: Experience and Expression*. Provo, UT: Heinneman.

Boenisch, Ed, & Haney, Michele. (2003). *The Stress Owner's Manual; Meaning, Balance, and Health in Your Life*. Atascadero, CA: Impact Publishers.

Borg, Marcus J. (1997). *The God We Never Knew*. San Francisco: Harper.

Borg, Marcus J. (2001). *Reading the Bible Again for the First Time*. San Francisco: Harper.

Borysenko, Joan. (2001). *Inner Peace for Busy People: Simple Strategies for Transforming Your Life*. Carlsbad, CA: Hay House.

Borysenko, Joan. (2005). *Meditations for Relaxation and Stress Reduction*. (Audiobook). Carlsbad, CA: Hay House.

Carter, Jimmy. (1996). *Living Faith*. New York: Times Books.

Chittister, Joan D. (2003). *Scarred by Struggle, Transformed by Hope*. Grand Rapids, MI: Eerdmans.

Chopra, Deepak. (2007). *The Seven Spiritual Laws of Success: A Pocketbook Guide to Fulfilling Your Dreams*. (Abridged). San Rafael, CA: Amber-Allen.

Chopra, Deepak, & Simon, David. (2001). *Grow Younger, Live Longer: Ten Steps to Reverse Aging.* New York: Three Rivers Press.

Cosby, Bill. (2002). *Cosbyology: Essays and Observations from the Doctor of Comedy.* New York: Hyperion.

Covey, Steven R. (1989). *The 7 Habits of Highly Effective People.* New York: Simon and Schuster.

Dangerfield, Rodney. (2004). *It's Not Easy Bein' Me: A Lifetime of No Respect but Plenty of Sex and Drugs.* New York: HarperCollins.

Ellis, Albert, & Velten, Emmett. (1992). *When AA Doesn't Work for You: Rational Steps to Quitting Alcohol.* Fort Lee, NJ: Barricade Books.

Ellis, Albert, & Tafrate, Raymond Chip. (1997). *How to Control Your Anger. Before It Controls You.* New York: Citadel Press.

Ferlo, Roger. (2002). *Sensing God.* Lanham, MD: Cowley.

Foxworthy, Jeff. (1996). *No Shirt, No Shoes . . . No Problem!* New York: Hyperion.

Girzone, Joseph F. (1998). *A Portrait of Jesus.* New York: Doubleday.

Gomes, Peter J. (1996). *The Good Book: Reading the Bible with Mind and Heart.* New York: HarperCollins.

Gupta, Sonjay. (2007). *Chasing Life: New Discoveries in the Search for Immortality to Help You Age Less Today.* New York: Warner Wellness.

Hallum, A. M. (1996). *Beyond Missionaries. Toward an Understanding of the Protestant Movement in Central America.* New York: Rowman and Littlefield.

Hanh, Thich Nhat. (1999). *Going Home: Jesus and Buddha as Brothers.* New York: Riverhead Books.

Hine, James R., & Peate, Wayne F. (1998). *On the Serendipity Road.* Tucson, AZ: Development Publications.

Horvath, A. Thomas. (2004). *Sex, Drugs, Gambling and Chocolate: A Workbook for Overcoming Addictions* (second edition). Atascadero, CA: Impact Publishers.

Keck, Robert L. (2000). *Sacred Quest: The Evolution and Future of the Human Soul.* West Chester, PA: Chrysalis Books.

Küng, Hans (2006). *Why I am Still a Christian.* NY: Continuum.

Küng, Hans (2008). *The Beginning of All Things: Science and Religion.* NY: Eerdmans.

Kushner, Harold S. (2001). *Living a Life That Matters.* New York: Alfred A. Knopf.

Lewis, C. S. (1996). *Mere Christianity.* New York: Simon and Schuster.

May, Gerald. (1994). *Simply Sane: The Spirituality of Mental Health.* New York: Crossroad.

McKay, Gary D., & Dinkmeyer, Don. (2002). *How You Feel Is Up to You* (second edition). Atascadero, CA: Impact Publishers.

McKay, Gary D., & Maybell, Steven A. (2004). *Calming the Family Storm: Anger Management for Moms, Dads, and All the Kids.* Atascadero, CA: Impact Publishers.

Meyers, Robert J., & Wolfe, Brenda L. (2004). *Get Your Loved One Sober: Alternatives to Nagging, Pleading, and Threatening.* Center City, MN: Hazelden.

Morris, Kathleen. (1998). *Amazing Grace: A Vocabulary of Faith.* New York: Riverhead Books.

Peate, Wayne F. (2002). *Native Healing: Four Paths to Health.* Tucson, AZ: Rio Nuevo.

Preston, John. (2004). *You Can Beat Depression* (fourth edition). Atascadero, CA: Impact.

Quinn, Daniel. (1995). *Providence: The Story of a Fifty-Year Vision Quest.* New York: Bantam.

Savage, Alan M. & Nicholl, Sheldon W. (Eds.) (2003). *Faith, Hope and Charity as Character Traits in Adler's Individual Psychology. With Related Essays in Spirituality and Phenomenology.* NY: University Press of America.

Schweitzer, Albert (1981). *Civilization and Ethics: The Philosophy of Civilization.* New York: Prometheus.

Seinfeld, Jerry. (1993). *Seinlanguage.* New York: Bantam.

Spong, John Shelby. (2001). *A New Christianity for a New World.* San Francisco: Harper.

Steinberger, Henry (Ed.). (2004). *SMART Recovery Handbook* (second edition). Mentor, OH: SMART Recovery.

Stokes, Kenneth. (1994). *Faith Is a Verb: Dynamics of Adult Faith Development.* New London, CT: Twenty-Third Publications.

Thompson, Marjorie J. (1995). *Soul Feast: An Invitation to the Christian Spiritual Life.* Louisville, KY: Westminster John Knox Press.

Trimpey, Jack. (1996). *Rational Recovery: The New Cure for Substance Addiction.* New York: Pocket Books.

Tutu, Desmond. (1999). *No Future without Forgiveness.* New York: Doubleday.

Volpicelli, Joseph, & Szalavitz, Maia. (2000). *Recovery Options: The Complete Guide.* New York: John Wiley and Sons.

Weil, Andrew. (2004). *Natural Health, Natural Medicine: The Complete Guide to Wellness and Self-Care for Optimum Health.* Boston: Houghton Mifflin.

Weil, Andrew. (2005). *Healthy Aging: A Lifelong Guide to Your Physical and Spiritual Well-Being.* New York: Knopf Publishing Group.

Weil, Andrew. (2006). *Eight Weeks to Optimum Health: A Proven Program for Taking Full Advantage of Your Body's Natural Healing Power* (revised edition). New York: Knopf Publishing Group.

Yancey, Philip. (1995). *The Jesus I Never Knew*. Grand Rapids, MI:
    Zondervan.
Yancey, Philip. (1997). *What's So Amazing about Grace*. Grand Rapids, MI:
    Zondervan.
Yancey, Philip. (2000). *Reaching for the Invisible God*. Grand Rapids. MI:
    Zondervan.
Yount, David. (1994). *Growing in Faith: A Guide for the Reluctant
    Christian*. New York: Penguin Books.
Yount, David. (1997). *Spiritual Simplicity*. New York: Simon and Schuster.

Recommended Websites

Addiction
Addiction Recovery Guide: http://www.addictionrecoveryguide.org
Addicts in Recovery Anonymous quiz: http://www.foodaddicts.org/quiz.html
Al-Anon-Alateen: http://www.al-anon.alateen.org
Alcoholics Anonymous: http://www.alcoholics-anonymous.org
Food Addiction: http://www.foodaddicts.org
Gamblers Anonymous: http://www.gamblersanonymous.org
Mental Help.net: http://mentalhelp.net/poc/view_doc.php?type=docandid
    =1860andcn=14.
Narcotics Anonymous: http://www.na.org
Nicotine: http://www.smokefree.gov/quit-smoking/nicotine_addiction.asp
Open Recovery Project: http://www.dmoz.org/Health/Addictions
Rational Recovery: http://www.rational.org
Sexaholics Anonymous: http://www.sa.org
Smart Recovery: http://www.smartrecovery.org

Aging and Chronic Illnesses
Alzheimer's Association: http://www.alz.org
American Association of Retired Persons: http://www.aarp.org
American Cancer Society: http://www.cancer.org
American Diabetes Association: http://www.diabetes.org
American Heart Association: http://www.americanheart.org
American Lung Association: http://www.lungusa.org
Arthritis.com: http://www.arthritis.com
Arthritis Association: http://www.arthritis.org
Center for Disease Control and Prevention: http://www.cdc.gov/aging
Everyday Health: http://www.everydayhealth.com
National Council on Aging: http://www.ncoa.org
National Institute on Aging: http://www.nia.nih.gov
American Pain and Wellness: "Pain Management: Fighting Back."
    http://www.painandwellness.com/pain_management_fighting_back_3.html

Diet, Exercise, Vitamins, and Minerals

Dietary Supplements: http://dietary-supplements.info.nih.gov/Health_
    Information/Health_Information.aspx
Familydoctor.org: http://familydoctor.org
Federal Food and Drug Administration: http://fda.org
National Academy of Sciences-National Research Council (NAS-NRC).
    "Recommended Dietary Allowance RDA." 2004. http://www.iom.edu/
    Object.File/Master/21/372/0.pdf
National Institutes of Health, Office of Dietary Supplements: Vitamin and
    Mineral Fact Sheets: http://ods.od.nih.gov/Health_information/Vitamin_
    and_Mineral_Supplement_Fact_Sheets.aspx
President's Council on Physical Fitness and Sports: http://www.fitness.gov
Science Daily: http://www.sciencedaily.com
United States Department of Agriculture: http://www.mypyramid.gov

Domestic Violence and Child Abuse

Child Abuse: Childhelp USA National Child Abuse Hotline (serves the
    United States, Canada, U.S. Virgin Islands, Puerto Rico, and Guam):
    http://www.childhelpusa.org
Domestic Violence: The National Domestic Violence Hotline: http://www.
    ndvh.org
The Hot Peaches Organization: http://www.hotpeachpages.net/a/countries.html
Intervention Specialists, Intervention Referral: http://www.intervention-
    referral.com

Golden Rule

Religious Tolerance.org: http://www.religioustolerance.org/reciproc.htm
Teaching Values.com: http://www.teachingvalues.com/goldenrule.html
Unification Net, World Scripture: http://www.unification.net/ws/theme
    015.htm

Holistic Health

American Holistic Health Association: http://ahha.org
Andrew Weil: http://www.drweil.com
Free Inquiry: http://www.freeinquiry.com
Holistic Online: http://www.holisticonline.com

Mattie Stepanek's Website

Information on Mattie's poetry, books and his foundation:
    www.mattieonline.com

Spirituality

Beliefnet: http://www.beliefnet.com
Deepak Chopra: http://www.chopra.com
Global Ethics Foundation: http://www.weltethos.org/dat-english/index.htm

Stress, Anger, and Depression

About.com, Depression: http://depression.about.com/

About.com, Stress Management: http://stress.about.com/

American Psychological Association: http://www.apa.org/topics/
controlanger.html

Cognitive Therapy and Anger Management: http://www.habitsmart.com/
anger.html

Depression.com: http://www.depression.com

National Institute of Mental Health: http://www.nimh.nih.gov/
healthinformation/depressionmenu.cfm

Optimal Health Concepts: http://www.optimalhealthconcepts.com/Stress

Therapist Locators

Albert Ellis Institute: http://www.albertellis.org/aei/find_therapist_a_list.html

American Counseling Association: http://www.counseling.org/Resources/
CounselorDirectory/TP/Home/CT2.aspx

American Psychological Association: http://locator.apa.org

For Therapy.com Network: http://www.4therapy.com/locator/index.php

Network Therapy Find a Therapist: http://www.networktherapy.com/
directory/find_therapist.asp

North American Society of Adlerian Psychology: http://www.alfredadler.org
(See office information at bottom of this web page and contact office for
information.)

Psychology Today Find a Therapist: http://therapists.psychologytoday.com/
ppc/prof_search.php?iorb=476

REFERENCES

2 Hearts Network, Inc. "Serenity Prayers." http://www.2heartsnetwork.org/serenity.htm

Abraham Lincoln Research Site. "Depressed? Read Abraham Lincoln's Words." http://home.att.net:80/~rjnorton/Lincoln84.html

Adler, Alfred. (2005). *The Collected Clinical Works of Alfred Adler, Volume 7: Journal Articles: 1931–1937: Birth Order & Early Memories, Social Interest & Education, Technique of Treatment*. Henry Stein (Ed.). San Francisco: Alfred Adler Institute.

Adler, Alfred. (1964). *Problems of Neurosis*. P. Mairet (Ed.). New York: Harper & Row. (Original work published 1929).

Allen, Paul. Neurosciencegateway. "Brain Atlas." http://www.brainatlas.org/aba

Alzheimer's Association. "Alzheimer's Disease Facts and Figures 2007." http://www.alz.org/national/documents/report_alzfactsfigures2007.pdf

"An Interview with Deepak Chopra, MD." http://www.intouchmag.com/chopra.html

Anandappa, Geoff in Tim Radford. The Guardian. "Scientists Close in on World's Funniest Joke." http://education.guardian.co.uk/higher/humanities/story/0,9850,622310,00.html

Ansbacher, Heinz. (1956). *The Individual Psychology of Alfred Adler*. New York: Basic Books.

"As It Were: The Ruminations of Topher1kenobe." http://derosia.com/phlog/non-seq

Barrish, Harriet H., & Barrish, I. J. (1989). *Managing and Understanding Parental Anger* (revised edition). Leawood, KS: Barrish and Barrish.

Bauhofer, A., & Torossian, A. (2007). Mechanical vagus nerve stimulation — a new adjunct in sepsis prophylaxis and treatment? *Crit Care Med* 35(12): 2868–2869.

Baur, Joseph A., Pearson, Kevin J., Price, Nathan L., Jamieson, Hamish A., Lerin, Carles, Kalra, Avash, et al. (2006). Resveratrol improves health and survival of mice on a high-calorie diet. *Nature* 444: 337–342.

Bengtsson, Sara L., Nagy, Z., Skare, S., Forsman, L., Forssberg, H., & Ullén, F. (2005). Extensive piano practicing has regionally specific effects on white matter development. *Nature Neuroscience* 8(9):1148–1150.

Bergin, P. L. (2002). *Holy War, Inc. Inside the Secret World of Osama bin Laden.* New York: Simon & Schuster.

Bristol University Press. "Does the Lack of Sleep Make You Fat?" Press Release December 7, 2004. http://www.bris.ac.uk/news/2004/582

Booth, L. (1992). *Breaking the Chains: Understanding Religious Addiction and Religious Abuse.* Philadelphia: J. P. Tarcher.

Broach, Dana, & Schroeder, David J. (2005). *Relationship of Air Traffic Control Specialist Age to En Route Operational Errors.* Washington, DC: Office of Aerospace Medicine.

Carey, B. (2006). "Long-Awaited Medical Study Questions the Power of Prayer." *New York Times.* http://www.nytimes.com/2006/03/31/health/31pray.html?pagewanted=1

"Catholic Dictionary." http://www.geocities.com/good_clean_fun_2/cath-1.htm

Centers for Disease Control and Prevention. "2007 National Immunization Survey — Adults Only." http://www.cdc.gov/vaccines/stats-surv/imz-coverage.htm#nisadult

Centers for Disease Control and Prevention. http://www.cdc.gov/mmwr/preview/mmwrhtml/mm5641a7.htm?s_cid=mm5641a7_e

Channel Five Broadcasting. "The Woman with Half a Body." http://www.five.tv/programmes/extraordinarypeople/womanwith

Cherkas, Lynn, Hochberg, Fran, MacGregor, Alex J., Snieder, Harold, & Spector, Tim D. (2000). Happy families: a twin study of humour. *Twin Research* 3(1): 17–22.

Chödrön, P. (2000). *When Things Fall Apart. Heart Advice for Difficult Times.* Boston: Shambhala.

Clark, Andrew, & Lelkes, Orsolya. European Center for Social Welfare Research, BBC News. "Religion 'linked to happy life.'" http://news.bbc.co.uk/2/hi/health/7302609.stm.

Conger, Krista. (2005). "Pain's stronghold: it's all in your head." *Stanford Medicine Magazine.* (Fall). http://stanmed.stanford.edu/2005fall/pain.html

Cousins, Norman. (1991). *Anatomy of an Illness as Perceived by the Patient.* New York: Bantam Dell.

Coyle, D. (2007). How to grow a super athlete. *Play Magazine, New York Times Sports.* March 4.

Davidson, Richard. (2005). *Neuroplasticity.* Madison, WI: University of Wisconsin Press.

DeMello, A. (1992). *The Way to Love. The Last Meditations of Anthony de Mello.* New York: Image Pocket Classics.

"Developing A Positive Attitude." http://www.recoverymedicine.com/developing_a_positive_attitude.htm

Dinkmeyer, Don Sr., McKay, Gary D., McKay, Joyce L., & Dinkmeyer, Don Jr. (1998). *Parenting Teenagers.* Bowling Green, KY: Step Publishers.

Dreikurs, Rudolf. (1958). A reliable differential diagnosis of psychological or somatic disturbance. *International Record of Medicine* 171:238–242.

Dreikurs, Rudolf. (1962). Can you be sure the disease is functional? *Consultant* (Smith, Kline and French Laboratories).

Dreikurs, Rudolf. (1967). *Psychodynamics, Psychotherapy, and Counseling.* Chicago, IL: Alfred Adler Institute.

Drug and Alcohol Resource Center. "Recognizing the Signs of Alcoholism." http://www.addict-help.com

Ellis, Albert. (1998). *A Guide to Rational Living.* North Hollywood, CA: Wilshire Books.

Ellis, Albert, & Becker, Irving. (1982). *A Guide to Personal Happiness.* North Hollywood, CA: Wilshire Books.

Ellis, Albert, & Velten, Emmett. (1992). *When AA Doesn't Work for You: Rational Steps to Quitting Alcohol.* Fort Lee, NJ: Barricade Books.

Emery, Gary. (1988). *Getting Undepressed: How a Woman Can Change Her Life through Cognitive Therapy.* New York: Simon and Shuster.

Erikson, E. H. (1950). *Childhood and Society.* New York: Norton.

Erikson, E. H. (1950). *The Life Cycle Completed.* New York: Norton.

Erikson, E. H. (1959). *Identity and the Life Cycle.* New York: Norton.

Erikson, E. H. (1964). *Insight and Responsibility.* New York: Norton.

Extraordinary People. "RoseMarie (Rose) Siggins: The Woman with Half a Body." http://www.mymultiplesclerosis.co.uk/misc/rosesiggins.html

Faith, S.A., Sweet, T. J., Bailey, E., Booth, T., & Docherty, J. J. (2006). Resveratrol suppresses nuclear factor-kappaB in herpes simplex virus infected cells. *Antiviral Research.* July 14.

Fields, R. Douglas. (2005). Myelination: An Overlooked Mechanism of Synaptic Plasticity? *Neuroscientist*, 11(5):528–531.

Fields, R. Douglas. (2008). White water matters. *Scientific American.* 298(3): 42–49.

Fields, Wayne. (1996). *What the River Knows: An Angler in Midstream.* Chicago: University of Chicago Press.

Fisher H. E., Aron, A., & Brown, L. L. (2006). Romantic love: a mammalian brain system for mate choice. *Philos Trans R Soc Lond B Biol Sci.* 361(1476):2173–2186.

Fowler, J. (1981). *Stages of Faith. The Psychology of Human Development and the Quest for Meaning.* New York: HarperCollins.

Frankl, Viktor E. (2000). *Man's Search for Meaning.* Boston: Beacon Press.

Frederickson, B. L. (2004). The broaden-and-build theory of positive emotions. *Philosophical Transactions: Biological Sciences (The Royal Society of London).* 359:1367–1377.

Fund-raiser speech at La Paloma Country Club, Tucson, AZ, May 21, 2007.

Goldin, J. (1957). *The Living Talmud. The Wisdom of the Fathers.* New York: Mentor Books.

Goleman, Daniel. (1995). *Emotional Intelligence*. New York: Bantam Books.

Gordon, Thomas. (2000). *Parent Effectiveness Training: The Proven Program for Raising Responsible Children*. Pittsburgh, PA: Three Rivers Press.

Gottlieb, Daniel J., Punjabi, N. M., Newman, A. B., Resnick, H. E., Redline, S., Baldwin, C.M., et al. (2005). Association of sleep time with diabetes mellitus and impaired glucose tolerance. *Archives of Internal Medicine*. 165(8):863–867.

Graham, H. N. (1992). Green tea composition, consumption, and polyphenol chemistry. *Preventive Medicine*. 21(3):334–350.

Grof, S., & Grof, C. (1989). *Spiritual Emergency. When Personal Transformation Becomes a Crisis*. Los Angeles: J. P. Tarcher.

Haddad, Y. Y., & Lummis, A. T. (1987). *Islamic Values in the United States. A Comparative Study*. Oxford: Oxford University Press.

"Half Body: A Woman's Courage." Discovery Channel, March 21, 2007.

Hallum, A. M. (1996). *Beyond Missionaries. Toward an Understanding of the Protestant Movement in Central America*. New York: Rowman & Littlefield.

Harvard Health Publications. "Harvard Heart Letter Examines the Costs of Not Getting Enough Sleep." http://www.health.harvard.edu/press_releases/sleep_deprivation_problem.htm

Hasler, G., Buysse, J. D., Klaghofer, R., Gamma, A., Ajdacic, V., Eich, D., et al. (2004). The association between short sleep duration and obesity in young adults: a 13-year prospective study. *Sleep* 27(4):661–666.

Hayashi, T., Urayama, O., Hori, M., Sakamoto, S., Nasir, U. M., Iwanage, S., et al. (2007). Humor has many health benefit including helping with diabetes control. *Journal of Psychosomatic Research* 62(June):703–706.

The Health Clock: When Will You Die? "Rodney Dangerfield." http://www.findadeath.com/Deceased/d/Dangerfield/rodney_dangerfield.htm

Hellwig, Jennifer Pitzi. "Empty Nest Syndrome: How to Cope When the Kids Leave Home." http://www.beliefnet.com/healthandhealing/getcontent.aspx?cid=13475

Helminiak, Daniel A. (2001). Treating spiritual issues in secular psychotherapy. *Counseling and Values*. 45:163–189.

Hillman, J. (1994). *Healing Fiction*. New York: Continuum.

Hobson, J. A., & McCarley, R. (1977). The brain as a dream state generator: an activation-synthesis hypothesis of the dream process. *American Journal of Psychiatry* 134:1335–1348.

Hommer, Daniel W. (2003). Male and female sensitivity to alcohol-induced brain damage. *Alcohol Research & Health* 27(2):181–185.

Horton, Amy. (1996). Teaching anger management skills to primary-age children. *Teaching and Change* 3(3):281–296.

"Humor and Laughter: Health Benefits and Online Sources." http://www.helpguide.org/life/humor_laughter_health.htm

Huston J. M., Gallowitsch-Puerta, M., Ochani, M., Ochani, K., Yuan, R., Rosas-Ballina M., et al. (2007). Transcutaneous vagus nerve stimulation reduces serum high mobility group box 1 levels and improves survival in murine sepsis. *Critical Care Medicine* 35(12):2762–2768.

"Interview with Mattie Stepanek," *Larry King Live*, CNN, February 17, 2003. http://transcripts.cnn.com/transcripts/0302/17/lkl.00.html

Ironson, Gail, Solomon, G. F., Balbin, E. G., O'Cleirigh, C., George, A., Kumar, M., et al. (2002). The Ironson-Woods spirituality/religiousness index is associated with long survival, health behaviors, less distress, and low cortisol in people with HIV/AIDS. *Annals of Behavioral Medicine* 24:34–48.

Jang, M., Cai, L., Udeani, G. O., Slowing, K. V., Thomas, C. F., Beecher, C. W., et al. (1997). Cancer chemopreventive activity of resveratrol, a natural product derived from grapes. *Science* 275(5297):218–220.

Jenkins, Roy. (2002). *Churchill: A Biography*. New York: Plume.

"Just Riddles and More." http://www.justriddlesandmore.com

Kasl, Charlotte D. (1992). *Many Roads, One Journey. Moving beyond the 12 Steps*. New York: Harper Collins.

Kawachi, Ichiro, Sparrow, David, Kubzansky, Laura D., Spiro, Avron III, Vokonas, Pantel S., & Weiss, Scott T. (1998). Prospective study of a self-report type A scale and risk of coronary heart disease test of the MMPI-2 type A scale. *Circulation* 98(5):405–412.

Kiecolt-Glaser, Preacher, Kristopher, J., MacCallum, Robert C., Atkinson, Cathie, Malarkey, William B., & Glaser, Ronald. (2003). Chronic stress and age-related increases in the proinflammatory cytokine IL-6. *Proceedings of the National Academy of Sciences of the United States of America* 100(15): 9090–9095.

Knutson, Brian, & Wimmer, G. E. (2007). Splitting the difference: how does the brain code reward episodes? *Annals of the New York Academy of Sciences* 1104:54–69.

Koenig, Harold G., McCullogh, Michael E., & Larson, David B. (2001). *Handbook of Religion and Health*. New York: Oxford University Press.

Koman, Kathleen. (2005). The science of hurt: medical researchers and doctors work to close the "gates" on pain. *Harvard Magazine* 108(2):46–54.

Küng, H. (1976). *On Being a Christian*. Translated by E. Quinn. New York: Doubleday. (Original work published 1974).

Küng, H. (1984). *Eternal Life? Life after Death as a Medical, Philosophical and Theological Problem*. Translated by E. Quinn. Garden City, New York: Doubleday. (Original work published 1982).

Küng, H. (2003). *My Struggle for Freedom. Memoirs*. Translated by J. Bowden. Grand Rapids, MI: Eerdmans Publishing.

Kushner, Harold S. (1981). *When Bad Things Happen to Good People*. New York: Schocken Books.

Lambert, C. (2007). The science of happiness: psychology explores humans at their best. *Harvard Magazine* 109(3):21–23.

Lambert, G. W., Kaye, D. M., Jennings, G. L., & Esler, M. D. (2002). Effect of sunlight and season on serotonin turnover in the brain. *The Lancet* 360(9348):1840–1842.

Larimore, W. L., Parker, M., & Crowther, M. (2002). Should clinicians incorporate positive spirituality into their practices? What does the evidence say? *Annals of Behavioral Medicine* 24:69–73.

Larry King Live. (April 22, 2005). http://transcripts.cnn.com/TRANSCRIPTS/0504/22/lkl.01.html

Levin, Jeffrey S., & Chatters, Linda M. (1998). Religion, health, and psychological well-being in older adults. *Journal of Aging and Health* 10:504–531.

Levin, Jeffrey S., Chatters, Linda M., & Taylor, R. J. (2006). Religious factors in health and medical care among older adults. *South Medical Journal* 99(10):1168–1169.

Levinas, E. (1996). Emmanuel Levinas: Basic Philosophical Writings. A. T. Peperzak, S. Critchley, and R. Bernasconi (Eds.). Bloomington, IN: Indiana University Press.

Limb, Charles, & Braun, Allen. NIH, *Jazz Musician.* March 11, 2008.

Malkin, Michelle. (2005). "The Cartoons Islamists Don't Want You to See." http://michellemalkin.com/2005/10/22/the-cartoons-islamists-dont-want-you-to-see

Marmot, Michael. (2003). Understanding social inequalities in health. *Perspectives in Biological Medicine* 46(3 supplement S9–S23):136.

Matthews, D. (2008). Possible link between periodontal disease and coronary heart disease. *Evidence-Based Dentistry* 9(1):8.

May, Gerald G. (2004). *The Dark Night of the Soul: A Psychiatrist Explores the Connection between Darkness and Spiritual Growth.* San Francisco: Harper.

Mayo Clinic. "Suicide: Understand Causes, Signs and Prevention." http://www.mayoclinic.com

McAuley, Edward, Morris, K. S., Motl, R. W., Hu, L., Konopack, J. F., & Elavsky, S. (2007). Long-term follow-up of physical activity behavior in older adults. *Health Psychology* 26(3): 375–380.

McCain, John, with Mark Salter. (2004). *Why Courage Matters: The Way to a Braver Life.* New York: Random House.

McGinnis, & Foege, W. H. (1993). Actual causes of death in the United States. *Journal of the American Medical Association* 270(18):2207–2212.

McKay, Gary D., & Dinkmeyer, Don, Sr. (2002). *How You Feel Is Up to You* (second edition). Atascadero, CA: Impact Publishers.

McKay, Gary D., & Maybell, Steven A. (2004). *Calming the Family Storm: Anger Management for Moms, Dads and All the Kids.* Atascadero, CA: Impact Publishers.

McKay, Gary D., McKay, Joyce L., Eckstein, Daniel, & Maybell, Steven A. (2001). *Raising Respectful Kids in a Rude World: Teaching Your Children the Power of Mutual Respect and Consideration*. New York: Random House.

McPherson, Miller, Smith-Lovin, Lynn, & Cook, James M. (2001). Birds of a feather: homophily in social networks. *Annual Review of Sociology* 27: 415–444.

Mehren, Elizabeth. "A Mormon in the White House?" (October 15, 2006). *Daily Herald*, Provo, UT, A1.

Meyers, Robert J., & Wolfe, Brenda L. (2004). *Get Your Loved One Sober: Alternatives to Nagging, Pleading, and Threatening*. Center City, MN: Hazelden.

Miller, Michael, et al. Study presented at the Scientific Session of the American College of Cardiology on March 7, 2005 in Orlando, FL.

Miller, Scott, & Berg, Insoo Kim. (1995). *The Miracle Method*. New York: W.W. Norton.

Moody, R. A. (1975). *Life After Life*. London: Bantam Books.

"Morris K. Udall Quotes." http://thinkexist.com/quotes/Morris_K._Udall

Mosak, Harold H. (1987). *Ha Ha and Aha: The Role of Humor in Psychotherapy*. Muncie, IN: Accelerated Development.

Mosak, Harold H. (1995). Adlerian Psychotherapy. In R. J. Corsini and D. Wedding (Eds.). *Current Psychotherapies*. Itasca, IL: F. E. Peacock, 51–94.

Mosak, Harold H., & Maniacci, Michael P. (1998). *Tactics in Counseling and Psychotherapy*. Itasca, IL: F. E. Peacock.

Naqvi, Nasir H., Rudrauf, David, Damasio, Hanna, & Bechara, Antoine. (2007). Damage to the Insula Disrupts Addiction to Cigarette Smoking. *Science* 315(5811): 531–534.

National Cancer Institute. "Radon and Cancer: Questions and Answers." http://www.cancer.gov/cancertopics/factsheet/Risk/radon

National Institute on Drug Abuse. "Research Report Series — Methamphetamine Abuse and Addiction." http://www.drugabuse.gov/ResearchReports/methamph/methamph2.html#what

National Sleep Foundation. "Let Sleep Work for You." http://www.sleep foundation.org/site/c.huIXKjM0IxF/b.2421185/k.7198/Let_Sleep_Work_for_You.htm

"New Attitude on Successful Aging." http://www.seniorresource.com/ageproc.htm#strategy

Oser, Fritz K., & Gmund, Paul. (1991). *Religious Judgment. A Developmental Perspective*. Birmingham, AL: Religious Education Press.

Osho, R. (1994). *Osho Zen Tarot*. New York: St. Martin's Press.

Paulson, Terry. (1989). *Making Humor Work: Take Your Job Seriously and Yourself Lightly*. Menlo Park, CA: Crisp Publishing.

Peate, Wayne F. (2002). *Native Healing: Four Sacred Paths to Health*. Tucson, AZ: Rio Nuevo.

Peate, Wayne. F., & Hine, James R. (1997). *On the Serendipity Road*. Tucson, AZ: Development Publications.

Peterman, Amy, Fitchett, G., Brady, M. J., Hernandez, L., & Cella, D. (2002). Measuring Spiritual Well-Being in People with Cancer: The Functional Assessment of Chronic Illness Therapy-Spiritual Well-Being Scale (FACIT-Sp). *Annals of Behavioral Medicine* 24:49–58.

Pierson, Vicki R., & Cloe, Renee. "The Motivation to Move." http://primusweb.com/fitnesspartner/library/activity/motomove.htm

Postgraduate Medicine Online. (2002). "Sleep Deprivation." *Postgraduate Medicine*. 112(4). http://www.postgradmed.com

Powers, R. L. (2003). Robert L. Powers' original contribution to "Spirituality in the Adlerian Forum." *The Journal of Individual Psychology*, 29:84–85.

Pratt, J. B. (1920). *The Religious Consciousness. A Psychological Study*. New York: Macmillan Co.

Proceedings of the National Academy of Sciences; 2005

"Quotations Page." http://www.quotationspage.com/quote/3251.html

Rausch, Thomas P. (2000). *Radical Christian Communities*. Eugene, OR: Wipf and Stock Publishers.

Read, Bryan F. "Sleep Deprivation." http://www.apa.org/ed/topss/bryanread.html

Reeves, Richard. The President's Been Shot: What Really Happened to Ronald Reagan? *Reader's Digest* December 2005. 168–184.

Rennard, S. I. (2008). Update on smoking cessation interventions for the primary care physician. Introduction. *American Journal of Medicine* 121(4 Suppl 1): S1–S2.

Ricoeur, P. (1978). *Freud and Philosophy: An Essay on Interpretation*. Princeton, NJ: Yale University Press. (Original work published 1970).

Riddles.com. http://www.riddles.com

Rosenbloom, Margaret, Sullivan, Edith V., & Pfefferbaum, Adolf. (2003). Using magnetic resonance imaging and diffusion tensor imaging to assess brain damage in alcoholics. *Alcohol Research & Health* 27(2): 146–152.

Salt of the Earth. "Modern Slavery." http://salt.claretianpubs.org/stats/2000/05/sh0005.html

Sawyer, G. J., Deak, Vicktor, Sarmiento, Esteban, & Milner, Richard. (2007). *The Last Human: A Guide to Twenty-Two Species of Extinct Humans*. New Haven, CT: Yale University Press.

Schneiders, S. M. (1989). The study of Christian spirituality: Contours and dynamics of a discipline. *Christian Spirituality Bulletin* 6:1, 3–12.

Shakespeare, William. *Coriolanus*. Act 1, Scene 1, Lines 159–161.

Sipe, A. W. R. (1995). *Sex, Priests, & Power. Anatomy of a Crisis.* Philadelphia: Brunner-Routledge.

Smart Recovery. "Four Point Program." http://www.smartrecovery.org

Snowdon, David. (2001). *Aging with Grace: What the Nun Study Teaches Us about Leading Longer, Healthier, and More Meaningful Lives.* New York: Bantam Dell.

Sperry, L. (2001). *Spirituality in Clinical Practice in Psychotherapy and Counseling.* New York: Psychology Press.

Sperry, L. (2001). *Spirituality in Clinical Practice. Incorporating the Spiritual Dimension in Psychotherapy and Counseling.* Philadelphia: Brunner-Routledge.

Stoll, D. (1991). *Is Latin America Turning Protestant? The Politics of Evangelical Growth.* Berkley, CA: University of California Press.

Stone, S. D. (1995). The myth of bodily perfection. *Disability & Society* 10:413–424.

Suarez, Edward. "Anger, Hostility and Depressive Symptoms Linked to High C-Reactive Protein Levels." *Duke University Medical Center: Dukemed News.* September 22, 2004. http://dukemednews.duke.edu/news/article.php?id=8164

Sultanoff, Steven M. (1999). Examining the research on humor: being cautious about our conclusions." (Originally published as the President's Column in *Therapeutic Humor* 13(3):3. American Association for Therapeutic Humor).

Tariq Khamisa Foundation. TKF Newsletter. Fall 2000. http://www.tkf.org

Thomas, Cliff. (2003). *Humor in Pharmacy.* Nemo Publishing.

"Tips for Coping with Chronic Illness." http://www.mindpub.com/art496.htm

Trimpey, Jack. "Rational Recovery." http://www.rational.org

Trimpey, Jack. (1996). *Rational Recovery: The New Cure for Substance Addiction.* New York: Pocket Books.

Trungpa, C. (2004). *Shambhala. The Sacred Path of the Warrior.* C. R. Gimian (Ed.). Boston: Shambhala. (Original work published 1984).

United States Department of Agriculture. "Steps to a Healthier You." http://www.mypyramid.gov

Utopia Home Care. "Ageism in America." Health Education Newsletter. Spring, 2007. http://www.utopiahomecare.com/dl/spring07.pdf

Vaillant, George E. (1983). *The Natural History of Alcoholism.* Cambridge, MA: Harvard University Press.

Van Cauter E., & Spiegel, K. (1999). Sleep as a mediator of the relationship between socioeconomic status and health: a hypothesis. *Annals of the New York Academy of Sciences.* 896:254–261.

Vanier, Jean. (2001). *Community and Growth: Our Pilgrimage Together.* Mahwah, NJ: Paulist Press.

Wall to Wall Television Ltd. (1998). "The Beast Within." *The Body Story*. DVD. The Discovery Channel.

Weber, M. (1956). *The Sociology of Religion*. Boston: Beacon Press. (Original work published 1922).

Weil, Andrew. "Living Longer, Better." http://www.cnn.com/2006/HEALTH/01/13/weil.interview/index.html

Wikpedia. "Twelve-step program." http://en.wikipedia.org/wiki/Twelve-step_program

Williams, Leanne M., Liddell, Belinda J., Kemp, Andrew H., Bryant, Richard A., Meares, Russel A., Peudto, Anthony S., et al. "Amygdala-prefrontal Dissociation of Subliminal and Supraliminal Fear." (August, 2006) *Human Brain Mapping*. 27 (8) 652–61.

Winzelberg, A. J., Classen, C., Alpers, G. W., Roberts, H., Koopman, C., Adams, R. E., et al. (2003). Evaluation of an Internet support group for women with primary breast cancer. *Cancer* 97(5):1164–1173.

Wong, Dean F., Maini, Atul, Rousset, Olivier, & Brasíc, James Robert. (2003). Positron emission tomography — a tool for identifying the effects of alcohol dependence on the brain. *Alcohol Research & Health* 27(2):161–173.

Wooten, T. C., Coker, J. W., & Elmore, R. C. (2003). Financial control in religious organizations: a status report. *Non-profit Management & Leadership* 13, 343–365.

Wulff, D. M. (1997). *Psychology of Religion. Classic & Contemporary* (second edition). New York: John Wiley & Sons.

Yokogoshi, H., Kobayashi, M., Mochizuki, M., & Terashima, T. (1998). Effect of theanine, r-glutamylethylamide, on brain monoamines and striatal dopamine release in conscious rats. *Neurochemical Research* 23(5):667–673.

Zager, Denny, and Evans, Rick. (1969). *In the Year 2525*. RCA Records.

"Zen Sarcasm: Words to live by..." http://toilette-paper.com/jokes/miscellaneous/zensarcasm.html

INDEX

AA (Alcoholics Anonymous), 187–88
Acceptance, 61–62, 225–26, 242
Act As If technique, 178
Acupuncture, 189
Addictions
  choice and, 195–97
  detox programs, 194–95
  of friends/family, 205–7
  identifying, 199–200
  physical effects of, 188–94
  purposes of, 198–99
  questions to consider, 217
  techniques for conquering, 197–98
  types of, 131, 186–87
  "vitamins" for, 219–20
Addictive Voice Recognition Techniques
    (AVRT), 203–5
Adler, Alfred, 39, 49, 65, 198
Adulthood crises, 272
Adversity, smiling at, 109
Aerobic exercise, 27
Affirmations, 270
Aggression
  controlling, 137–44, 154–55
  Nazi anecdote, 133–34
  pervasiveness of, 134
  physical effects, 153–54
  roots of, 135, 154–55
  spiritual perspectives on, 144–49, 156
  "vitamins" for, 158
  web resources, 289
  See also Anger
Aging
  attitude and, 264–66, 269–70
  exercise and, 18–19, 261–62
  improvements with, 259–60
  overview, 255–56
  physical ills and, 262–63

rules for, 260–61
spiritual steps to, 278–80
stages of, 271–74
transitions to, 274–78
"vitamins" for, 283–84
working and, 261
Ahmann, Frederic, 252–53
Alcohol addiction, 191–92, 194–95, 199
Alcoholics Anonymous (AA), 187–88
Alfie, 7
Alzheimer's disease, 18–19, 256–58
Alzhemed, 258
Anaerobic exercise, 27
Anger
  alternative behaviors, 139–44
  chemical pathways, 6
  chronic illness and, 236
  controlling, 136–38, 139–44, 156–57, 260
  depression and, 166, 180–81
  directions of, 146–47
  emotions leading to, 138–39
  physical effects, 150–52, 156
  roots of, 135–36
  spiritual perspectives on, 144–49, 156
  "vitamins" for, 158
  web resources, 290
  See also Aggression
Ansbacher, Heinz, 223
Anticipation, 116–17
Antidepressants, 170–71, 181–82
Antipsychotics, 195
Anxiety and alcohol, 199
Apply vitamin, 87, 168
Approval, need for, 179
Aron, Arthur, 262
Articles/books, recommended, 285–88

Ask vitamin, 86, 168
Assisted-living facilities, 277–78
Ativan, 195
Attitude
    addiction and, 187–88
    aging and, 256, 264–66, 269–70
    chronic illness and, 239–42
    healing, 172–75
Aupumut, 281
AVRT (Addictive Voice Recognition Techniques), 203–5
Awareness, 78–80, 85
AWARE vitamins, 86–88, 168, 280–81

"The Beast," 204
Behavior
    changing, 49–55, 180
    disease and, 16
    stress and, 115
Bennett, Arnold, 180
Benzodiazepams, 195
Benzodiazepine, 195
Berde, Charles, 19–20
Berg, Insoo Kim, 214–15
"Big picture" perspective, 3–4
Big Questions/Answers, 68–70
Binocular vision, 77
Black dog days, 173–74
Blame, 47–48
Blind drive theory, 76
Bombeck, Erma, 89
Books/articles, recommended, 285–88
Booth, Leo, 213
Brain health
    aging and, 259–60
    chemicals and depression, 169–71
    diet and, 18
    drugs' effects on, 191–94
    exercises for, 17–18, 257
    fMRI and, 21–23
Breathing exercises
    for grief, 131–32
    for stress, 52–53, 116
    tonglen practice, 149
Broken ways and addiction, 208–10
Buddhist perspectives, 22–23, 108
Buddies for exercising, 29
Burns, George, 261

Calming the Family Storm, 138, 269
Cancer, 259
    See also Chronic illness
Cardiovascular exercises, 17
Caregivers for chronically ill, 235–38
Carey, Benedict, 225
Caring virtue, 272
Catholic humor, 106–7
Celebrate Recovery group, 201
Chatters, Linda M., 275
Child abuse, 289
Children
    coming to know the world, 71–75
    feeling little, 75–79
    leaving home, 267–68
    psychological vitamins for, 56–57
    stress and, 119–20
Chödrön, Pema, 124–25
Choices, 55, 195–97
Chopra, Deepak, 65, 264
Christianity
    Jesus's righteous anger, 148
    light/dark schema of, 209–11
    recovery groups and, 201
Chronic illness
    acceptance, 225–26
    attitudes toward, 222–23, 239–42,
        243, 245–46
    firefighter anecdote, 221–22
    living with, 231–39
    management techniques, 242–46
    as reward/punishment, 223–25
    support guidelines, 235–38
    "vitamins" for, 247
Churchill, Winston, 173–74, 175
Cloe, Renee, 29–30
Cocaine addiction, 193–94
Codependence, 209
Community and Growth, 278
Community focus, 83
Community Reinforcement and Family
        Training (CRAFT), 206
Complaints, 238
Concerned Significant Others (CSOs), 206
Conjunctive faith, 274
Consciousness-change practice, 124–25
Control, 91–92, 212
Cook, Marilyn, 11–12

Cooperation, 81–82, 134, 154–55
Country music, 47
Couple meetings, 268–69, 276
Courage, 245–46
CRAFT (Community Reinforcement and Family Training), 206
C-reactive protein (CRP), 151
Cree Shield, 11–12
Crowther, M., 226
CRP (C-reactive protein), 151
CSOs (Concerned Significant Others), 206

Dark Night experiences, 161–63, 167–68
Davidson, Richard, 22
Decisions and addiction, 187–88
Deep breathing, 57–60
Delirium tremens (DTs), 194–95
Demands, reevaluation of. *See* REAL thoughts
DeMello, Anthony, 125–26
Depression
    alcohol and, 199
    anger and, 166, 180–81
    AWARE vitamins for, 168
    Dark Nights compared to, 161–63, 167–68
    diagnosis/treatment of, 172, 181–82
    effects of, 159–60, 165–66
    of family/friends, 183
    purposes of, 179–80
    roots of, 168–71, 176–78
    suicide, 182–83
    web resources, 290
Descartes, Rene, 36
Detoxification programs, 194–95
Diazepam, 195
Diet
    brain health and, 18
    food pyramid, 24
    sleep and, 33
    stress and, 117
    supplements to, 25–26
    See also Vitamins/minerals
Disappointments, 47
Discouraged Negative Attitude (DNA) anecdote, 43–44
Domestic violence, 289
Dopamine, 262

Drach, George, 250–52
Dreikurs, Rudolf, 49, 56, 92, 126–27, 145
DTs (delirium tremens), 194–95
DUMB thoughts, 45–46, 49–50, 120, 136, 265

Ecstasy (drug), 192
Either/or thinking, 210
Elder care, 277–78
    See also Aging
Ellis, Albert, 4, 46, 96–97, 121, 196–97
Emotional Intelligence, 236–37
Emotions
    as domain of well-being, 230–31
    reasons for, 48–49
    sharing, 54, 139–40, 245
    universality of, 144–45
    See also specific emotions
Empathy, 230
Empty nest syndrome, 267–68
Encouragement vitamin, 56
Endorphins, 27, 189, 190–91
Erikson, Erik, 271–73
Espirit, 76
European Union, 155
Excuses, 47
Exercise
    aging and, 261–62
    benefits, 26–27, 115–16, 131, 156, 245
    brain health and, 17–18, 257
    buddies for, 29
    emotions and, 54
    motivation for, 28–30
    types, 27–28, 30–31
    web resources, 289
    See also Breathing exercises
Expectations, 178–79
Experience vitamin, 87–88, 168
Expert knowledge, 259–60

Face/freeze responses, 145
Failure, 118
Faith development, 273–74
Families
    chronic illness and, 235–38
    as domain of well-being, 229–30
    influences on children, 72

Families *(cont'd.)*
  loss of life partner, 277
  meetings with, 268–69
  See also Children; Social connections
Fat-soluble vitamins, 25
Fear, 6, 199
Feng shui for the brain, 46–48
Fighting with others/one's self, 146–47
  See also Aggression
Fight or flight response, 6
Firefighter anecdotes, 130–32, 221–22
Fisher, Helen, 262
Fixes and addiction, 209
Flashbacks, 153–54
Flexibility exercises, 27–28
Flexible confidence, 82–83
fMRI (functional magnetic resonance
    imaging), 21–23, 191, 239
Foege, Bill, 16
Folic acid, 25
Food pyramid, 24
Fowler, James, 273–74
Frankl, Viktor, 153
Fredrickson, Barbara, 4
Friends. *See* Social connections
Frustrations and humor, 90–91
Functional domain of well-being,
    228–29
Functional magnetic resonance imaging
    (fMRI), 21–23, 191, 239
Fundamentalism, 66
Future plans, 266–68

Gender differences, 181, 233
Geographic influences on children, 72–73
Get Your Loved One Sober, 206
Gifting, 276
God
  as drug, 208
  Hines on, 250–53
  prayers to, 128–29, 225–26
  spirituality and, 65
  See also Spirituality; *specific religions*
Golden Rule, 156, 289
Goleman, Daniel, 236–37
Gratefulness, 129
Grief, 130
Group exercise programs, 29

Group recovery approaches, 191
Guilt, 126

Haldol, 195
Haloperidol, 195
Handbook of Religion and Health, 226
Happiness, 16, 23, 36–37
Healing from surgery, 57–60
Health
  answering questions about, 238
  disease prevention, 16–17
  happiness as dependent on, 16
  humor and, 99–100
  religious beliefs and, 67
  stress and, 115
  "vitamins" for, 40
Heart and courage, 245–46
Heart attacks, 99, 150–52
Helminiak, Daniel, 224–25
Hillman, Bill, 41
Hinduism perspective on aging, 278
Hine, James R., 249–53
Holistic health, 289
Holy humor, 104–9
Hope, Bob, 89
HOPE acronym, 177
Humble humor, 104–9
Humility, 230–31
Humor
  benefits, 89, 97–103, 116
  chronic illness and, 243–44
  combating discouraging beliefs with,
      91–93
  depression and, 177
  funny songs, 96–97
  reframing with, 52, 90–91
  religion and, 104–9
  techniques for developing, 93–97
  types, 98
  "vitamins" for, 110

Illness, 57–62, 67
  See also Chronic illness
Imagery techniques, 54, 57–60, 130–32,
    198, 244–45
I-messages, 139–40, 151
Immune systems, 258–59
Immunizations, 16–17

Imperfections (physical), 72
Individual recovery process, 203
Inflammatory reflex, 259
Insight meditation, 116
Integration, 82–83, 84, 280
Interleukin 6, 152
International politics, 155–56
Interrelationships, 3–4
Interventions, 206–7
Inward movement, 8, 227–31
Ironson, Gail, 226
Isaiah, 148
Islam, 103–4, 109, 209–11, 278
Isolation, 153

Journals, 119–20
Joy, 230
Judaism
    anger in scriptures, 148
    humor and, 89
    light/dark schema of, 209–11
    Sabbath, 154

Kasl, Charlotte Davis, 215–17
Keep Learning pyramid, 19–20
Keep Moving pyramid, 30
Keillor, Garrison, 107
Khamisa, Azim, 69–70
Kibra gene, 258
Kicanas, Gerald, 101
Knowing and not knowing, 75–80, 86
Knutson, Brian, 116–17
Kushner, Harold, 223

Labyrinth exercise
    movement into, 66–70
    movement out of, 78–85
    overview, 41–42, 65
    sacred center, 71–78
La Mance, Thomas, 46
Langer, Ellen, 262
Larimore, W. L., 226
Laughter, 52
    See also Humor
"Let it be," 125
Levin, Jeffrey S., 275
Levy, Becca, 269
Librium, 195

Life partners, loss of, 277
Lincoln, Abraham, 174–75
Littleness, 209
Livingston, Bill, 259–60
Logan, Mac, 91–93
Loss and grief, 161–64, 277
Love relationships, 262, 268–69, 277
Lung cancer, 237

Man's Search for Meaning, 153
Many Roads, One Journey, 215–17
Marmot, Michael, 35–36
Massage, 116
May, Gerald G., 161
Mazes. *See* Labyrinth exercise
McAuley, Edward, 115–16
McCain, John, 100, 245–46
McGinnis, Mike, 16
Meaning, pondering of, 55, 64, 68–70
    See also Spirituality
Medications, 235, 258
    See also specific medications
Meditation, 22–23, 41–42, 116, 259
Memory and exercise, 17
Mental exercises, 17–18, 257
Methamphetamine addiction, 193
Meyers, Robert J., 206
Miller, Emmett E., 57, 244
Miller, Michael, 99
Miller, Scott, 214–15
Minerals. *See* Vitamins/minerals
Minibreaks, 116
The Miracle Method, 214–15
Mirror neurons, 237
Mission as antidepressant, 174–75
Modernitis, 4–5, 31–32, 114
Motivation for exercise, 28–30
Music, 6, 22, 96–97

Narcotics. *See* Addictions
Natural highs, 190–91
Near-death experiences, 165
Negative thoughts, 4, 118–19, 120
    See also DUMB thoughts
Negotiations, 142–44
New roads, 215–17
Newton, John, 155
Norepinephrine, 151–52, 259

Novel experiences, 262
Numbness, 153
Nun Study, 257
Nursing homes, 277–78

Old age crises, 272–73
One-liners, 94–95
Opiate addiction, 192, 194
Optimism, 222–23, 269–70
Oral hygiene, 34
Organization and stress, 119–20
Oser, Fritz, 273–74
Osteoporosis, 263
OTC (over the counter) medications, 235
Outward movement, 8, 227–31
Oxazepam, 195

Pain, 39–40, 59, 234–35
Parker, M., 226
Passive thinking, 47
Past-life experiences, 165
Path of spirituality, 8
    See also Labyrinth exercise
Patience, 229
Peak experiences, 165
Peate, Marlea "Molly," 256, 260–61
Perceptions, 6–7, 34–37
Perfection and humor, 92–93
Personal hygiene, 34
Peterman, Amy, 227
Petitions, 128–29
Physical addictions, 188–94
Physical domain of well-being, 228
Physical exams, 16
Physical influences on children, 72
Pierson, Vicki R., 29–30
Placebo effects, 190
Plans for the future, 266–68
Plasticity, 22
Pleasers, 93
Politics, 155–56
Positive addictions, 131
Positive Imagery for People with Cancer, 244
Positive perceptions, 6–7, 34–37
    See also REAL thoughts
Possession states, 165
Postures of spiritual nourishment, 86–88

Powers, Bob, 77
Practices for spiritual nourishment, 86–88
Prayer, 128–29, 225–26
Predispositions for addiction, 190
Pregnancy, 25–26
Prevention of disease, 16–17
Priorities and stress, 119–21
Process of questioning, 70
Procrastination, 118
Production orientation, 277
Professions, making light of, 95–96
Psychological addiction, 186–87
Psychological DNA, 45–46, 50, 55–62
Psychological vitamins, 55–57
Psychosocial and physical health, 35–37
Psychosomatic pain, 39–40
Pyramids
    food, 24
    Keep Learning, 19–20
    Keep Moving, 30
    Stay Connected, 37–39

Quality of life, 225, 227–31
Question about pain, 39
Questioning and knowing, 68–70, 75–80, 86, 217
Quiet time, 86–87

Radical Christian Communities, 278
Rapid eye movement (REM) sleep, 31–32
Rational emotive behavior therapy (REBT), 196–97
Rational Recovery, 204
Rausch, Thomas P., 278
REAL thoughts, 46–48, 50, 121, 136–37, 240, 265–66
REBT (rational emotive behavior therapy), 196–97
Recommended books/articles, 285–88
Recovery groups, 201
Reeves, Richard, 98
Reflective listening, 140–42
Reflect vitamin, 87, 168
Reframing techniques
    for addiction, 197–98
    for aging, 266
    benefits, 51–52
    chronic illness and, 60, 243

grief and, 131
prayer as, 128–29
vexations and, 125–26
Refuse-to-leavers, 68
Regeneration, 154
Relationships. *See* Families; Social
connections
Relaxation, 53–54, 57–60, 117
See also Breathing exercises
Religion
addictions to, 208–19
arguments about, 63–64
chronic illness and, 223–25, 226
faith development, 273–74
fundamentalism, 66
humor and, 103–9
influence on children, 73
spirituality compared to, 227
See also Spirituality; *specific religions*
Research, health-related, 238–39
Responsibility, 56–57
Resveratrol, 258
Retirement, 261
Revenge, 133–34, 136
Rheumatoid arthritis, 34–35
Riddles, 257
Righters, 92–93
Role reversals, 237
Roller coaster of chronic illness, 234
Romney, Mitt, 100–101

Sabbath, need for, 154
Sacred center, 71–78
Schweitzer, Albert, 175
Seasons, stages of, 271–74
Self-deprecating humor, 104–406
Self-esteem, 211–12
Self-management and recovery training
(SMART) programs, 201–3, 206
Self-pity, 38
Self-talk, 270
Self-tests for addiction, 199–200
Self-transcendence, 83
Serax, 195
Serenity Prayer, 62
Service to others, 84–85, 174–75, 234,
266
Sharma, Vijai P., 242

Short-term successes, 234
Sick humor, 97
Siggins, Rose, 241–42
Sleep, 18, 31–33, 117
Sloan, Richard, 226
SMART (self-management and recovery
training) programs, 201–3, 206
Social connections, 37, 73–74, 81–82,
117, 229–30, 235–38
See also Families
Solitary confinement, 9
Somatic pain, 39–40
Songs, 96–97
Soulful influences on children, 74–75
Spiritual domain of well-being, 227–28
Spirituality
aggression and, 144–49
aging and, 278–80
children and, 74–75
crises compared to emergencies,
163–65
definitions, 8–9
depression and, 161–63
god and, 65
humor and, 103–9
religion compared to, 66–67, 227
stress and, 122–30
"vitamins" for, 86–88
web resources, 289
wellness continuum and, 80–85
Stay Connected pyramid, 37–39
Steadfastness, 82
Stepanek, Mattie J., 1–2, 47, 241, 289
Stinking thinking, 197
Stop, Think, and Act technique, 137–38,
151
Straub, Vicki, 57–60, 239–40, 244
Strength training, 27
Stress
causes, 113–15, 118–19, 259
firefighter anecdote, 130–32
managing, 6, 115–17, 122–30, 290
responses to, 5, 117–18
Strivings, 76, 81–82, 280
Struthers, Lucia, 261
Stuttering, 22
Successful Surgery and Recovery, 57
Suicide, 182–83

Sunova, Ludmila, 261–62
Sunshine and vitamin D, 34
Superiority and humor, 92
Supplements, 25–26
Support groups, 61, 263
Surgery recovery, 57–60

Tang, William, 231–33
Team orientation, 81–82
Terminal illnesses, 60–61
TGen (Translational Genomics Research
    Institute), 258
Therapist locators, 290
Thomas, Cliff, 103–4
Tibetan practice, 149
Tobacco addiction, 192
To Do lists, 119–20
Tonglen practice, 149
Tracey, Kevin, 259
Tragedies, 69–70
Transcendence, 280
Translational Genomics Research Institute
    (TGen), 258
Treatment for addiction, 200–205
Triggers for addiction, 196
Trimpey, Jack, 203–5
Trungpa, Chögyam, 149
Twelve-step programs, 200–201,
    215–17
Type A personalities, 150

Udall, Mo, 100
Ultimate value, 80, 84
Universal emotions, 144–45
"Use it or lose it," 18–20

Vaccinations, 16–17
Vaillant, George, 212–13
Valium, 195
Vanier, Jean, 278
Vegetarian/vegan diet, 26
Vexations of the spirit, 123–26
Vitamin D, 34
Vitamins as food for thought
    addiction, 219–20
    aggression/anger, 158
    aging and tomorrow, 283–84

AWARE, 86–88, 168, 280–81
    chronic illness, 247
    depression, 168, 184
    humor, 110
    mind, 55–57, 62
    physical health/body, 40
    spirituality, 86–88
    stress, 132
    whole health introduction, 10
Vitamins/minerals
    in detox programs, 195
    for physical health, 5
    supplements, 25–26
    types, 25
    web resources, 289
Voltaire, 89
Volunteers/volunteering, 234, 266

Wait vitamin, 86–87, 168
Water-soluble vitamins, 25
Weber, Max, 277
Web resources
    addiction, 199–200, 202, 204, 288
    aging, 288
    chronic illness, 243, 288
    domestic violence/child abuse, 289
    exercise, 289
    golden rule, 289
    holistic health, 289
    negative emotions, 290
    riddles, 257
    spirituality, 289
    Stepanek (Mattie), 289
    vitamins/minerals, 289
Weight-bearing exercises, 28
Weil, Andrew, 264
"We'll see about that!", 239–42
Why Courage Matters, 245–46
Williams, Leanne, 260
Win-win world, 154–56
Wisdom, 273
Wolfe, Brenda L., 206
Women and chronic illness, 233
Worry, 118–19
Wulff, David M., 273–74, 274

Zen sarcasm, 108